W9-BRN-500

a LANGE medical book

Medical
Epidemiology

second edition

a LANGE medical book

Medical Epidemiology

Second Edition

Raymond S. Greenberg, MD, PhD
Vice President for Academic Affairs and Provost
Medical University of South Carolina
Charleston

Stephen R. Daniels, MD, PhD
Professor
University of Cincinnati School of Medicine
Cincinnati

W. Dana Flanders, MD, DSc
Professor
Rollins School of Public Health
Emory University
Atlanta

John William Eley, MD, MPH
Associate Professor
Rollins School of Public Health
Emory University
Atlanta

John R. Boring, III, PhD
Professor
Rollins School of Public Health
Emory University
Atlanta

APPLETON & LANGE
Norwalk, Connecticut

Notice: The authors and the publisher of this volume have taken care to
make certain that the doses of drugs and schedules of treatment are correct
and compatible with the standards generally accepted at the time of
publication. Nevertheless, as new information becomes available, changes in
treatment and in the use of drugs become necessary. The reader is advised to
carefully consult the instruction and information material included in the
package insert of each drug or therapeutic agent before administration.
This advice is especially important when using new or infrequently used drugs.
The publisher and author disclaim any liability, loss, injury, or damage incurred as
a consequence, directly or indirectly, or the use and application of any of
the contents of the volume.

Copyright © 1996 by Appleton & Lange
A Simon & Schuster Company
Copyright © 1993 by Appleton & Lange

All rights reserved. This book, or any parts thereof, may not be used or
reproduced in any manner without written permission. For information,
address Appleton & Lange, Four Stamford Plaza, 107 Elm Street, Stamford, Ct 06902

96 97 98 99 / 10 9 8 7 6 5 4 3 2 1

Prentice Hall International (UK) Limited, *London*
Prentice Hall of Australia Pty. Limited, *Sydney*
Prentice Hall Canada, Inc., *Toronto*
Prentice Hall Hispanoamericana, S.A., *Mexico*
Prentice Hall of India Private Limited, *New Delhi*
Prentice Hall of Japan, Inc., *Tokyo*
Simon & Schuster Asia Pte. Ltd., *Singapore*
Editora Prentice Hall do Brasil Ltda., *Rio de Janeiro*
Prentice Hall, Englewood Cliffs, *New Jersey*

ISBN: 0-8385-6206-X
ISSN: 1064-1025

Acquisitions Editor: John Dolan
Production Editor: Chris Langan
Managing Editor: Gregory Huth
Development Editor: John Dinolfo
Illustrator: Linda F. Harris
Art Coordinator: Becky Hainz-Baxter

PRINTED IN THE UNITED STATES OF AMERICA

ISBN 0-8385-6206-X
N82I
90000

9 780838 562062

In loving memory of
John Rutledge Boring, Jr., June Gibson Daniels, Hubert Wayne Eley, Sr.,
William Dana Flanders, Jr., and Bernard George Greenberg

Table of Contents

Preface

The authors of *Medical Epidemiology* are grateful for the positive response generated by the first edition of this book. In this new version, the text has been expanded with the addition of two new chapters, one on genetic epidemiology and one on clinical decision-making. Moreover, the revised book includes new material on current topics such as emerging infections, as well as the latest available surveillance data.

Medical Epidemiology introduces the principles and methods of epidemiology. Although this text is written primarily with the needs of medical students in mind, students of other health professions such as nursing, dentistry, pharmacy, and veterinary medicine should find it suitable for their needs as well. Epidemiology often is taught in conjunction with biostatistics, and this book is designed to complement *Basic and Clinical Biostatistics* (Dawson-Saunders and Trapp, 1994). References to the Dawson-Saunders text are provided throughout *Medical Epidemiology* to facilitate using the two books together. The reader who is interested in a more focused introduction to epidemiology should find the present work to be a self-contained, independent reference, however.

OBJECTIVES

The aim of this book is to provide the reader with an appreciation for the role of epidemiology in medicine. The authors have emphasized how epidemiology can be used to achieve the following objectives:

- Measure disease frequency
- Describe patterns of disease occurrence
- Investigate disease outbreaks
- Assess diagnostic test accuracy
- Evaluate treatment effectiveness
- Identify causes of disease development
- Predict disease prognosis
- Select from among alternative treatment strategies.

Upon completion of this book, the reader should be able to calculate and interpret basic epidemiologic measures, recognize the strengths and limitations of various study designs, understand the concepts of variability and bias, and critique published epidemiologic studies.

APPROACH & FEATURES

The guiding principle in the development of this book is the presentation of epidemiology in a manner that is both understandable and interesting to the reader. This text incorporates the following features:

- The scope of topics is limited to core principles and concepts, thus reducing the overall length of the text.
- Attention is devoted to both the descriptive and comparative roles of epidemiology. In contrast to most other introductory books, chapters are included on medical surveillance

and investigation of disease outbreaks.

- Each chapter begins with a Patient Profile—a clinical vignette that helps to relate the epidemiologic topic to the practice of medicine.
- Data and references are drawn from up-to-date sources, thus emphasizing relevance to current applications.
- Clinical examples are drawn from content areas such as cancer, ischemic heart disease, diabetes mellitus, Alzheimer's disease, infectious diseases, and perinatal disorders, thereby demonstrating the diverse settings in which epidemiologic methods can be employed.
- Only essential formulas and equations are included in the text with illustrative calculations. Where appropriate, more complicated mathematical relationships are described in appendices.
- Figures are used extensively to promote comprehension and retention of the material.
- Important concepts and principles are highlighted for emphasis.
- A summary of essential information is provided at the end of each chapter for the benefit of the reader.
- Each chapter is followed by an updated set of multiple-choice questions in standardized test format to facilitate self-assessment and preparation for examinations.
- An integrative chapter on the critical review of published medical literature is included.
- A glossary is provided as a guide to the correct use of epidemiologic terminology.

The authors, all of whom are practicing epidemiologists and medical educators, have attempted to infuse the text with the excitement of discovery that epidemiology has brought to their lives. To the extent that the reader is engaged by a similar sense of discovery, this book will have been faithful to its subject.

Raymond S. Greenberg, MD, PhD
Charleston, South Carolina
October 1995

Acknowledgments

The second edition of this book was made possible through the dedicated efforts of many individuals. John Dolan, Senior Medical Editor at Lange Medical Publications, was a strong advocate for this project. Gregory R. Huth, Managing Editor, oversaw the revision process, and John Dinolfo spent countless hours improving the text. Becky Hainz-Baxter coordinated the artwork, and Linda Harris composed the figures.

Many publishers and authors kindly allowed their work to be cited in this book. Several sources of current data were particularly useful and warrant special acknowledgment: the *Morbidity and Mortality Weekly Report* of the Centers for Disease Control (Editor, Dr. Richard Goodman); the *Cancer Statistics Review* of the Surveillance Program of the National Cancer Institute (Director, Dr. Benjamin Hankey); and the *Monthly Vital Statistics Report* of the National Center for Health Statistics (Director, Dr. Manning Feinleib). The authors are grateful to J. Virgil Peavy, MS, who provided information and data about the disease outbreak described in Chapter 5.

The comments and suggestions of several anonymous reviewers were helpful in refining the style and contents of this book. In addition, Dr. Beth Dawson-Saunders and Dr. Paul Levy provided valuable advice in the initial developmental process. The didactic approach used in this book was developed largely through the experience of teaching epidemiology to medical students at Emory University and the University of Cincinnati. We have learned a great deal from these students, and we hope that their suggestions are adequately represented in the pages that follow.

The authors have had the good fortune to study under and to work with a number of outstanding epidemiologists. In writing an introductory text, we were inevitably drawn back to the teachers who first attracted us to the field. The influences of former mentors can be found throughout this book. Of particular note are the teachings of Dr. Philip Cole at the School of Public Health of the University of Alabama-Birmingham, Dr. Kenneth Rothman at Boston University, Dr. David Kleinbaum, formerly of the University of North Carolina and now of Emory University, and Dean Michel Ibrahim at the School of Public Health of the University of North Carolina.

The support and encouragement of our respective institutions was essential for the completion of this project. With the transition of Dr. Greenberg to the Medical University of South Carolina, he is particularly grateful to President James B. Edwards for his support of this undertaking. We also thank Dean Jeffrey Houpt of the Emory University School of Medicine for promoting strong educational and research linkages with the faculty of the Rollins School of Public Health. Dr. Charles Hatcher, Jr., Vice President for Health Affairs at Emory University, provided the resources and environment necessary for epidemiology and public health to develop at that institution. We also thank former Emory University President James T. Laney for his vision of the role of public health in serving human needs.

Ms. Essie Mills spent many long hours in the preparation of the manuscript. For her extraordinary tolerance in dealing with countless revisions, erratic work schedules, and urgent deadlines, the authors will remain forever in her debt.

This book could not have been completed without the understanding and support of our wives and families. Time and again, precious hours at home were preempted by writing tasks, and we are grateful for the sacrifices that were made by our loved ones.

Authors

John R. Boring, III, PhD
Professor and Director, Division of Epidemiology, Rollins School of Public Health, Emory University, Atlanta; formerly Epidemic Intelligence Service Officer, Centers for Disease Control, Atlanta.

Stephen R. Daniels, MD, PhD
Professor of Pediatrics and Environmental Health, University of Cincinnati College of Medicine, Cincinnati.

John William Eley, MD, MPH
Associate Professor, Rollins School of Public Health, Assistant Professor, Winship Cancer Center, Senior Associate, Department of Medicine, Emory University, Atlanta.

W. Dana Flanders, MD, DSc, MPH
Professor, Rollins School of Public Health, Emory University, Atlanta.

Raymond S. Greenberg, MD, PhD
Vice President for Academic Affairs and Provost, Professor of Biometry and Epidemiology, Medical University of South Carolina, Charleston.

Introduction to Epidemiology

PATIENT PROFILE

A 29-year-old previously healthy man was referred to the University of California at Los Angeles (UCLA) Medical Center with a history of fever, fatigue, lymph node enlargement, and weight loss of almost 25 lb over the preceding 8 months. He had a temperature of 39.5°C, appeared physically wasted, and had swollen lymph nodes. Laboratory evaluation revealed a depressed level of peripheral blood lymphocytes. The patient suffered from simultaneous infections involving Candida albicans *in his upper digestive tract, cytomegalovirus in his urinary tract, and* Pneumocystis carinii *in his lungs. Although antibiotic therapy was administered, the patient remained severely ill.*

INTRODUCTION

Epidemiology is a fundamental medical science that focuses on the distribution and determinants of disease frequency in human populations. Specifically, epidemiologists examine patterns of illness in groups of people and then try to learn why certain individuals develop a particular disease whereas other persons do not.

Knowledge about who is likely to develop a particular condition and under what circumstances is central to the daily practice of medicine. To prevent an illness, health care providers must be able to identify persons who are at high risk and then intervene to reduce that risk. This type of knowledge emerges in many cases from epidemiologic research.

This book serves as an introduction to epidemiologic methods and the ways in which they can be used to answer key medical questions. This chapter begins with consideration of a single disease, as described in the Patient Profile. Confining our attention to this one disease enables us to demonstrate the important contribution of epidemiology to current knowledge about this condition. While the focus here is on a single disease entity, it must be emphasized that epidemiologic methods can be applied to a wide spectrum of conditions ranging from acute infectious diseases to chronic conditions such as cancer and heart disease.

The man in the Patient Profile was referred to the UCLA Medical Center in June 1981. At the time, there was no obvious explanation why a healthy young man would suddenly develop concurrent infections of three different organ systems involving three different microorganisms. More surprising still was the nature of the infections that were present. In particular, the parasite *P carinii* was known to cause illness only in persons with impaired immune responses. The young man described in the Patient Profile, however, did not have any obvious underlying causes of immune dysfunction. For example, he did not have cancer, severe malnutrition, and he did not use immune-suppressing drugs. Why then was his body overwhelmed by the infections? This question was given a heightened sense of urgency by the severity of the patient's illness.

This patient was not the first to be referred to the UCLA Medical Center with this clinical presentation. Three other patients had been examined within the preceding 6 months, all of them previously healthy young men with recent histories of weight loss, fever, and lymph node enlargement. All had *P carinii* pneumonia and *C albicans* infections.

Why were four such patients appearing at about the same time in the same location? Suspicious that the illnesses in these four patients might be related in some way, the UCLA physicians notified public health officials and prepared a descriptive report of their findings for publication.

Was this new appearance of a rare and life-threatening form of pneumonia confined to UCLA Medical Center, or were physicians elsewhere observing similar patients? If the experience at UCLA was unique, then the entire episode might be regarded as a medical curiosity—unusual, but not a reason for great public health concern. On the other hand, if patients similar to those at UCLA were turning up in clinics or medical offices elsewhere, this episode could not be easily dismissed. Within a matter of weeks, public health authorities received reports of outbreaks of *P carinii* pneumonia among previously healthy young men in San Francisco and New York City.

In the United States, the federal agency that is responsible for monitoring unusual patterns of disease occurrence is the Centers for Disease Control and Prevention (CDC). Recognizing the potential for widespread emergence of this new, unexplained, and debilitating condition, the CDC established a special task force to collect more detailed information on the affected persons. In addition, a formal request to report such patients was issued by the CDC to all state health departments. Between June and November 1981, a total of 76 instances of *P carinii* pneumonia were identified in persons who did not have known predisposing illnesses and were not taking immune-suppressing medications. A few months later, the disease that afflicted these patients was named the acquired immune deficiency syndrome (AIDS).

PERSON, PLACE, & TIME

The UCLA physicians played a crucial role in establishing the presence of a new disease in their community. The story of the first few AIDS patients—also called "sentinel cases"—is particularly dramatic because of the severity of the illness and the extent and speed with which the disease spread to affect others. In 1981, no one could have predicted that almost 350,000 persons in the United States would be diagnosed with this syndrome during the following dozen years. Over that same period, about 200,000 deaths from AIDS would be reported. By 1992, AIDS had become the most common cause of death among men aged 25–44 in the United States.

Looking back to 1981, it is instructive to consider the features of the sentinel cases that suggested a possible connection between them. All the AIDS patients who presented to the UCLA clinicians suffered from the same rare opportunistic infections. Had the infections involved more conventional human pathogens—or less severe symptoms—then the entire episode might have gone unnoticed for some time.

Beyond their clinical similarities, the sentinel cases shared other features, as summarized in Table 1–1. All four patients were previously healthy homosexual men in their early 30s (personal characteristics) who resided in Los Angeles (place) and first became ill in the 9 months ending in June 1981 (time). These three dimensions—**person, place,** and **time**—are the features traditionally used to characterize patterns of disease occurrence, as discussed in Chapter 3.

THE EPIDEMIOLOGIC APPROACH

Epidemiology is concerned with the distribution and determinants of disease frequency in human populations. Interest in disease frequency or occurrence derives largely from a basic tenet of epidemiology, ie, that disease does not develop at random. In essence, this means that all persons are not equally likely to develop a particular disease. Certain persons are at comparatively high risk by virtue of their personal characteristics and environment.

Table 1–1. Characteristics of sentinel cases of AIDS in Los Angeles, 1981.

Characteristic of Sentinel Cases	Personal Attributes
Age	Early 30s
Gender	Male
Prior health	Good
Sexual preference	Homosexual
Place of occurrence	Los Angeles
Time of occurrence	October 19, 1980 to June 19, 1981

As applied to the outbreak of AIDS, for instance, it is highly unlikely that each of the first four cases in Los Angeles would have occurred in homosexual males if the disease was striking at random. At the time, the repeated occurrence of AIDS in homosexual men suggested that this segment of the population had an increased risk of AIDS. Other high-risk groups for AIDS were identified soon thereafter, including hemophiliacs and injecting drug users. On the surface, these three subgroups seemed to have little in common. Upon closer examination, however, it became evident that they all had an increased risk of exposure to the blood of other persons.

Most contemporary medical research is devoted to investigating the biologic elements of disease development. For example, in the study of AIDS, a microbiologist tends to focus on the infectious agent, human immunodeficiency virus (HIV). An immunologist might concentrate on the primary target of HIV infection, the CD4+ T-lymphocyte, that coordinates a number of immune functions. The epidemiologist, on the other hand, views a disease from both a biologic and a social perspective. It is not enough to know that HIV is transmitted primarily through contaminated blood. The epidemiologist must be able to understand the circumstances of HIV transmission among humans. Here, the influence of social factors is undeniable. One cannot fully appreciate the spread of AIDS in human populations without recognizing the role of certain behaviors, such as sexual practices or injecting drug use.

The desire to study social factors that impinge upon health has definite implications for how epidemiologic research is conducted. In most instances, this research involves observations of phenomena that occur naturally within human populations. Such an approach is unique among the medical sciences. The features that distinguish the epidemiologic approach are: (1) the focus on human populations, and (2) a heavy reliance on nonexperimental observations.

At first thought, the focus on human populations may not seem at all distinctive. Ultimately, all medical research is motivated by a desire to prevent or control human illnesses. The process leading to that goal, however, may take various routes. Laboratory scientists, eg, often rely upon experiments that involve nonhuman animals or in vitro preparations. While these studies offer important advantages to the investigator, such as precise control over the experimental conditions, certain limitations must also be recognized. Obviously, a laboratory environment may not accurately reflect the actual conditions of exposure in the external world. Of equal importance is the recognition that animals of different species may have dissimilar responses to experimental manipulations. One cannot assume, eg, that biologic effects detected in rodents will necessarily apply to humans.

Epidemiologists avoid these concerns by attempting to study people directly in their natural environments. With this approach, one does not need to make assumptions about similarity of effects either across species or across doses and routes of exposure. The epidemiologist actually observes the patterns of exposure and disease development as they naturally occur within human populations. Without such information, one could never reach a definitive conclusion about the extent of disease related to a particular agent.

As with any scientific method, the epidemiologic approach has inherent constraints. In observational research, which comprises much of epidemiology, the investigator merely watches the phenomena under study. That is, the epidemiologist has no control over the events that occur. It is often difficult, therefore, to sort out any possible contribution to causation from the exposure of interest from contributions from other background influences in the population. Even direct measurement of the degree of exposure may not be possible in some settings, thereby forcing the epidemiologist to rely upon indirect estimates.

The epidemiologist's perspective of the relationship between exposure to risk factors and the development of disease in human populations may appear rather crude in comparison to the exacting research performed at the molecular level. Indeed, epidemiology has limited utility for characterizing the precise biologic mechanisms of disease development. More often than not, the epidemiologist sees only the net effect of different levels of exposure upon the likelihood of disease acquisition.

One must realize, however, that medical progress often is best advanced when the subcellular and molecular basic sciences work in tandem with the population-oriented science of epidemiology. For example, as bench scientists struggle to characterize the molecular properties of HIV, epidemiologists already have recognized that AIDS is a contagious disease that is spread through certain interpersonal behaviors. As the painstaking search continues for improved treatment, or even a cure or vaccine, public health professionals have recommended measures to prevent the spread of HIV by reducing the frequency of high-risk practices; those recommended measures include the avoidance of (a) casual, unprotected sex and (b) sharing needles among injecting drug users.

THE APPLICATIONS OF EPIDEMIOLOGY

Epidemiologic methods can be used for a number of distinct purposes. In the following sections, these areas of application are specified, with corresponding illustrations drawn from the literature on AIDS.

Disease Surveillance

Perhaps the most basic question that can be asked about a disease is "What is the frequency with which the disease occurs?" To address this question, one must know the number of persons who acquire the disease (cases) over a specified period of time and the size of the unaffected population. Measures of disease frequency, described in Chapter 2, are used to characterize the patterns of disease occurrence described in Chapter 3 and the medical surveillance discussed in Chapter 4. Typically, the criteria used to define the occurrence of a disease depend on current knowledge about the disease; such criteria may become more refined as the causes of a disease are delineated and new diagnostic tests are introduced. For example, in 1982, the CDC created an initial, relatively simple surveillance definition for AIDS:

> A disease, at least moderately indicative of a defect in cell-mediated immunity, occurring in a person with no known cause for diminished resistance to that disease.

A more specific definition became possible once the causative agent, HIV, was identified and tests for the detection of antibodies to the virus were developed. In 1987, the CDC surveillance definition was expanded to incorporate clinical conditions that are indicative of AIDS. A 1993 revision further expanded the surveillance definition on the basis of three additional indicator conditions (pulmonary tuberculosis, recurrent pneumonia, or invasive cervical cancer), or the presence of a severely depressed CD4+ T-lymphocyte count.

Such changes in diagnostic criteria can have a profound effect on the apparent frequency of a disease. The expanded definition of AIDS introduced in 1987 increased the number of reported AIDS patients by about 50% during the next 2 years. The 1993 revision more than doubled the number of persons who met the surveillance definition. Most of the latter increase was attributable to persons made eligible on the basis of reduced CD4+ T-lymphocyte counts and HIV infection. Accordingly, analysis of trends in disease occurrence over time must account for the possible effects of any temporal changes in diagnostic criteria.

The identification of patients with a disease can occur through various mechanisms, most commonly by physician and laboratory reporting. In the United States, a number of diseases, including AIDS, must be reported to public health authorities. Collection of this information serves mainly to identify unusual patterns of occurrence. A rapid and dramatic increase in the frequency of a disease within a particular population is referred to as an **epidemic.** Early recognition of an epidemic may draw attention to the problem and help to define features of high-risk groups.

For surveillance purposes, the size of the source population from which cases arise usually is estimated from census data. The frequency of disease occurrence is then expressed as the number of new cases developing within a specified time among a standard number of unaffected individuals. For example, in the United States during 1993, 40.2 cases of AIDS were reported for every 100,000 persons. This measure of the rapidity of disease occurrence is referred to as an **incidence rate.** More information on incidence rates is presented in Chapter 2.

To characterize patterns of disease occurrence, incidence rates may be determined for subgroups defined by geographic area. For example, in Figure 1–1 annual incidence rates for AIDS are presented by place of residence in the United States. During 1993, the incidence rate for the District of Columbia was the highest observed, with 274.0 cases for every 100,000 residents. At the other extreme, North Dakota experienced the lowest annual incidence rate (1.7 cases per 100,000). In other words, AIDS occurred in the District of Columbia over 160 times more frequently than in North Dakota (274.0/1.7 = 161.2). Why are persons in the District of Columbia so frequently diagnosed with AIDS; conversely, why are North Dakotans so infrequently affected?

Answers to such questions typically do not derive from surveillance information alone. Surveillance data usually are limited to general characteristics of affected persons, such as their age, race, gender, and place of residence. While variations in incidence rates according to these demographic features can lead to the identification of high-risk groups, explanations of these patterns generally call for more in-depth investigation into personal characteristics, behaviors, and environments.

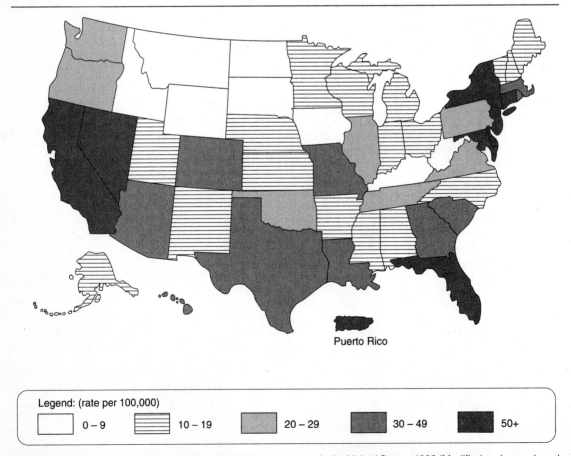

Puerto Rico

Legend: (rate per 100,000)

| | 0 – 9 | | 10 – 19 | | 20 – 29 | | 30 – 49 | | 50+ |

Figure 1–1. The incidence rates of AIDS per 100,000 person-years in the United States, 1993 (Modified and reproduced from CDC: Summary of notifiable diseases, United States, 1993. MMWR 1993;**42**:17.)

Searching for Causes

To study personal and environmental characteristics, epidemiologists often rely upon interviews, record reviews, and laboratory examinations. Through such sources of information, a profile of characteristics that accompany the disease can be generated. Associations between these characteristics and the occurrence of disease can arise by coincidence, by noncausal linkages to other features, or by cause-and-effect relationships. Of course, the epidemiologist is primarily interested in the last category, ie, determinants of disease development, also known as **risk factors.** Identification of risk factors can result in a better understanding of the pathways leading to disease acquisition and, consequently, better preventive strategies.

Again, returning to the AIDS example, early epidemiologic studies played an important role in determining the cause of this disease. Within the first 5 months after recognition of this syndrome, the CDC had received reports on 70 patients in four urban centers. Of these individuals, 50 homosexual male AIDS patients were interviewed as well as 120 unaffected homosexual male comparison subjects. Persons who are affected with a disease are referred to by epidemiologists as **cases,** and unaffected comparison persons are called **controls.** Comparison of the responses from cases and controls revealed that the AIDS patients had a higher number of sexual partners. This type of investigation is referred to as a **case-control study,** and the basic design of such a study is illustrated in Figure 1–2.

In essence, this study is an attempt to look backward in time to identify characteristics that may have contributed to disease development. The increased number of sexual partners—as well as a greater frequency of syphilis among cases—suggested that AIDS resulted from a sexually transmitted infectious agent, later discovered to be the HIV virus. Case-control studies are described in Chapter 9.

Comparison of historical exposures reported by cases and controls can provide suggestive evidence of a cause-and-effect relationship. This type of information, however, may be distorted or **biased** by differing abilities of cases and controls to recall earlier exposures. Such bias could be avoided by using a **cohort study** design in which exposure is assessed among unaffected persons, and subjects are then observed for subsequent development of illness. To collect such data, a cohort of 2507 homosexual men without antibodies to HIV (seronegative) were questioned about their sexual practices and then followed for development of antibodies to HIV (seroconversion). Within 6 months, 95 men (3.8%) seroconverted, and the likelihood or **risk** of developing HIV antibodies was found to be related to receptive anal intercourse. The basic design of this cohort study is illustrated schematically in Figure 1–3. Cohort studies are discussed in Chapter 8.

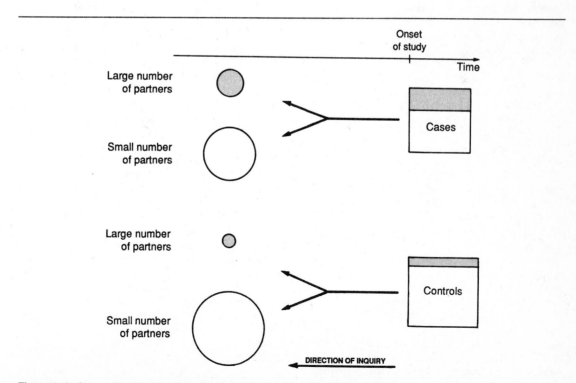

Figure 1–2. Schematic diagram of a case-control study of the association between the number of male sexual partners of homosexual men and the risk of AIDS. Shaded areas represent subjects with a large number of sexual partners and unshaded areas represent subjects with a small number of sexual partners.

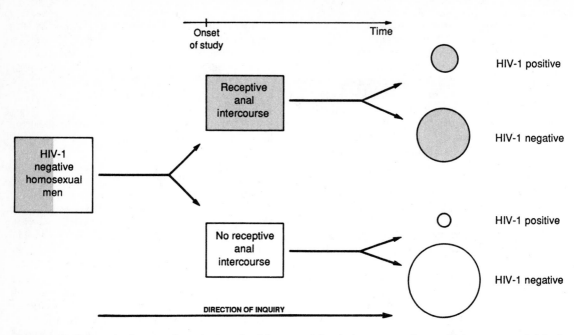

Figure 1–3. Schematic diagram of a cohort study of the association between receptive anal intercourse and risk of HIV-positivity. Shaded areas indicate subjects who practice receptive anal intercourse and unshaded areas represent subjects who do not.

Although roughly half of all AIDS cases in this country still occur among homosexual/bisexual men, the proportion is declining over time. By 1991, the incidence rate of AIDS among homosexual/bisexual men in the United States began to fall—presumably a consequence of reduction in high-risk behavior. Indeed, surveys conducted over time within established cohorts of homosexual/bisexual men have indicated a trend toward avoidance of high-risk behaviors. Whether these changes are sustainable is unclear, however, since recent studies have shown that high-risk behaviors occur frequently among young homosexual/bisexual men.

HIV transmission through heterosexual intercourse continues to increase in the United States and is the leading mode of transmission worldwide. The ability of safe sexual practices to prevent the transmission of AIDS among heterosexuals was demonstrated clearly in a recently published cohort study (de Vincenzi I, 1994). That European study included heterosexual couples in which only one partner was HIV seropositive at the outset. Couples were followed for an average of almost 2 years to determine the relationship between certain sexual practices and the risk of HIV transmission to the uninfected partner. Condom use was found to be an effective barrier to HIV transmission. There were no episodes of seroconversion of uninfected partners among 124 couples who consistently used condoms. Among 121 couples whose condom use was inconsistent, however, there were 12 seroconversions of initially uninfected partners.

The difficulty of changing human sexual behavior is well illustrated by this European cohort study. In that investigation, where one partner was known to be HIV seropositive, and each couple received counseling on safe sexual practices, only one-half of the couples consistently used condoms. One might anticipate even greater resistance to the use of condoms among persons in the general population who are likely to perceive themselves to be at low risk of contacting the virus and who have not received personal counseling about safe sexual practices.

Diagnostic Testing

The purpose of diagnostic testing is to obtain objective evidence of the presence or absence of a particular condition. This evidence can be obtained to detect disease at its earliest stages among asymptomatic persons in the general population, a process referred to as **screening.** In other circumstances, diagnostic tests are used to confirm a diagnosis among persons with existing signs or symptoms of illness. Ideally, a diagnostic test would correctly distinguish affected persons from unaffected persons without any mistakes. Unfortunately, as is true of most diagnostic tests, assays for HIV infection are not perfect.

Occasionally, a test will incorrectly suggest that infection is present (positive test result) in an unaffected person. This type of outcome is referred to as a **false positive,** because the positive test result was in error. Obviously, a false-positive finding for HIV infection could be devastating to the tested individual, so every effort must be made to keep such mistakes to a minimum. A test with a very low percentage of false-positive results is said to have **high specificity.**

Another type of error is committed when a test incorrectly suggests that infection is not present (negative test result) in an affected person. This type of outcome is referred to as a **false negative,** because the negative test result was in error. A false-negative finding for HIV infection could provide inappropriate reassurance to an infected person, thereby delaying the start of treatment and perhaps increasing the risk of spread to other persons. A test with a very low percentage of false-negative results is described as having **high sensitivity.** More detail on measures of test accuracy is presented in Chapter 6.

A number of different tests for the presence of HIV infection are available. The screening approach used most widely is to look for antibodies to the virus. The logic of this strategy requires two assumptions: (1) that HIV-infected persons have detectable antibodies, and (2) that persons with detectable HIV antibodies are infected with HIV. In practice, these assumptions appear to be reasonably valid among patients who are beyond the first few months of infection. The time required to mount an antibody response sufficient for detection (seroconversion) varies across patients, but the vast majority seroconvert in less than 6 months following initial HIV infection.

The performance of an enzyme-linked immunosorbent assay (ELISA) test for antibodies to HIV was first reported in 1985. Among 74 patients who met the CDC clinical surveillance definition for AIDS and had unequivocal ELISA test results, 72 (97%) had detectable antibodies. In other words, a false-negative outcome was observed for only 2 patients (3%). Among 261 healthy blood donors with unequivocal ELISA test results, 257 (98%) had no detectable antibodies (ie, a false-positive outcome was found for 4 persons [2%]). Thus, the ELISA test was judged to be both sensitive and specific, and it has become the most widely employed screening test for HIV infection.

A number of different ELISA kits are commercially available. When false-negative ELISA results occur among high-risk individuals, the most likely explanation is that the test was performed prior to the development of detectable antibody levels in the immediate post-infection period. False-positive ELISA test results have been observed among patients with medical conditions unrelated to HIV, such as autoimmune disorders, hematologic malignancies, and infections with viruses other than HIV. Patients recently vaccinated against hepatitis B or influenza, or those who have received immune globulin, also may have false-positive ELISA tests. Technical or human errors in performing the ELISA test also can produce false-positive results.

In light of the potential for error, it is recommended that a positive ELISA test should be repeated in duplicate. If either of the follow-up tests is positive, a supplementary test should be performed. The most widely used confirmatory test is referred to as a Western blot. This type of test is not recommended for screening purposes, because Western blot can produce a substantial proportion of equivocal results among persons who are negative to all other HIV tests.

The presence of infection with HIV can be detected through other approaches. An antigen of the virus, p24, can be detected intermittently in the serum or plasma of infected patients. Since this antigen can be detected in only 20–30% of symptomatic patients, it is not recommended for screening purposes; but it may be useful for evaluating antibody-negative individuals with suspected recent infection. In the research laboratory, the polymerase chain reaction (PCR) has been used to amplify viral genetic material so that HIV can be detected in minute concentrations. Although not yet widely available for clinical application, PCR is sensitive and specific, and it eventually could replace the Western blot test for confirmatory purposes.

Determining the Natural History

In the clinical setting, one of the questions that patients ask most frequently is, "What will happen to me?" This question cannot be answered with certainty, because of variation in outcome from one individual to another. Usually, the best guidance for predictions is the experience of other patients who are similar to the patient in question. Even when the ultimate outcome can be predicted with some confidence, the actual sequence of events can vary widely among patients.

Consider, for example, the situation of a patient newly diagnosed as being HIV-positive. In this instance, the chances for avoiding clinical AIDS and ultimately death are virtually nil, so concern focuses on issues such as quality of life and the anticipated duration of survival. In attempting to address these questions, the physician might consult published research on the progression of HIV-related illness. Usually these data are collected on large groups of patients. By noting the timing of critical events for each patient (eg, dates of diagnosis, development of further manifestations, and death), the progression of disease can be subdivided into phases. When summarized over many patients, precise and accurate estimates of the typical sequence of events—ie, the natural history of the illness—can be constructed. Some authors restrict the use of the descriptor "natural" to situations in which medical treatment is unavailable or ineffective. Others use the term more broadly to indicate the typical course of an illness, regardless of whether it can be treated effectively.

There are several ways to characterize the natural history of an illness. One simple measure is the **case fatality,** which represents the percentage of patients with a disease who die within a specified observation period. For example, among all 10,233 reported adolescent and adult AIDS patients diagnosed prior to 1985 in the United States, 9248 were known to have died before 1991. In other words, the case fatality was:

$$\frac{9248}{10,233} \times 100\% = 90.4\%$$

The approach to determining the case fatality is illustrated schematically in Figure 1–4.

Another method of characterizing the natural history of a disease is to estimate the typical duration from diagnosis to death (**survival time**). As an illustration, a study was conducted of two groups of homosexual men in San Francisco diagnosed with clinical AIDS. These patients were followed to determine whether they had died by February 1993. The results were arrayed in two different but related formats. First, the investigators ordered the survival times sequentially from shortest to longest and identified the duration that was exceeded by half of the patients as the **median survival time**. Among men with clinical AIDS, the median survival time was found to be about 16 months. Next, the investigators estimated the percentages of subjects who survived to various fixed time intervals after clinical diagnosis. Overall, about 30% of patients remained alive 2 years following clinical diagnosis, with only about 10% surviving at least 3 years.

The time from clinical diagnosis of AIDS to death may not be the best indicator of the natural history of this disease. HIV infection may exist for a prolonged period of time prior to the development of symptoms that lead to a clinical diagnosis of AIDS. Recognition of the presence of infection during this preclinical phase clearly is dependent upon the availability of an effective screening test, the sensitivity of the test to detect early infection, and the extent to which the screening test is applied in the population. One would expect, therefore, that in the earliest years of the AIDS epidemic, prior to the development and widespread application of screening tests for HIV, patients tended to be diagnosed at comparatively advanced stages of infection, when symptoms already were evident.

Regional and international comparisons of the survival experience of AIDS patients also might be distorted by differences in the extent to which screening for HIV and CD4+ T-lymphocyte counts are employed in the different locations.

Changes over time in the diagnostic criteria used for AIDS also could alter the apparent survival experience of patients with this disease. For example, analysis of Italian patients with HIV registered between July 1987 and December 1991 revealed a median survival of 24 months for 1220 patients who met the 1987 CDC case definition for AIDS. When the broadened 1993 CDC case definition was retrospectively applied to this same population, not only did a larger number of patients meet the definition, but the median survival was found to exceed 57 months.

Yet another possibility is that the introduction of measures to prevent or treat opportunistic infections among HIV-seropositive persons might delay symptoms, and thereby postpone the clinical diagnosis of AIDS. To minimize the impact of the various factors affecting the timing of the clinical diagnosis of AIDS, it would be desirable to estimate survival from a more definitive and consistent starting point. Ideally, one might want to estimate natural history from the time of initial HIV infection. Unfortunately, the exact time of infection is unlikely to be known for most HIV-seropositive patients. An alternative strategy is to estimate natural history from the time of initial biologic effect. For HIV infection, a suitable marker of early biologic impact on the host is reduction in the CD4+ T-lymphocyte count.

The investigators of the previously cited cohort of homosexual men in San Francisco examined survival from the time that CD4+ T-lymphocyte counts fell

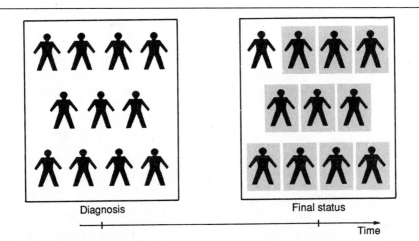

Figure 1–4. Schematic diagram of the concept of case fatality. Shaded figures represent patients who are deceased and unshaded figures represent patients who are alive.

below a defined level. Median survival increased by about 1 year from the earliest patients to the most recent ones. Most of the gain in survival time was observed for patients with *P carinii* pneumonia. From these data, it appears that the most noteworthy impact on the natural history of AIDS over time has come from the treatment of opportunistic infections, rather than from therapy directed against the HIV infection itself.

Searching for Prognostic Factors

Survival analysis can be employed to identify subgroups of patients with unusually favorable (or unfavorable) clinical outcomes. Characteristics that relate to the likelihood of survival are referred to as **prognostic factors.** Saah and colleagues conducted a study of prognostic factors for AIDS. Using data collected from the Multicenter AIDS Cohort Study of homosexual men in five urban areas of the United States, the investigators evaluated factors related to the duration of time from AIDS diagnosis to death. The design of this study is depicted schematically in Figure 1–5. This diagram shows that the study design is similar to that of the cohort study (Figure 1–3), except that, in the former study, the focus is on predicting survival rather than determining risk factors for the onset of disease.

In the Saah study, many potential prognostic factors were assessed, including demographic characteristics (eg, the patient's age and race), clinical manifestations at diagnosis (eg, presence of *P carinii* pneumonia, fever, or oral candidiasis), and laboratory test results (eg, white blood cell count, total lymphocyte count, CD4+ T-lymphocyte count, CD8+ T-lymphocyte count, and hemoglobin). When these factors were evaluated individually, all were found to be related to survival, with the exception of race. When the factors were assessed collectively and adjustment was made for the type of treatments that were administered, however, certain characteristics appeared more important than others. The independent predictors of survival are shown in Table 1–2.

Patients who were 37 years of age or older experienced almost a 30% higher death rate than younger patients. Several aspects of the initial diagnosis appeared to have prognostic importance. Patients with more than one manifestation at diagnosis had a 64% higher rate of death than those with just one manifestation. Those who had a single manifestation other than Kaposi's sarcoma or *P carinii* pneumonia had almost a 50% elevation in death rate, and those who presented with fever or oral candidiasis had a 31% increased rate of death. Loss of CD4+ T-lymphocytes was a particularly strong predictor of death; to a lesser extent, anemia, as reflected by declining hemoglobin levels, also predicted poor survival.

Testing New Treatments

In the United States, all new medications must be proved effective before they can be introduced into routine clinical care. The standard approach used to evaluate treatment effectiveness is the **randomized**

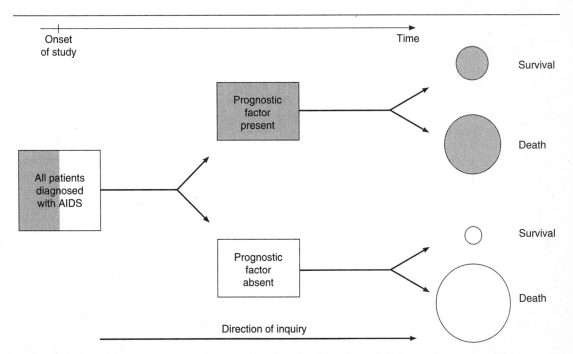

Figure 1–5. Schematic diagram of a study to evaluate prognostic factors for AIDS patients. The shaded areas represent patients with the prognostic factor of interest and the unshaded areas represent patients without the prognostic factor of interest.

Table 1–2. Independent prognostic factors for AIDS.

Factor	Poor Prognosis Level
Age	37 years or older
Initial presentation	Multiple diagnoses
Single diagnosis other than Kaposi's sarcoma or *P carinii* pneumonia	Thrush
CD4+ T-lymphocytes	Low
Hemoglobin	Low

controlled clinical trial. The term "controlled" means that patients (experimental subjects) who receive the new medication are compared against patients (control subjects) who receive either an inactive substance (placebo) or a standard treatment if one exists. "Randomized" refers to a method of assignment of subjects to either the experimental or control group that is determined by chance rather than patient preference or physician selection. This type of allocation system is desirable because it tends to result in study groups that are comparable with respect to important prognostic factors. Randomized controlled clinical trials are discussed in Chapter 7.

The principles of randomized controlled clinical trials can be demonstrated by a study of the effectiveness of zidovudine, formerly referred to as AZT (azidothymidine), in the treatment of AIDS. Zidovudine is a thymidine analog with the ability to inhibit the replication of HIV in laboratory tests. In early 1986, investigators at 12 medical centers in the United States enrolled 282 patients with AIDS or a related complex

of symptoms in a randomized controlled clinical trial comparing zidovudine to a placebo. The basic design of the trial is depicted in Figure 1–6.

Randomized assignment resulted in the allocation of 145 patients to zidovudine and 137 to the placebo. The two study groups were similar with respect to most clinical characteristics at the onset of treatment. After an average of about 4 months of observation, the trial was terminated because of a dramatic difference in the survival experience of the two groups. Among the zidovudine-treated patients, only 1 death occurred, whereas there were 19 deaths among the placebo-treated patients.

The short-term treatment benefit of zidovudine was clear, and therefore, continuation of a study that would deny effective therapy to the patients randomized to placebo would have been unethical. Nevertheless, the rapid termination of this trial left open the question of whether the benefit of zidovudine therapy was sustainable over longer periods of time. Subsequent research suggested that the survival benefit of zidovudine treatment primarily is confined to the first year of therapy. Other clinical trials have shown further survival advantage when additional antiviral agents, such as didanosine (ddI) or zalcitabine (ddC), are added to the zidovudine treatment regimen.

A randomized placebo-controlled clinical trial demonstrated that zidovudine treatment can delay the clinical progression of disease in asymptomatic HIV-infected patients with low CD4+ T-lymphocyte counts. Again, this effect was dramatic enough to cause the investigators to terminate the clinical trial

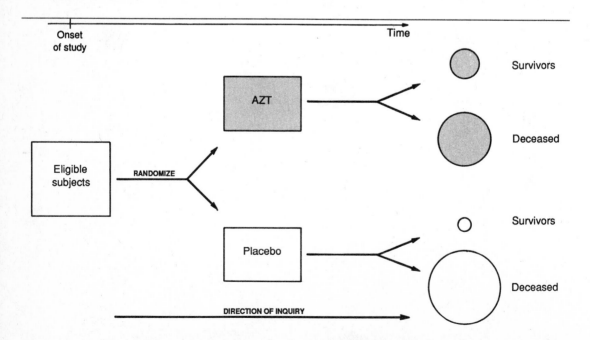

Figure 1–6. Schematic diagram of a randomized placebo-controlled clinical trial of zidovudine (AZT) treatment for AIDS patients. The shaded area indicates patients randomized to receive AZT treatment.

early, thereby allowing all enrolled patients to receive zidovudine. Subsequent research suggests that the benefit of ziduvidine treatment in these patients declines over time and lasts for about 2 years. The reasons for this diminishing benefit are unknown, but may reflect the development of HIV resistance to zidovudine, or some other adaptation of the virus to treatment. Further research is underway to determine optimal treatment regimens for asymptomatic and symptomatic HIV infection.

SUMMARY

In this chapter, we have seen how epidemiologic research has contributed to basic knowledge about AIDS:

(1) The techniques of surveillance were used to determine the patterns of HIV-infection and AIDS occurrence by person, place, and time.
(2) Comparisons of affected and unaffected persons led to the identification of risk factors and ultimately the suspicion that an infectious agent was responsible.
(3) Evaluation of tests for antibodies to HIV allowed improved diagnosis and prevention of spread by contaminated blood products.
(4) Studies of natural history helped to define the clinical course of the illness.
(5) Prognostic factors were determined through comparison of patients with favorable and unfavorable outcomes.
(6) Finally, improvement in treatment was demonstrated through randomized controlled clinical trials.

The story of HIV and AIDS is especially dramatic because it involves a devastating disease that emerged rapidly in the population and developed with minimal advance warning. It is an unfinished story because new cases are still occurring with alarming frequency, and a cure has not yet been identified. Epidemiology will continue to play an important role in monitoring progress in the prevention and treatment of HIV-related illness and AIDS.

Epidemiologic research has been pivotal in gaining insight into many different diseases. From infectious illnesses, to heart disease, to cancer, to congenital malformations, epidemiology has provided insights into patterns of disease occurrence and underlying causal factors. Ultimately, this information can be used to help control the impact of diseases either through preventive measures or improved clinical management.

STUDY QUESTIONS

Questions 1–5: For each measure described in the numbered statements below, select the most appropriate numerical value from the following lettered

options. Each option can be used once, more than once, or not at all.

A. .05	**E.** 2.5
B. .10	**F.** 50
C. .25	**G.** 80
D. .50	**H.** 98

1. What is the annual incidence rate (per 1000 persons) of colon cancer, if it is diagnosed in 5 patients per year within a community of 10,000 unaffected individuals, assuming that half of affected individuals die from the condition?

2. What is the 5-year cumulative risk (in %) of developing colon cancer in the community described in (1), assuming that there are no migrations in or out of the community, and that there are no deaths from other causes?

3. What is the case fatality (in %) of colon cancer in the community described in (1)?

4. A screening test is applied to all residents of the community described in question (1). What is the sensitivity (in %) of the screening test, if it detects 4 of the colon cancers and correctly determines that 9800 of the unaffected persons do not have colon cancer?

5. What is the specificity (in %) of the test described in question (4)?

Questions 6–9: For each numbered situation below, select the most appropriate measure from the following lettered options. Each option can be used once, more than once, or not at all.

A. Incidence rate	**D.** Sensitivity
B. Risk	**E.** Specificity
C. Case fatality	

6. What is the best measure to characterize the prognosis of patients with adult respiratory distress syndrome?

7. What is the best measure to estimate the rapidity with which new cases of non-insulin dependent diabetes mellitus develop within a health maintenance organization patient population?

8. What is the best measure to estimate the cumulative 5-year probability of developing a stroke within a population of elderly hypertensive patients?

9. What is the best measure to estimate the likelihood that children without otitis media will have a normal otoscopic examination?

Questions 10–12: For each numbered objective below, select the most appropriate epidemiologic approach from the following lettered options. Each option can be used once, more than once, or not at all.

A. Surveillance
B. Case-control study
C. Screening test evaluation
D. Prognostic evaluation
E. Randomized controlled clinical trial

10. Which approach is used to compare the relative benefits of two alternative pharmacologic treatments for peptic ulcer disease?

11. Which approach is used to evaluate factors suspected of contributing to the development of intrauterine growth retardation?

12. Which approach is used to assess trends in the rate of occurrence of measles?

13. An epidemiologist was asked to investigate an outbreak of a respiratory illness among children attending a day care facility. Of the 48 children at the facility, 26 developed the illness over a 2-week period. The epidemiologist plotted the days of onset as shown in Figure 1–7. The sentinel cases were indicated by the letter:

A. A
B. B
C. C
D. D
E. E

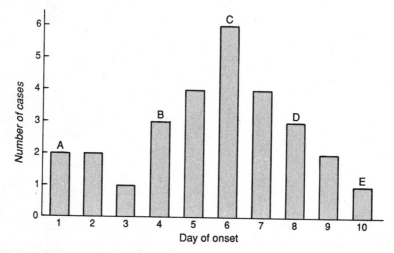

Figure 1–7. Distribution of patients with a respiratory illness at a day care facility, grouped by day of onset.

FURTHER READING

Brookmeyer R, Gail MH: *AIDS Epidemiology: A Quantitative Approach.* Oxford Univ Press, 1994.

REFERENCES

Patient Profile
Gottlieb MS et al: *Pneumocystis carinii* pneumonia and mucosal candidiasis in previously healthy homosexual men. N Engl J Med 1981;**305:**1425.

Introduction
MacMahon B, Pugh TF: *Epidemiology: Principles and Methods.* Little, Brown, 1970.

Person, Place, & Time
CDC: Mortality attributable to HIV infection/AIDS– United States, 1981–1990. MMWR 1991;**40:**40.

The Epidemiologic Approach
Stallones RA: To advance epidemiology. Ann Rev Public Health 1980;**1:**69.

Disease Surveillance
CDC: 1993 Revised classification system for HIV infection and expanded surveillance case definition for AIDS among adolescents and adults. MMWR 1992; **41**(No. RR-17):1.
CDC: Summary of notifiable diseases, United States, 1993. MMWR 1993;**42:**17.
CDC: Update: Impact of the expanded AIDS surveillance case definition for adolescents and adults on case reporting—United States, 1993. MMWR 1994;**43:**160.

Searching for Causes
Jaffe HW et al: National case-control study of Kaposi's sarcoma and *Pneumocystis carinii* pneumonia in homosexual men: Part 1, epidemiologic results. Ann Intern Med 1983;**99:**145.

Kingsley LA et al: Risk factors for seroconversion to human immunodeficiency virus among male homosexuals. Lancet 1987;**1**:345.

Lemp GF et al: Seroprevalence of HIV and risk behaviors among young homosexual and bisexual men. JAMA 1994;**272**:449.

McKusick L et al: Longitudinal predictors of reductions in unprotected anal intercourse among gay men in San Francisco: the AIDS Behavioral Research Project. Am J Public Health 1990;**80**:978.

de Vincenzi I, for the European Study Group on Heterosexual Transmission of HIV: A longitudinal study of human immunodeficiency virus transmission by heterosexual partners. N Engl J Med 1994;**331**:341.

Diagnostic Testing

Phair JP, Wolinsky S: Diagnosis of infection with the human immunodeficiency virus. Clin Infect Dis 1992;**15**:13.

Proffitt MR, Yen-Lieberman B: Laboratory diagnosis of human immunodeficiency virus infection. Infect Dis Clin North Am 1993;**7**:203.

Weiss SH et al: Screening test for HTLV-III (AIDS agent) antibodies. JAMA 1985;**253**:221.

Determining the Natural History

Osmond D et al: Changes in AIDS survival time in two San Francisco cohorts of homosexual men, 1983 to 1993. JAMA 1994;**271**:1083.

CDC: HIV/AIDS Surveillance Report, February 1991:1.

Vella S et al: Differential survival of patients with AIDS according to the 1987 and 1993 CDC case definitions. JAMA 1994;**271**:1197.

Establishing the Prognosis

Saah AJ et al: Factors influencing survival after AIDS: Report from the Multicenter AIDS Cohort Study (MACS). J Acquir Immune Defic Syndr 1994;**7**:287.

Testing New Treatments

Abrams DI et al: A comparative trial of didanosine or zalcitabine after treatment with zidovudine in patients with human immunodeficiency virus infection. N Engl J Med 1994;**330**:657.

Fischl MA et al: The efficacy of azidothymidine (AZT) in the treatment of patients with AIDS and AIDS-related complex. N Engl J Med 1987;**317**:185.

Kahn JO et al: A controlled trial comparing continued zidovudine with didanosine in human immunodeficiency virus infection. N Engl J Med 1992;**327**:581.

Lundgren JD et al: Comparison of long-term prognosis of patients with AIDS treated and not treated with zidovudine. JAMA 1994;**271**:1088.

Volberding PA et al: The duration of zidovudine benefit in persons with asymptomatic HIV infection. JAMA 1994;**272**:437.

Epidemiologic Measures

2

PATIENT PROFILE

A 60-year-old previously healthy female research chemist recently developed shortness of breath and nosebleeds. On physical examination, the patient was pale and her pulse was elevated at 110 beats per minute. Her hematocrit was 20% (low), indicating anemia, her white blood cell count was 20,000/μL (elevated), her platelet count was 15,000/μL (low), and examination of her peripheral blood smear revealed atypical myeloblasts. The patient was hospitalized for suspected acute myelogenous leukemia. The diagnosis was confirmed by examination of a bone marrow aspirate and biopsy. Chemotherapy was started and about 3 weeks later, the patient's temperature rose abruptly to 39°C, and her neutrophil count dropped to 100/μL (abnormally low). Although no source of infection was apparent, cultures were obtained of her blood and urine, and antibiotics were administered to cover a wide range of potential infections. These cultures confirmed the presence of Staphylococcus aureus *in the blood.*

CLINICAL BACKGROUND

Acute myelogenous leukemia (AML), also known as acute nonlymphocytic leukemia, is a heterogeneous group of disorders involving uncontrolled proliferation of primitive blood-forming cells. AML accounts for about one-fourth of all leukemias, with almost 7000 patients newly diagnosed each year in the United States. This disease tends to occur in later life, with a median age at onset of 67 years. Males are at a slightly higher risk.

Although the cause of AML is unknown for most patients, a number of risk factors have been identified, including exposure to ionizing radiation, benzene, certain drugs, and perhaps cigarette smoke. This disease also occurs with unusual frequency among patients with certain congenital disorders—such as Down syndrome.

Patients with AML may present with a variety of symptoms, including weakness, fatigue, unexplained weight loss, infection, and bleeding. On physical examination, these patients often are pale with multiple

bruises, and they have fevers, with evidence of localized infections. In some instances, enlargement of the lymph nodes, spleen, or liver may be found. Examination of blood specimens reveals anemia, low platelet counts, and markedly elevated leukocyte counts, with immature granulocytes abnormally appearing in the circulating blood. The bone marrow of these patients tends to be packed densely with cells, including a high proportion of immature cells.

The clinical management of AML involves an attempt to induce remission with chemotherapy. The likelihood of achieving remission is reduced for patients who are older, obese, have impaired renal function, or pre-existing medical conditions, especially prior disorders of the bone marrow. Remissions may be induced in two-thirds or more of patients, with remission failures most commonly attributable to death from infection or hemorrhage. Even among patients in remission, about 75% will eventually relapse, and only 10% of patients can be expected to live 5 years beyond the time of diagnosis.

The complications of infection and bleeding among these patients are directly related to chemotherapy-induced suppression of the bone marrow, with consequent reductions in the circulating levels of neutrophils and platelets. Patients with very low neutrophil counts are susceptible to a wide variety of bacterial infections, primarily those caused by *S aureus*, *S epidermidis*, *Viridans streptococci*, *Escherichia coli*, *Enterobacter*, *Pseudomonas* and *Klebsiella* species. *Candida albicans* and other fungi can also cause infections among these patients. Treatment with broad-spectrum antibiotics has reduced the risk of life-threatening infections in these individuals.

INTRODUCTION

The importance of risk assessment is evident in the Patient Profile. Antibiotics were administered to the patient even before an infectious cause of fever was identified. In this situation, the attending physician concluded that the potential risk of complications from delayed antibiotic treatment outweighed the likelihood of harm from treatment administered before the cause of the fever is determined. Virtually every treatment decision involves a counterbalancing of risks and benefits. In this chapter, emphasis will be placed on how epidemiologic measures can be used to assess outcomes and thereby guide decision-making.

MEASURES OF DISEASE OCCURRENCE

In this chapter, three basic measures to assess the frequency of health events are introduced. These measures, which play key roles in medicine, epidemiology, and public health, are **risk,** (the likelihood that an individual will contract a disease), **prevalence** (the amount of disease already present in a population), and **incidence rate** (how fast new occurrences of disease arise). In addition, these measures can be used to assess the prognosis and mortality of patients with disease.

Risk

Risk, or cumulative incidence, is a measure of the occurrence of new cases in the population. More precisely, *risk is the proportion of unaffected individuals who, on average, will contract the disease of interest over a specified period of time.* Risk is estimated by observing a particular population for a defined period of time—the risk period. The estimated risk *(R)* is a proportion; the numerator is the number of newly affected persons *(A),* called cases by epidemiologists, and the denominator is the size *(N)* of the unaffected population under observation:

$$R = \frac{\textbf{New cases}}{\textbf{Persons at risk}} = \frac{A}{N}$$

All members of the population, or cohort, are free of disease at the start of observation. Risk, which has no units, lies between 0 (when no new occurrences arise) and 1 (when, at the other extreme, the entire population becomes affected during the risk period). Alternatively, one can express risk as a percentage by multiplying the proportion by 100.

A hypothetical study of six subjects in Figure 2–1 illustrates the calculation of risk. This study began in 1986 and concluded in 1995. The timing of when individual subjects entered the study varied, but each participant was free of the disease of interest at the time of enrollment. All subjects were followed for at least 2 years. For example, Patient A was enrolled in 1986, was diagnosed with the disease just prior to 1988, and then was followed until death in 1993. Patient B was enrolled in 1988, was followed until 1990 without developing the disease, and then discontinued participation in the study. Patient C was enrolled in 1990, was

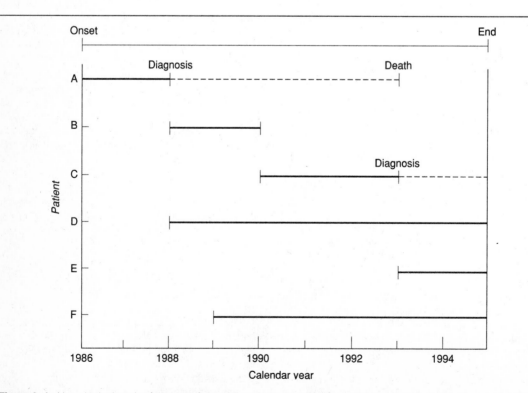

Figure 2–1. Hypothetical study of a group of six subjects between 1986 and 1995. The solid horizontal lines indicate time observed while the subjects are at risk for developing the disease of interest. The dashed horizontal lines indicate time observed after the subjects are diagnosed.

diagnosed with the disease just prior to 1993, and then survived through the end of observation in 1995. Patients D through F entered the study in 1988, 1993, and 1989, respectively; each patient was followed through 1995 without developing the disease.

Of the six subjects under observation $(N = 6)$, only one $(A = 1)$ developed the disease within 2 years of entry into the study. The 2-year risk of disease, therefore, is estimated by:

$$R = \frac{A}{N} = \frac{1}{6} = 0.17 = 17\%$$

These same data also can be summarized as in Figure 2–2, where the time scale on the horizontal axis represents the duration of observation for each subject. In other words, observation of a particular individual begins at time zero and continues until that person dies, is lost from the study, or the study is concluded. The format used in Figure 2–2 is sometimes preferred as a matter of convenience, because it may be easier to visualize the actual relative lengths of observation of individual subjects. The following example further illustrates the use of risks and how they are estimated.

Example 1. In deciding whether to treat the patient in the Patient Profile with antibiotics prior to defining the cause of the fever, the clinician faced this key question: How likely is it that the patient has a bacterial infection? The answer can be based upon experience with similar patients. For example, to estimate a cancer patient's risk of acquiring an infection in the hospital (a nosocomial infection), a study was conducted of more than 5000 patients admitted to a comprehensive cancer center. These investigators carefully defined a nosocomial infection as one that (a) is documented by cultures, (b) was not incubating at admission, (c) occurred at least 48 hours after admission, and (d) occurred no more than 48 hours following discharge (somewhat longer for surgical wound infections). Of the 5031 patients, 596 developed an infection that met these criteria. The risk was:

$$R = \frac{596}{5031} = 0.12 = 12\%$$

In this example, the risk period for each patient began 48 hours after hospitalization and ended 48 hours after discharge. The above result indicates that about 12% of cancer patients similar to those studied will develop a nosocomial infection during or soon after hospitalization. The risk is greater than would be expected for the average hospitalized patient, suggesting that cancer patients are at unusually high risk of developing a hospital-acquired infection.

A broad range of hospitalized cancer patients were involved in this study. The woman in the Patient Profile, however, had a fever and a low granulocyte count. A more refined estimate of the likelihood of infection could be derived from a study of patients with similar conditions. In one such study, 1022 cancer patients with fever and granulocytopenia were studied according to a defined protocol. Of these patients, 530 had a

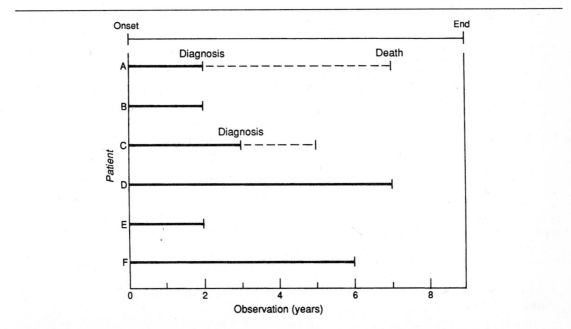

Figure 2–2. Restructuring of observations in a hypothetical study. Times along the horizontal axis reflect years of observation for each subject, rather than calendar years.

clinically or microbiologically documented bacterial infection. Thus, the risk of infection in granulocytopenic, febrile cancer patients is estimated to be:

$$R = \frac{530}{1022} = 0.52 = 52\%$$

This result suggests a very high risk of a bacterial infection in patients similar to the one described in the Patient Profile, thus supporting the decision to treat with antibiotics even before an infection is diagnosed.

Prevalence

Prevalence indicates the number of existing cases in a population. Specifically, the point prevalence *(P)* is the proportion of a population that has the disease of interest at a particular time, eg, on a given day. This value is estimated by dividing the number of existing affected individuals, or cases *(C)*, by the number of persons in the population *(N)*:

$$P = \frac{C}{N}$$

Prevalence, like risk, ranges between 0 and 1 and has no units. The calculation of prevalence can be illustrated using the data summarized in Figure 2–1. For example, to calculate the prevalence of the disease of interest in 1992, two pieces of information are needed: (1) the number of persons under observation in 1992 and (2) the number of affected individuals. First, four persons are under observation in 1992 (Patients A, C, D, and F) *(N* = 4). Second, one of these persons (Patient A) is affected *(C* = 1). Thus, the prevalence in 1992 is:

$$P = \frac{C}{N} = \frac{1}{4} = 0.25 = 25\%$$

Example 2. An important question in deciding whether to administer antibiotics to the patient described in the Patient Profile is the type of infection involved. As indicated earlier, individuals with low neutrophil counts are susceptible to a wide variety of bacterial infections. Therefore, broad spectrum antibiotics are used empirically in these patients until the specific infecting organism is identified.

These bacteria often can be cultured from persons without symptomatic illness. For example,the prevalence of *S aureus* skin colonization was estimated among 96 people attending an outpatient clinic for the first time. Patients with skin infections were excluded from the study. *S aureus* was cultured from specimens from 62 patients. The prevalence of *S aureus* colonization in this group was:

$$P = \frac{62}{96} = 0.65 = 65\%$$

From this prevalence, it is estimated that in a group of patients similar to those studied, about 65% will have skin colonization with *S aureus*.

Incidence Rate

The incidence rate *(IR)*, like risk, reflects occurrence of new cases of disease. *This rate measures the rapidity with which newly diagnosed disease develops.* To estimate the incidence rate, one observes a population, counts the number of new cases of disease in that population *(A)*, and measures the net time, called person-time *(PT)*, that individuals in the population at risk for developing disease are observed. A subject at risk of disease followed for 1 year contributes 1 person-year of observation. The incidence rate is:

$$IR = \frac{A}{PT}$$

To illustrate calculation of person-time and incidence rate, consider the small hypothetical cohort illustrated schematically in Figure 2–2. Patient A developed the disease 2 years after entry into the study. Since subjects contribute person-time only while eligible to develop the disease, the person-time for Patient A was 2 years. Similarly, Patients B, C, D, E, and F contributed 2, 3, 7, 2, and 6 years, respectively. Patients A and C developed disease. Thus, *A* (the number of new cases of disease in the population) = 2, the total *PT* = 2 + 2 + 3 + 7 + 2 + 6 = 22 person-years, and the incidence rate is:

$$IR = \frac{A}{PT} = \frac{2}{22} = 0.09 \text{ cases/person-year}$$

Notice that the total person-years of observation are obtained by simple addition of the years contributed by each subject. Alternatively, this rate can be expressed as 9 cases/100 person-years by multiplying the numerator and denominator by 100. Although these two expressions are equivalent, the latter might be preferred since it does not require use of decimal points.

Example 3. Returning to the study cited in Example 1, the incidence rate of nosocomial infections can be calculated from additional data reported in that investigation. The 5031 patients remained under observation for a total of 127,859 patient-days (or an average length of stay of 127,859/5031 = 25.4 days). Since 596 patients developed an infection that met the definition for a hospital-acquired infection, the incidence rate can be estimated as:

$$IR = \frac{596}{127,859} = 0.0047 \text{ cases/patient-day}$$

$$= 4.7 \text{ cases/1000 patient-days}$$

This means that one would expect, on average, about 0.47% of patients per day to develop a nosocomial infection among patients similar to those studied.

Calculation of incidence rates for a large population, such as that in a city, by separately enumerating the person-years at risk for each individual as described above, would require a tremendous amount of work. Fortunately, one can often calculate person-time for a large population by multiplying the average size of the population at risk by the length of time the population is observed:

PT = (Average size of population at risk)
× (Length of observation)

In many instances, relatively few people in the population develop the disease, and the population undergoes no major demographic shifts during the time period of observation. In such situations, the average size of the population at risk can be estimated by the size of the entire population, using census or other data. One can often estimate the person-time of a large, stable population by:

PT = (Size of entire population)
× (length of observation)

Example 4 illustrates calculation of incidence rates using this alternative approach to estimating person-time.

Example 4. In four metropolitan areas (Atlanta, Detroit, San Francisco-Oakland, and Seattle) and five states (Connecticut, Hawaii, Iowa, New Mexico, and Utah) collectively covered by a network of National Cancer Institute-supported registries, 1308 females were newly diagnosed with acute myelocytic leukemia between 1986 and 1990. An estimated 11,802,416 females lived in these combined areas on average during this 5-year period. Thus, the woman-years of observation for this population were: 11,802,416 women × 5 years = 59,012,080 woman-years. The average annual incidence rate of acute myelocytic leukemia among females, therefore, was:

$$IR = \frac{1308 \text{ cases}}{59,012,080 \text{ woman-years}}$$
$$= 0.000022 \text{ cases/woman-year}$$
$$= 2.2 \text{ cases/100,000 woman-years}$$

DIFFERENCES BETWEEN RISK, PREVALENCE, & INCIDENCE

As summarized in Table 2–1, incidence rates, risk, and prevalence differ in at least three important ways. First, the measures have different units. Incidence rates have units of newly diagnosed patients per unit of person-time, whereas risk and prevalence have no units. Second, these measures reflect different aspects of disease. Incidence rates and risks describe occurrence of new disease, whereas prevalence reflects already existing disease. Third, these measures are

calculated differently. In Figure 2–1, the prevalence in 1992 was 0.25, the 2-year risk was 17%, and the incidence rate was nine cases per 100 person-years. These differences imply that the three measures cannot be compared directly with one another.

In light of these inherent differences, the measures have different applications. Risks are most useful if interest centers on the probability that an individual will become ill over a specified period of time. Incidence rates are preferred if interest centers on the rapidity with which new cases arise (the time period may be long or unspecified). Prevalence is preferred if interest centers on the number of existing cases or the proportion of cases of a given type. Example 5 illustrates some of the differences between these measures.

Example 5. The use of an antibiotic, norfloxacin, was studied for prevention of gram-negative bacterial infections in patients with acute leukemia who had treatment-related low neutrophil counts. All 35 patients who received norfloxacin developed fever. The 35 patients were observed for a total of 220.5 person-days before first developing fever; each day, on average, about 28% of the patients had a fever. Thus, the risk of developing a fever was 35/35 = 1 in this group of patients, the incidence rate was 35/220.5 = 0.16 cases/person-day = 16 cases/100 person-days, and the average prevalence was 28%.

The risk of 1 suggests that treatment with norfloxacin does not ultimately prevent infectious fevers or reduce risk of fever development. On the other hand, the incidence rate in the norfloxacin-treated group was lower than that in a group of similar patients who did not receive norfloxacin, suggesting that treatment slowed or delayed the onset of fever. Furthermore, prevalence of fever was lower in the norfloxacin group, which indicates that treated patients are less likely to be febrile on an "average" day.

SURVIVAL

Survival is the probability of remaining alive for a specific length of time. For a chronic disease such as cancer, 1-year survival and 5-year survival are often used as indicators of the severity of disease and the prognosis. For example, the 5-year survival for acute myelocytic leukemia is about 0.10, indicating that only 10% of patients with acute myelocytic leukemia survive at least 5 years after diagnosis.

In simple situations, one estimates survival (S) as:

$$S = \frac{A - D}{A}$$

where D is the number of deaths observed in a specified period of time and A is the number of newly diagnosed patients under observation. Survival for at least 2 years after diagnosis can be determined from the data in Figure 2–3. Observation of each patient begins at

Table 2-1. Characteristics of risk, prevalence, and incidence rate.

Characteristic	Risk	Prevalence	Incidence Rate
What is measured	Probability of disease	Percent of population with disease	Rapidity of disease occurrence
Units	None	None	Cases/person-time
Time of disease diagnosis	Newly diagnosed	Existing	Newly diagnosed
Synonyms	Cumulative incidence	—	Incidence density

diagnosis (time = 0), and continues until death, survival for 5 years, or follow-up ceases (the subject is "censored"). A patient is censored when follow-up ends prior to death or completion of a full period of observation. Follow-up could end for one of several reasons: (1) the patient decides to discontinue participation, (2) the patient is "lost" to follow-up, or (3) the study ends. Five of the six people under observation ($N = 6$) in Figure 2–3 survive at least 2 years. Thus, the 2-year survival is:

$$S = \frac{5}{6} = 0.83 = 83\%$$

Calculation of survival indicates the probability of surviving a specified length of time and is inversely related to the risk of death. Survival estimates provide a useful way to summarize prognosis, as illustrated in Example 6.

Example 6. The patient described in the Patient Profile has acute myelogenous leukemia. Data collected by the National Cancer Institute for patients diagnosed with this disease between 1983 and 1989 in the United States indicate that only about 10% of patients survived for at least 5 years from the time of diagnosis. For persons who were under 65 years of age at diagnosis, the 5-year survival rate (17%) was higher than that for those who were 65 or older at diagnosis (2%). Nevertheless, it can be concluded from these data that, regardless of age, patients with acute myelogenous leukemia have an extremely poor prognosis.

Life Table and Other Survival Analyses

When studying survival and risk, problems can arise if the investigator cannot follow some subjects for the entire risk period. This situation may result if some subjects move away or miss a follow-up appointment. In Figure 2–3, for example, observation of Patients B and E stopped after 2 years (censored). If one wishes to determine the survival for a 5-year period, observation of Patients B and E is incomplete. One knows only that these individuals survived for at least 2 years; we do not know if they survived a full 5 years. It might seem, therefore, that these patients do not contribute any useful information toward the estimation of a

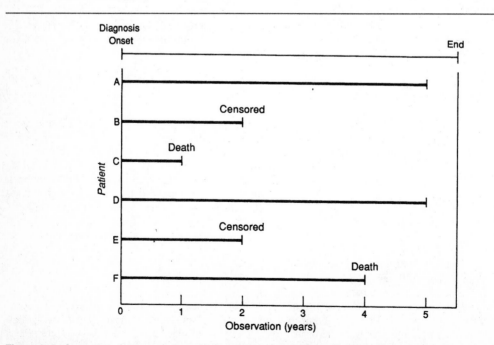

Figure 2-3. Survival experience of a hypothetical group of six patients. The time of observation for each subject, beginning with diagnosis, is measured in years.

5-year survival probability. In the absence of information about what happened to these patients, we might consider two extreme scenarios. In the first scenario, both Patients B and E survive the full 5 years. The overall 5-year survival estimate in this situation would be:

$$S = \frac{4}{6} = 0.67 = 67\%$$

In the second scenario, neither Patient B nor E survive for the full 5 years. The overall 5-year survival estimate in this situation would be:

$$S = \frac{2}{6} = 0.33 = 33\%$$

Clearly, these two extreme assumptions lead to very different estimates of the 5-year probability of survival. Since the observations are incomplete, we do not know which, if either, of these two calculations is correct. In this case, the inability to estimate survival probabilities points to the need for analytic methods to handle censored observations.

Statisticians have developed special techniques, called survival analyses, to account for such incomplete observations. Two particularly useful methods of survival analysis are life table analysis and Kaplan-Meier analysis. Life table and Kaplan-Meier analyses allow calculation of risks even if some of the observations are incomplete. Descriptions of these and other methods of survival analysis can be found in *Basic and Clinical Biostatistics,* (Dawson-Saunders and Trapp, 1994).

The results of a survival analysis can be presented graphically, as shown in Figure 2–4. The information portrayed in this graph relates to the survival experience of patients diagnosed in the United States during 1986 with any type of leukemia. Along the horizontal axis, time in years since diagnosis is plotted (0 = time of diagnosis). Along the vertical axis, the percentage of patients who are alive is plotted. The survival curve begins at the time of diagnosis, when 100% of patients are alive. During the first year following diagnosis, 36% of the patients die (or equivalently, 100% − 36% = 64% survive). During the next year, another 10% of patients die (cumulative survival = 64% − 10% = 54%). The process of attrition to death continues through the end of the 5-year observation period.

The survival curve can be used to determine basic summary measures about the prognosis of leukemia in adults. For example, one may wish to know the percentage of patients who survive to some fixed period of time following diagnosis. Typically, cancer prognosis is assessed by determining the percentage of patients who survive for at least 5 years after diagnosis. The approach to estimating this percentage is depicted in Figure 2–5. Beginning on the horizontal axis at 5 years, a line is drawn to the survival curve (Step A). From the point of intersection with the survival curve, a line is drawn across to the vertical axis (Step B). The percentage of survivors (40%) is then read from the vertical axis.

Another summary measure of prognosis is the median survival time, which is the time following diagnosis at which one-half of the patients remain alive. The approach to estimating the median survival time is shown in Figure 2–6. Beginning on the vertical axis

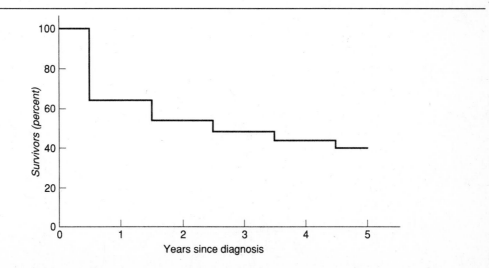

Figure 2–4. Survival curve for patients diagnosed in the United States during 1986 with any type of leukemia. (Adapted from Ries LAG et al: *SEER Cancer Statistics Review,* 1973–1991. National Cancer Institute. NIH Publication No. 94-2789, 1994.)

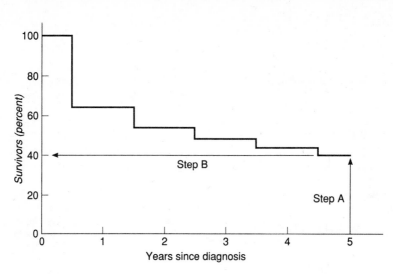

Figure 2–5. Approach to estimating the survival 5 years after diagnosis for patients diagnosed in the United States during 1986 with any type of leukemia. (Adapted from Ries LAG et al: *SEER Cancer Statistics Review,* 1973–1991. National Cancer Institute. NIH Publication No. 94-2789, 1994.)

at the 50% (median) survival level, a line is drawn across to the survival curve (Step A). From the point of intersection with the survival curve, a line is drawn down to the horizontal axis (Step B). The median survival time in this example is estimated to be about 2.5 years.

Case Fatality

The propensity of a disease to cause the death of affected patients is referred to as the **case fatality.** The terms "rate" and "ratio" are sometimes associated with "case fatality," although mathematically this is not ap-

propriate since case fatality is a proportion. Case fatality (CF) is estimated by:

$$CF = \frac{\text{Number of deaths}}{\text{Number of diagnosed patients}} = \frac{D}{A}$$

The resulting estimate can be left as a proportion or multiplied by 100 to convert it to a percentage. Notice that this formula is analogous in structure to that previously described for risk, or cumulative incidence. The difference between these two measures is the phase of illness to which they are applied. Risk of dis-

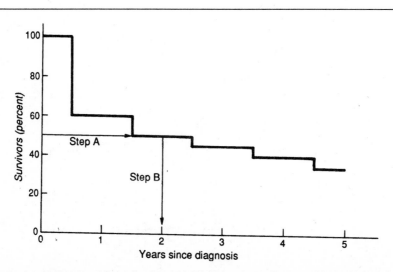

Figure 2–6. Approach to estimating the median survival time for patients diagnosed in the United States during 1986 with any type of leukemia. (Adapted from Ries LAG et al: *SEER Cancer Statistics Review,* 1973–1991. National Cancer Institute. NIH Publication No. 94-2789, 1994.)

ease refers to the initial development of the condition, and case fatality refers to the likelihood of death among persons diagnosed with the disease. Both measures require specification of some time period over which events are counted.

The relationship between risk and case fatality is depicted schematically in Figure 2–7. The initial population at risk of disease consists of 15 women ($N = 15$), five of whom develop the condition of interest ($A = 5$). Risk, or cumulative incidence, therefore, is:

$$R = \frac{A}{N} = \frac{5}{15} = 0.33 = 33\%$$

Only two ($D = 2$) of the affected women ($A = 5$) subsequently die from the condition. The case fatality, therefore, is:

$$CF = \frac{D}{A} = \frac{2}{5} = 0.40 = 40\%$$

The case fatality can range from 0, when no patients die from the disease, to 1 (or 100%), when all patients die from the disease. Since the case fatality represents the proportion of persons affected with a disease who die from it, the case fatality may be thought of as the complement to survival. In other words, for a given period of observation, the case fatality and survi-

val should sum to 100%. Returning to Figure 2–7, survival is:

$$S = \frac{(A - D)}{A} = \frac{(5 - 2)}{5} = \frac{3}{5} = 0.60 = 60\%$$

Thus, the case fatality ($CF = 40\%$) and the survival ($S = 60\%$) total 100%.

SUMMARY

Five of the basic descriptive measures used in epidemiology have been introduced in this chapter. Although other indicators of disease frequency and prognosis exist, these five measures are central to the descriptive function of epidemiology. Key points to remember are listed below.

(1) **Risk,** or cumulative incidence, is the proportion of unaffected persons who develop the disease of interest in a specified period of time.
(2) **Prevalence** is the number of persons affected by the disease of interest at a particular time.
(3) **Incidence rate** measures the rapidity with which unaffected persons develop a particular disease.

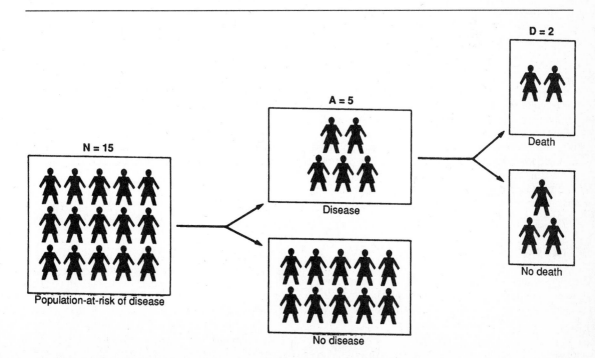

Figure 2–7. Schematic diagram of the natural history of an illness, indicating the population at risk of disease (N), incident cases (A), and deaths from the disease (D).

(4) Survival is the proportion of persons affected by the disease of interest who live for at least a specified period of time.

(5) Case fatality is the proportion of persons affected by a particular disease who die from it within a specified period of time.

Survival and case fatality represent mutually exclusive outcomes, and together must account for all individuals affected with the disease who have known vital status.

Application of these measures to the questions raised by the Patient Profile result in the following conclusions:

(1) Hospitalized cancer patients have a substantial risk ($R = 0.12$, or 12%) of developing an infection during hospitalization.

(2) The infectious agents that cause bloodstream infections (eg, *S aureus*) in cancer patients, are commonly cultured from the skin of healthy persons (prevalence [P] = 0.65, or 65%).

(3) The incidence rate of infection among hospitalized cancer patients is appreciable ($IR = 4.7$ cases per 1000 patient-days), but the corresponding incidence rate for patients with impaired immune systems is more than 30 times greater ($IR = 160$ cases per 1000 patient-days).

(4) The 5-year survival for adult patients with acute myelogenous leukemia is extremely low ($S = 0.10$, or 10%).

(5) Based upon the survival data, it can be concluded that 90% of patients with acute myelogenous leukemia die from this disease or its complications within 5 years of diagnosis.

With this information in mind, the physician in the Patient Profile can conclude that the patient is at unusually high risk for a life-threatening nosocomial bacterial infection. Rapid initiation of broad spectrum antibiotic therapy is warranted, even before the results of culture specimens are known. When the results of pre-treatment cultures and antibiotic susceptibilities become available, the antibiotic regimen can be modified, if necessary. By appropriate use and interpretation of standard epidemiologic measures such as risk and incidence rate, the physician can make informed and potentially life-saving treatment decisions.

STUDY QUESTIONS

Questions 1–4: For each numbered measure below, select the most appropriate numerical value from the following lettered options. Each lettered option can be used once, more than once, or not at all.

A. 0.015
B. 0.020
C. 0.024
D. 0.100
E. 0.118
F. 0.133
G. 0.150
H. 0.176
I. 0.750
J. 1.5
K. 7.5

1. Estimate the prevalence of hypertension for a health maintenance organization with 100,000 participants, for whom an initial review of all medical records reveals that 15,000 persons have hypertension. Follow-up of this population reveals 2000 new diagnoses each year.

2. Estimate the incidence rate (per person-year) of new case development in the population described in question (1), assuming no entries from—or losses of—patients and no deaths from other causes.

3. Estimate the 5-year cumulative risk of newly developing hypertension in the population described in question (1), assuming no entries from—or losses of—patients and no deaths from other causes.

4. Estimate the average duration (in years) of hypertension in the population described in question (1), given the incidence rate and prevalence estimated above.

Questions 5–8: For each numbered situation below, select the most appropriate measure from the following lettered options. Each option can be used once, more than once, or not at all.

A. Incidence rate
B. Prevalence
C. Risk
D. Median survival
E. Case fatality

5. Which is the best measure to estimate the typical duration of hospice services required for patients with pancreatic cancer?

6. Which is the best measure to estimate the proportion of newly-entering school children with auditory deficits?

7. Which is the best measure to estimate the likelihood of death for patients diagnosed with hantavirus pulmonary syndrome?

8. Which is the best measure to estimate the rapidity with which new cases of papilloma virus infection occur among students on a college campus?

Questions 9–12: For each numbered measure below, select the most likely direction of change from the following lettered options. Each option can be used once, more than once, or not at all.

A. Increase
B. Decrease
C. Stay the same
D. Cannot be determined from the information provided

9. What is the most likely effect on case fatality, as the probability of survival from childhood leukemia increases?

10. What is the most likely effect on prevalence, as the incidence rate of tuberculosis increases?

11. What is the most likely effect on prevalence, as the case fatality from renal failure decreases?

12. What is the most likely effect on risk, as the incidence rate of stomach cancer decreases?

Questions 13–14: A study about risk of stroke among elderly hypertensive patients was conducted between 1986 and 1991. The results of observations on six patients are depicted graphically in Figure 2–8.

13. The prevalence of stroke among these patients in 1988 was

A. 1/6 = 0.17
B. 2/6 = 0.33
C. 2/5 = 0.40
D. 3/6 = 0.50
E. 3/5 = 0.60

14. The 2-year risk of developing a stroke among these patients is

A. 1/6 = 0.17
B. 2/6 = 0.33
C. 2/5 = 0.40
D. 3/6 = 0.50
E. 3/5 = 0.60

Question 15: A survival curve for women with ovarian cancer is shown in Figure 2–9.

15. From this curve, the 5-year survival is estimated to be closest to

A. 45%
B. 55%
C. 65%
D. 75%
E. 85%

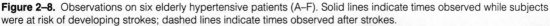

Figure 2–8. Observations on six elderly hypertensive patients (A–F). Solid lines indicate times observed while subjects were at risk of developing strokes; dashed lines indicate times observed after strokes.

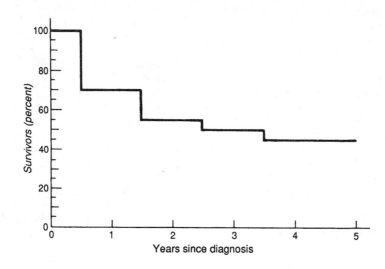

Figure 2–9. Survival curve for patients with ovarian cancer.

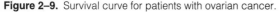

FURTHER READING

Elandt-Johnson RC: Definition of rates: Some remarks on their use and misuse. Am J Epidem 1975;**102:**267.

Flanders WD, O'Brien TR: Inappropriate comparisons of incidence and prevalence in epidemiologic research. Am J Pub Health 1989;**79:**1301.

REFERENCES

Clinical Background

Koll BS, Brown AE: The changing epidemiology of infections at cancer hospitals. Clin Infect Dis 1993;**17** (Suppl 2):S322.

Mitus AJ, Rosenthal DS: Adult leukemias. In: *American Cancer Society Textbook of Clinical Oncology.* Holleb AI, Fink DJ, Murphy GP (editors). American Cancer Society, 1991.

Verhoef J: Prevention of infections in the neutropenic patient. Clin Infect Dis 1993;**17**(Suppl 2):S359.

Risk

European Organization for Research and Treatment of Cancer International Antimicrobial Therapy Cooperative: Ceftazidime combined with a short or long course of amikacin for empirical therapy of gram-negative bacteremia in cancer patients with granulocytopenia. N Engl J Med 1987;**317:**1692.

Rotstein C et al: Nosocomial infection rates at an oncology center. Infect Control Hosp Epidemiol 1988;**9:**13.

Prevalence

Schimpff SC: Empiric antibiotic therapy for granulocytopenic cancer patients. Am J Med 1986;**80:**13.

Incidence Rate

Ries LAG et al: *SEER Cancer Statistics Review,* 1973–1991. National Cancer Institute. NIH Publication No. 94-2789, 1994.

Differences Between Risk, Prevalence, & Incidence

Karp JE et al: Oral norfloxacin for prevention of gram-negative bacterial infections in patients with acute leukemia and granulocytopenia. Ann Intern Med 1987; **106:**1.

Survival

Ries LAG et al: *SEER Cancer Statistics Review, 1973–91.* National Cancer Institute. NIH Publication No. 94-2789, 1994.

Life Table & Other Survival Analyses

Dawson-Saunders B, Trapp RG: *Basic and Clinical Biostatistics,* 2nd ed. Appleton & Lange, 1994.

Evans C et al: High-dose cytosine arabinoside and L-asparaginase therapy for poor-risk adult acute nonlymphocytic leukemia. Cancer 1990;**66:**2624.

Patterns of Occurrence

3

PATIENT PROFILE

A 34-year-old female domestic worker who had recently emigrated from Southeast Asia to the United States came to the emergency room with a 6-week history of cough, fever, night sweats, weakness, fatigue, and shortness of breath. Previously, she had been in good health with two uncomplicated pregnancies and deliveries, followed by a tubal sterilization. Cavitary lesions were visible on the patient's chest x-ray. A smear of a sputum specimen revealed acid-fast bacilli. Mycobacterium tuberculosis subsequently grew from cultures of the sputum, and these organisms were susceptible to all drugs tested. The patient was placed on an initial antibiotic regimen involving four drugs administered under direct observation by the health care provider. After 2 weeks of daily therapy, the patient improved clinically; she was switched to directly-observed, four-drug therapy twice each week for the next 6 weeks. The patient remained asymptomatic, and there was no evidence of bacilli in her sputum. Her treatment regimen was reduced to two drugs administered twice each week, and she remained under direct observation for an additional 16 weeks.

The patient resided with her husband and two young children in an apartment building. Tuberculin skin tests were administered to each of the family members at the time of the patient's initial diagnosis, and results were positive for the patient's husband and 3-year-old daughter. Although no evidence of clinically active tuberculosis was found in either the spouse or daughter, preventive therapy was administered to all three family members. Skin testing of 54 other residents of the apartment building revealed one other infected adult, who lacked evidence of active disease and received preventive antibiotic therapy. None of the tuberculin skin tests administered to the patient's contacts at work were positive.

CLINICAL BACKGROUND

Tuberculosis is caused by mycobacteria transmitted on small airborne particles that are created when an individual with pulmonary tuberculosis coughs or sneezes. Air currents circulate these particles throughout an entire room or building. When a susceptible person inhales these particles, tubercle bacilli may become established in the lungs and spread throughout the body. Usually the host's immune system contains this initial infection within a short period of time. A small proportion (5-10%) of patients will develop active clinical illness months-to-years later, when the mycobacteria begin to replicate and cause symptoms.

As shown in Table 3–1, environmental as well as personal factors affect the likelihood of tuberculosis transmission. Each of the environmental features listed tends to increase the concentration of mycobacteria in the air. Transmission also is promoted by (a) characteristics of the infected individual that contribute to greater release of mycobacteria and (b) characteristics of the susceptible person that diminish the immune response.

Public health officials in the United States have developed a strategic plan for the elimination of tuberculosis in this country by the year 2010. An effective plan for the control of tuberculosis requires that persons who are infectious with active tuberculosis be identified early, isolated from susceptible persons, and treated with adequate antibiotic therapy. Control strategies also include screening for the presence of asymptomatic infection within groups at high risk of tuberculosis, followed by antibiotic therapy to prevent the development of active disease. On the basis of epidemiologic data, a number of groups with an elevated risk of tuberculosis have been identified (Table 3–2).

The Patient Profile illustrates many important points about tuberculosis. Since the patient had recently left an area with an elevated prevalence of tuberculosis, she was a member of a high-risk group. The presence of symptoms, in conjunction with cavitary lung lesions and tubercle bacilli in the sputum, indicated that the patient was highly infectious. Although the infectious state may end after several weeks of appropriate antibiotic treatment, relapse may occur unless therapy is sustained for at least 6 months in persons without concurrent human immunodeficiency virus (HIV) infection, and 9 months in persons with HIV infection.

In recent years, the emergence of drug-resistant tuberculosis has complicated the clinical management of this disease. Drug-resistant strains of tubercle bacilli arise from spontaneous chromosomal mutations; different mutations affect susceptibility to different drugs. Under conditions where inadequate therapy is

Table 3–1. Factors that increase the probability of tuberculosis transmission.

Environment	Infectious Individuals	Susceptible Individuals
1. Close contact of infectious and susceptible people in small, enclosed spaces	1. Pulmonary or laryngeal disease (especially with bacilli in sputum or cavitary lesions in the lung)	1. Compromised immune system
2. Poor ventilation	2. Cough or other cause of forceful expiration; uncovered mouth when coughing	2. Presence of certain predisposing medical conditions (eg, silicosis, cancer)
3. Recirculation of contaminated air	3. Less than 2–3 weeks of appropriate antimicrobial therapy	3. Lack of adequate nutrition
		4. Injecting drug use or heavy alcohol intake

administered—as may occur when too few drugs are prescribed, the dosages are inadequate, or patient adherence to the prescribed regimen is poor—resistance to multiple antibiotic agents can arise. Recent surveillance data in the United States indicate that about 1 in 7 patients with tuberculosis has a strain resistant to one antibiotic. In some urban areas, the proportion of drug-resistant strains is much higher. For example, in New York City one-third of tuberculosis patients have a strain resistant to one drug, and 19% have strains resistant to both rifampin and isoniazid, two of the most effective antibiotics available to treat tuberculosis.

A number of outbreaks of multidrug-resistant tuberculosis have been observed in the past few years. These episodes tend to occur in institutional settings, such as hospitals and prisons, and often arise in groups where HIV infection is prevalent. Multidrug-resistant tuberculosis is a particularly virulent form of disease. This is especially true for patients coinfected with HIV, for whom median survival time from diagnosis of tuberculosis to death is only a few months. Transmission of multidrug-resistant tuberculosis to persons without HIV infection can occur in these settings, and other outbreaks have been reported among HIV-negative groups.

The treatment recommendations for tuberculosis have been modified in light of the rise in incidence of multidrug-resistant forms of the disease. These guidelines include:

- in vitro testing of isolated tubercle bacilli for drug resistance and reporting of these results to the health department;

- the use of a four antibiotic regimen for initial treatment of tuberculosis infections;
- and direct observation of initial therapy by a health care provider.

Directly observed therapy is intended to ensure adherence to the prescribed antibiotic regimen, and it involves antibiotic ingestion by the patient in the presence of the health care provider or another designated person.

Once a patient is diagnosed with clinically active tuberculosis, the patient's close personal contacts should be tested for tuberculosis. The husband and two children of the woman in the Patient Profile were considered close contacts. Since asymptomatic infection was demonstrated in the husband and one child, preventive therapy was administered. The other child showed no signs of infection. Guidelines for preventive therapy dictate that children who are close contacts should receive antibiotics until a negative skin test is repeated 12 weeks later. Residents of the patient's apartment building and her contacts at work also were considered to be at high risk and were investigated for infection. The single infected resident was treated with preventive antibiotics, in accordance with established guidelines.

DESCRIPTIVE EPIDEMIOLOGY

Broadly speaking, epidemiologic work can be divided into two main categories:

Table 3–2. Populations at high risk of tuberculosis.

Sub-sets of Individuals Composing the Population at High Risk for TB		
Individuals Who Have Daily Contact with a TB Patient	Individuals with Predisposing Medical Conditions	Other Individuals
1. Family members and close personal contacts of persons with tuberculosis	1. Persons with the human immunodeficiency virus (HIV)	1. Foreign-born persons from countries where the prevalence of tuberculosis is high
2. Health care workers	2. Persons with silicosis, hematologic disorders, cancer, chronic renal failure, or diabetes mellitus	2. Residents of long-term facilities, eg, correctional institutions, nursing homes, and mental institutions
	3. Medically underserved low-income populations	3. Alcohol and injecting drug users

(1) **descriptive epidemiology**, which includes activities related to characterizing the distribution of diseases within a population, and

(2) **analytic epidemiology**, which concerns activities related to identifying possible causes for the occurrence of diseases.

Both types of epidemiology are fundamental to the prevention and control of diseases and to the advancement of medical knowledge. Descriptive patterns of disease occurrence often lead to hypotheses about disease causation that are tested in analytic investigations. Analytic studies may yield findings that help to explain descriptive patterns and to improve surveillance efforts.

Measures of disease occurrence—the tools for descriptive epidemiology—were introduced in Chapter 2. In the present chapter, these tools are used to characterize the population distribution of tuberculosis. Toward that end, three basic questions can be asked:

(1) **Who** develops tuberculosis?
(2) **Where** does tuberculosis occur?
(3) **When** does tuberculosis occur?

Collectively, these three questions serve as the basis for a descriptive investigation of tuberculosis. Answers to these questions characterize the distribution of tuberculosis by **person, place,** and **time.** As shown schematically in Figure 3–1, these features are the standard dimensions used to track the occurrence of a disease.

Person

A basic tenet of epidemiology is that diseases do not occur at random. In other words, not all persons within a population are equally likely to develop a particular condition. Variation of occurrence in relation to personal characteristics may reflect differences in level of exposure to causal factors, susceptibility to the effects of causal factors, or both exposure and susceptibility.

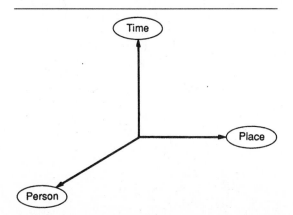

Figure 3–1. Schematic representation of the standard dimensions used to characterize disease occurrence.

Typically, the personal characteristics that are examined with respect to disease occurrence are age, race, and gender. Since such information is collected routinely on the affected persons (cases), as well as the unaffected population from which the cases develop, epidemiologists rely on these characteristics to a great extent. The use of other attributes of interest, such as level of education and income, marital status, and occupation, is contingent upon the availability of data.

The age distribution of cases of tuberculosis reported in the United States during 1992 is shown in Figure 3–2. It should be emphasized that these data are derived from information reported by physicians, laboratories, and other health care providers. Tuberculosis is one of 49 infectious diseases that currently are designated as notifiable at the national level within the United States. The Centers for Disease Control and Prevention (CDC) definition of a notifiable disease is:

A disease for which regular, frequent, and timely information on individual cases is considered necessary for the prevention and control of the disease.

The compulsory collection of information on selected infectious diseases was authorized at the national level in the United States and a number of other countries in the late 1800s. The list of nationally notifiable diseases is revised periodically. For example, the list of notifiable diseases in the United States was expanded to include *Haemophilus influenzae* and Lyme disease in 1991.

Reporting of notifiable diseases in the United States typically begins with a clinician forwarding basic information on a newly diagnosed patient to the designated local or state health department. On a weekly basis, state and territorial officials transmit information about individual or aggregated cases of nationally notifiable diseases to the CDC. These reports follow a standard format, including information on the age, sex, race, and date of occurrence of reported cases.

Although reporting of notifiable diseases is mandatory, and sanctions can be enforced for noncompliance, these sanctions rarely are applied. As a consequence, reporting often is incomplete, with wide ranging estimates of completeness for various notifiable diseases. A number of factors probably affect the likelihood that a notifiable disease will be reported:

(1) The clinical severity of the condition.
(2) Whether the affected individual consults a physician.
(3) The type of physician consulted (eg, private vs public provider, generalist vs specialist).
(4) Any social stigma associated with the condition.
(5) Level of interest in the condition among clinicians.

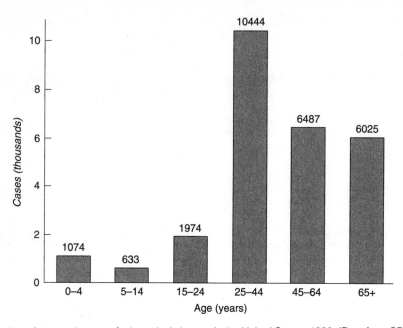

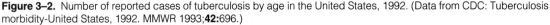

Figure 3–2. Number of reported cases of tuberculosis by age in the United States, 1992. (Data from CDC: Tuberculosis morbidity-United States, 1992. MMWR 1993;**42**:696.)

(6) The physician's knowledge of reporting requirements.

(7) Existence of an adequate definition of the condition for surveillance purposes.

(8) Availability and utilization of appropriate diagnostic laboratories.

(9) Availability of effective disease control measures.

(10) Interests and priorities of local and state health officials.

For a disease such as tuberculosis, in which clinical manisfestations can be serious, clear diagnostic criteria and effective treatments are available, and the risk of interpersonal transmission is high, complete reporting of diagnosed cases obviously is crucial. On the other hand, interpretation of reported numbers of cases must bear in mind the possibility of incomplete notification.

Returning to the data presented in Figure 3–2, and recognizing the possibility of incomplete reporting, it appears that the age group with the highest risk of tuberculosis is 25–44 years. This conclusion is incorrect, however, because it fails to take into account the varying sizes of the source populations across the different age groups. There were over 82 million persons in the 25 to 44-year-old age group, as compared with about 48 million persons in the 45 to 64-year-old category, and only about 32 million persons in the group aged 65 years or older. By calculating incidence rates, one can compensate for disparities in sizes of the source of populations. As illustrated in Figure 3–3, after the first

few years of life, the incidence of tuberculosis rises with age, reaching a level of 18.7 cases per 100,000 persons among those 65 years or older. The incidence among persons in the oldest age group is almost 50% higher than that for the 25 to 44-year-old group.

A number of factors contribute to the nonrandom relationship between tuberculosis incidence and age.

(1) The long latent period between infection and development of clinical symptoms means that the ages at detection of illness are expected to be skewed toward later life.

(2) Since elderly individuals lived through time periods when the disease was more common, they are more likely to have been infected than younger persons (**birth cohort effect**).

(3) Older persons are more likely to have other illnesses (eg, cancer, diabetes mellitus) that may make them more susceptible to tuberculosis.

(4) The decline in immune function associated with the normal aging process may increase susceptibility.

(5) Elderly persons are more likely to live in closed communal settings that are conducive to the spread of tuberculosis.

An equally striking nonrandom pattern of occurrence is seen when incidence is examined as a function of race or ethnicity (Figure 3–4). The highest incidence rate of tuberculosis in the United States is found among Asians and Pacific Islanders; it is more than 10 times greater than the rate for white non-Hispanics.

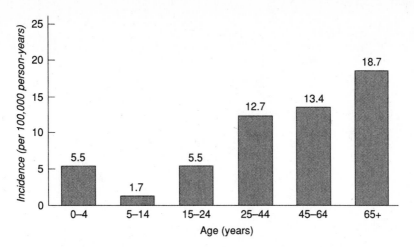

Figure 3–3. Incidence rates for reported tuberculosis, grouped by age, in the United States, 1992. (Data from CDC: Tuberculosis morbidity-United States, 1992. MMWR 1993;**42:**696.)

The vast majority of tuberculosis cases among Asians and Pacific Islanders in the United States occur among foreign-born persons. Most of these individuals, as exemplified by the subject of the Patient Profile, acquire the infection in the high-risk country of origin but do not develop symptomatic disease until they arrive in the United States. A high proportion of tuberculosis cases among Hispanics in the United States also occurs in foreign-born persons.

The high incidence rates of tuberculosis within other minority groups in the United States reflect the influences of other risk factors. Tuberculosis is a disease that is associated with socioeconomic disadvantage. The combination of crowded housing, poor nutrition, inadequate access to preventive and therapeutic medical services, alcoholism and injecting drug use, as well as any predisposing medical conditions, contributes to the high risk of tuberculosis among the poor. Since black and Native American/Alaskan Native populations in the United States have disproportionately large numbers of disadvantaged persons, the incidence of tuberculosis in these communities is elevated.

The distribution of tuberculosis by gender is shown in Figure 3–5. The incidence of tuberculosis is twice

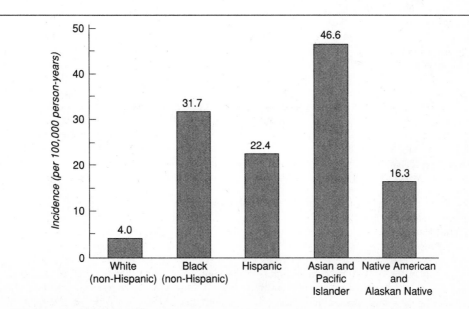

Figure 3–4. Incidence rates for reported tuberculosis, grouped by race/ethnicity, in the United States, 1992. (Data from CDC: Tuberculosis morbidity-United States, 1992. MMWR 1993;**42:**696.)

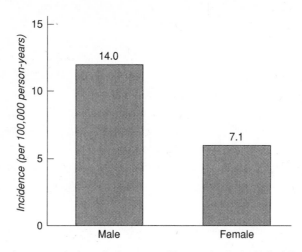

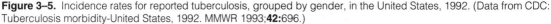

Figure 3–5. Incidence rates for reported tuberculosis, grouped by gender, in the United States, 1992. (Data from CDC: Tuberculosis morbidity-United States, 1992. MMWR 1993;**42:**696.)

as high among males as among females. The higher occurrence of tuberculosis among males probably is related to gender differences in certain high-risk behaviors (eg, heavy alcohol consumption), as well as predisposing diseases (eg, AIDS, silicosis).

Place

Variation in the place of occurrence of a disease can be evaluated at the national level (eg, across countries), at the regional level (eg, across states), or at the local level (eg, across communities). Certain countries, particularly those in the nonindustrialized parts of the world, have comparatively high rates of tuberculosis occurrence. The estimated incidence rates of this disease across various parts of the developing world during 1995 are shown in Figure 3–6.

Worldwide, it is estimated that 8.8 million people developed tuberculosis during 1995, with the annual number of new cases expected to reach 10.2 million by the year 2000. The corresponding incidence rates are 152 cases per 100,000 person-years in 1995 and 163 cases per 100,000 person-years in 2000. These numbers are estimates because the actual reporting of numbers of new cases of tuberculosis, as well as the sizes of the source populations, are incomplete in many nonindustrialized countries. Accordingly, this information must be interpreted with caution. Nevertheless, 95% of all new tuberculosis infections are thought to occur in the developing world.

The region of the world where the incidence rate of tuberculosis is rising most rapidly is Africa, which surpassed the previous leader, Southeast Asia, in 1995. The developing countries of the Eastern Mediterranean and the Americas have comparatively lower incidence rates, but even these rates are more than 10 times greater than the corresponding incidence in the United States and other industrialized countries. The

high rates of tuberculosis in the nonindustrialized nations are attributable to poverty, malnutrition, crowded living conditions, inadequate preventive and therapeutic programs, and particularly in sub-Saharan Africa, the high prevalence of infection with the human immunodeficiency virus (HIV). It is estimated that about two-thirds of the persons who have infections with both tuberculosis and HIV live in sub-Saharan Africa. By the year 2000, it is predicted that almost 14% of tuberculosis occurrence worldwide will be associated with HIV.

Even within an industrialized country like the United States, variation in the incidence of tuberculosis is observed (Figure 3–7). The highest rates occur in urban areas, eg, the District of Columbia (28 cases per 100,000 persons-years) and New York City (45 cases per 100,000 person-years). Comparatively low rates are found in rural states of the Midwest and mountain regions like North Dakota and Idaho (each has 1 case per 100,000 person-years). These geographic patterns reflect differences in the underlying demographic characteristics of the various populations, including such factors as racial/ethnic composition and representation of immigrants from developing countries. In addition, the geographic distribution of other risk factors—eg, poverty, malnutrition, crowded living conditions, injecting drug use, and infection with HIV—probably influence the pattern of tuberculosis occurrence.

Time

The overall annual incidence of tuberculosis between 1980 and 1992 in the United States is depicted in Figure 3–8. During the first part of the 1980s, a consistent downward trend was observed, continuing a pattern that began many decades earlier. Between 1984 and 1989, the incidence of this disease remained fairly constant, with a rising incidence thereafter.

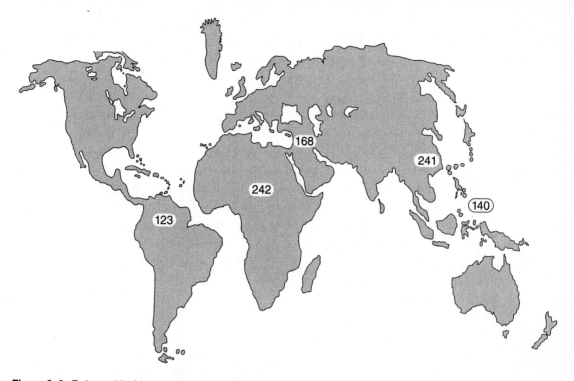

Figure 3–6. Estimated incidence rates per 100,000 person-years for tuberculosis in regions of the developing world in 1995. (Data from CDC: Estimates of future global tuberculosis morbidity and mortality. MMWR 1993;**42**:961.)

Another way to visualize this pattern is to compare the percentage change in incidence between the first and last years of 3-year time intervals (Figure 3–9). Between 1981 and 1983, the incidence of tuberculosis fell by 15%, with an 8% decrease from 1983 to 1985, and no change between 1985 and 1987. Between 1987 and 1989, the incidence increased by 2%, with a 9% increase in the last 3-year period.

When the percentage change in the incidence rate of tuberculosis in the United States between 1985 and 1992 is examined by age, a striking pattern becomes apparent (Figure 3–10). For each age group under 45 years, the incidence rate rose dramatically, with the greatest increase (38%) in the 25 to 44-year group. In contrast, for persons above 45 years of age, the incidence rates tended to decline, with a 16% fall among persons 65 years of age or older. The rise in the incidence rate of tuberculosis among persons aged 25 to 44-years is thought to be related to HIV infection. Surveys of tuberculosis clinics in the United States have shown that almost half of the U.S.-born patients between the ages of 25 and 44 are infected with HIV.

The usual rate of occurrence for a disease in a population is referred to as the **endemic rate**. A rapid and dramatic increase over the endemic rate is described as an **epidemic rate.** The development of an epidemic as a function of time is illustrated schematically in Figure 3–11. For an acute condition, such as a viral illness, the epidemic may develop over a matter of days or weeks. In contrast, for a chronic illness like lung cancer, the epidemic may emerge over a period of years to decades.

The time lag or latent period between exposure to a risk factor and diagnosis of a disease can be as short as a few hours (eg, staphylococcal food poisoning) to decades (eg, infection to clinically active tuberculosis). Obviously, the greater the time between the occurrence of an initiating event and recognition of disease, the more difficult it may be to establish the linkage between risk factor and disease occurrence. This task is made even more challenging if the risk factor is a weak determinant of the disease, or if multiple different risk factors are involved.

As noted earlier, the incidence rate of tuberculosis in the United States ended a long-term continuous decline in 1984. At the prior rate of decline, one would have expected almost 52,000 fewer new occurrences of tuberculosis between 1985 and 1992 (Figure 3–12). This increase in disease occurrence does not represent an epidemic in the conventional sense of a rapid rise in incidence. It does indicate a departure from the prior downward trend, however, and suggests that some new force began influencing tuberculosis incidence after 1984.

Several observations support the speculation that HIV influenced the observed trend in the incidence rate of reported tuberculosis:

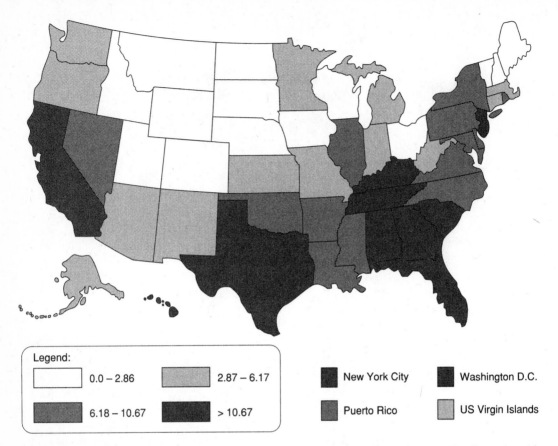

Legend:

☐	0.0 – 2.86	▨	2.87 – 6.17
▨	6.18 – 10.67	■	> 10.67

■ New York City ■ Washington D.C.

▨ Puerto Rico ▨ US Virgin Islands

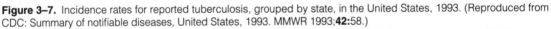

Figure 3–7. Incidence rates for reported tuberculosis, grouped by state, in the United States, 1993. (Reproduced from CDC: Summary of notifiable diseases, United States, 1993. MMWR 1993;**42:**58.)

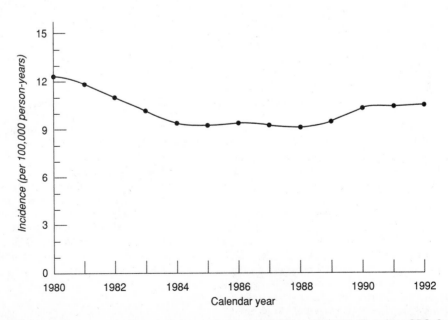

Figure 3–8. Incidence rates for reported tuberculosis by year in the United States, 1980–92. (Data from CDC: Summary of notifiable diseases, United States, 1993. MMWR 1993;**42:**68.)

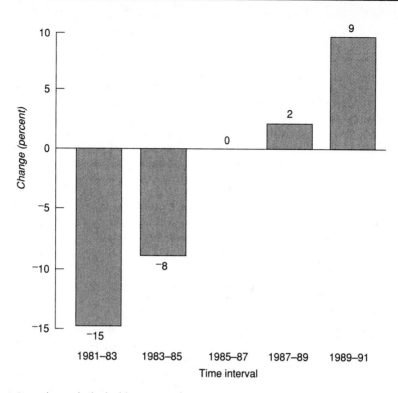

Figure 3–9. Percentage change in the incidence rates for reported tuberculosis, grouped by 3-year time intervals, in the United States, 1981–91. (Data from CDC: Summary of notifiable diseases, United States, 1993. MMWR 1993;**42:**68.)

(1) AIDS emerged at about the same time as the decline in tuberculosis incidence ended.

(2) The geographic areas with the highest incidence rates of AIDS also tend to have high incidence rates of tuberculosis.

(3) The age groups most affected by AIDS also have experienced the most dramatic increase in tuberculosis incidence.

(4) The incidence rates of both AIDS and tuberculosis have increased considerably in black and Hispanic populations since 1984.

(5) The immune dysfunction associated with HIV infection facilitates progression from latent to clinically active tuberculosis.

(6) Clinical studies have revealed that a high proportion of persons infected with HIV have a history of tuberculosis, and as already noted, a high proportion of tuberculosis patients in certain populations are seropositive for HIV.

The actual impact of HIV infection on the trends in tuberculosis morbidity is uncertain, because information on predisposing factors for tuberculosis, such as immunosuppression, has not been collected as a part of routine surveillance for tuberculosis in the United States until recently. Nevertheless, on the basis of the preceding evidence, it appears reasonable to conclude that HIV infection is responsible for a substantial pro-

portion of the observed resurgence of tuberculosis. It has been estimated that about half of the "excess" occurrences of tuberculosis since 1984 in the United States, as depicted in Figure 3–12, are related to HIV infection.

CORRELATIONS WITH DISEASE OCCURRENCE

To develop hypotheses about possible causes of disease occurrence, the presence of a suspected risk factor can be measured in different populations and compared with the incidence of a particular disease. This type of comparison is referred to as an **ecologic study** because the analysis is at the level of an entire population, rather than at the level of individual persons. Another name for this type of investigation is **correlation study,** since it seeks to determine the extent to which two characteristics (risk factor and disease occurrence) are related.

An example of ecologic data is shown in Figure 3–13. In this graph, the incidence rates of AIDS in 15 states of the United States during 1993 are compared with corresponding incidence rates of tuberculosis for that same year. The states included in this analysis (New York, Pennsylvania, Massachusetts, Virginia, Florida, Georgia, Kentucky, Texas, Illinois,

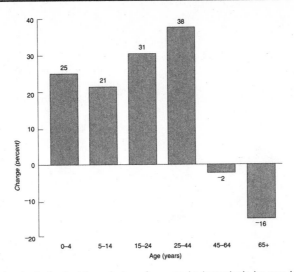

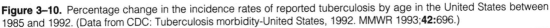

Figure 3–10. Percentage change in the incidence rates of reported tuberculosis by age in the United States between 1985 and 1992. (Data from CDC: Tuberculosis morbidity-United States, 1992. MMWR 1993;**42**:696.)

Kansas, Iowa, North Dakota, Utah, California, and Washington) were selected because they represent diverse geographic areas with varying demographic characteristics.

In general, the states that had a high incidence of AIDS also had a high incidence of tuberculosis (eg, New York and California). At the other extreme, states with a low incidence of AIDS also tended to have a low incidence of tuberculosis (eg, North Dakota, Iowa, Utah, Kansas). As a general rule, the incidence of AIDS was 3–5 times greater than the corresponding incidence of tuberculosis. A few exceptions occurred, such as Kentucky, where the incidence of AIDS (8.5 cases per 100,000 person-years) was less than the incidence of tuberculosis (10.7 cases per 100,000 person-years). An exception in the opposite direction was Massachusetts, where the incidence of AIDS (45.0 cases per 100,000 person-years) was over seven-fold greater than the incidence of tuberculosis (6.2 cases per 100,000 person-years).

To assess the strength of the relationship between AIDS and tuberculosis incidence, a correlation analysis was performed (see *Basic and Clinical Biostatistics,* [Dawson-Saunders and Trapp, 1994]). The correlation coefficient was 0.83, which indicates that the incidence of AIDS and tuberculosis in the study are strongly and positively related. The **coefficient of determination,** the square of the correlation coefficient, was 0.68. This means that about two-thirds of the variability in the incidence of tuberculosis could be accounted for by knowing the AIDS incidence.

A linear regression analysis of these data (see Dawson-Saunders and Trapp, 1994) yielded the following equation:

Tuberculosis IR = 2.6 + 0.18 × (AIDS IR)

The graph of this regression line is depicted in Figure 3–14. In this analysis, the effect of AIDS incidence in determining the incidence of tuberculosis is highly statistically significant. In other words, it is very unlikely that the observed relationship between AIDS and tuberculosis incidence rates occurred by chance alone. From the regression equation it also can be seen that in the absence of AIDS (AIDS incidence = 0 cases per 100,000 person-years), the expected incidence of tuberculosis is 2.6 cases per 100,000 person-years. For every increase of one case per 100,000 person-years in the AIDS incidence, the tuberculosis incidence is expected to increase by 0.18 cases per 100,000 person-years.

The relationship depicted in Figure 3–14 is very striking and suggests that the occurrence of AIDS may influence the development of tuberculosis. This type

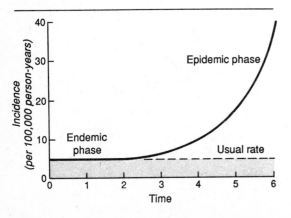

Figure 3–11. Schematic representation of the development of an epidemic of disease over time.

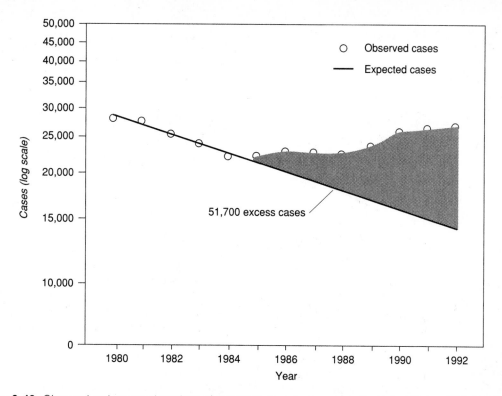

Figure 3–12. Observed and expected numbers of reported tuberculosis cases in the United States, 1980–92. (Reproduced from CDC: Tuberculosis morbidity-United States, 1992. MMWR 1993;**42:**696.)

of correlation analysis, however, is best viewed as a **hypothesis-generating study,** which means that it can help to formulate a hypothesis about the link between these two diseases, but it cannot establish a causal relationship between them. A correlation between AIDS and tuberculosis incidence could occur for reasons other than a cause-and-effect relationship. For example, risk factors for both diseases (eg, injecting drug use) might be the true reason for the apparent association between AIDS and tuberculosis.

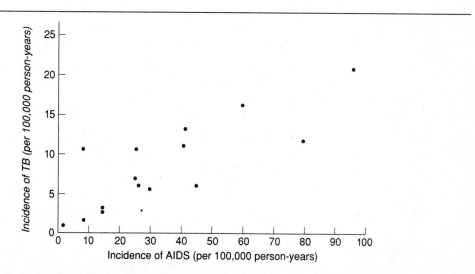

Figure 3–13. Scatterplot of the incidence rates of reported AIDS and tuberculosis (TB) in fifteen states of the United States, 1993. (Data from CDC: Summary of notifiable diseases, United States, 1993. MMWR 1993;**42:**4.)

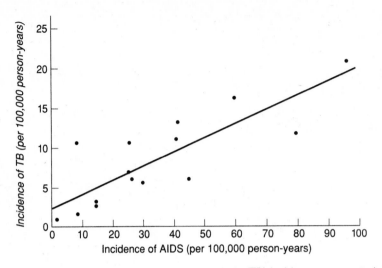

Figure 3–14. Regression line for regression of reported tuberculosis (TB) incidence on reported AIDS incidence in fifteen states of the United States, 1993. (Data from CDC: Summary of notifiable diseases, United States, 1989. MMWR 1993;**42**:4.)

Studies that are designed to test the likelihood of a cause-and-effect relationship between a risk factor and a disease are termed **hypothesis-testing** investigations. The two approaches most commonly employed to test associations between risk factors and disease are cohort and case-control studies. These research designs are described in Chapters 8 and 9, respectively. The effects of related variables, such as injecting drug use, can be considered in the design and analysis of these studies.

An important limitation on the epidemiologist's ability to infer a causal explanation from a correlation study is the **ecologic fallacy.** This problem may occur when a suspected risk factor and disease occurrence are associated at the population level, but not at the individual subject level. In other words, populations may have high incidence rates of AIDS (risk factor) and of tuberculosis (disease occurrence) without the same persons being affected by both conditions. This type of ecologic fallacy can be avoided only by making observations of risk factor and disease status on individual subjects. Methods of analytic epidemiology, such as cohort and case-control studies, involve observations on individuals, and thus are not subject to the hazards of ecologic reasoning.

MIGRATION & DISEASE OCCURRENCE

Another useful technique in descriptive epidemiology is the examination of the effects of migration on the rate of disease occurrence. Studies of this type can help to clarify whether a disease of unknown cause is determined principally by genetic inheritance or by environmental exposure. As depicted in Figure 3–15, migration from a high-risk population to a low-risk population should not affect the occurrence of a genetically determined disease among the migrants. In contrast, migration from a high-risk population to a low-risk population is expected to be associated with a reduction in occurrence of an environmentally determined disease. Expressed in another way, migration diminishes the likelihood of exposure to environmental risk factors, and accordingly, the occurrence of disease should decrease. Of course, for diseases with long latent periods, it may take many years for the reduced rate of occurrence to manifest.

If environmental exposures early in life are critical, then the rate of occurrence may not be reduced among the migrants themselves (who were exposed prior to their departure), but should be diminished among their offspring born in the new location. A dramatic change in disease incidence within a single generation could not be explained on the basis of genetic changes. Approaches to the study of diseases that are thought to have genetic predispositions are presented in Chapter 11.

A number of studies have indicated that a progressive decline over time in the incidence of tuberculosis occurs among persons who migrate from high-risk areas (eg, Asia) to low-risk areas (eg, the United States, Western Europe). The basic pattern of change in incidence is shown in Figure 3–16. The incidence of tuberculosis is highest at the time of migration and falls rapidly in the next few years. The decline continues for many years, with smaller increments of change over time. The incidence among migrants does not fall to the level of the general population, however, presumably because of latent infections acquired prior to

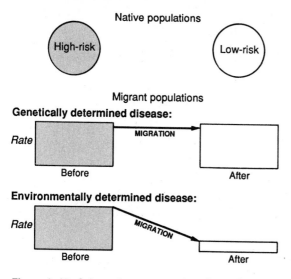

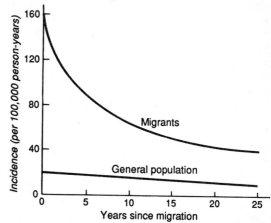

Figure 3–15. Schematic representation of the effects of migration on the rates of occurrence of genetically and environmentally determined diseases.

Figure 3–16. Comparison of the incidence of tuberculosis among migrants who moved from high- to low-risk countries with the incidence in the general population of the adopted country.

migration. Other factors that may contribute to the persistence of an elevated incidence of tuberculosis among migrants include:

(1) Residence in migrant communities, thus maintaining a comparatively high rate of disease transmission.
(2) Crowded housing conditions.
(3) Poor nutritional status.
(4) Inadequate access to preventive or therapeutic medical services.
(5) Noncompliance with therapy.
(6) Presence of tuberculosis that is resistant to conventional antibiotics.
(7) Reinfection upon return visits to the country of origin.

The overall decline in incidence of tuberculosis among migrants from high- to low-risk countries, however, provides strong circumstantial evidence about the importance of environmental determinants of this disease.

SUMMARY

In this chapter, the basic approaches to descriptive epidemiology are presented, with a focus on the patterns of occurrence of tuberculosis. Description in epidemiology begins with the assumption that diseases do not occur at random. Typically, three standard questions are posed to characterize the nonrandom distribution of a disease:

(1) **Who** gets the disease?
(2) **Where** does the disease occur?
(3) **When** does the disease occur?

These questions concern the elements of **person, place,** and **time,** respectively.

At a minimum, the personal attributes examined in relation to disease occurrence are the distributions by age, race, and sex. The incidence of tuberculosis in the United States increases with advancing age. The racial/ethnic groups with the highest occurrence of this disease are Asians and Pacific Islanders, blacks, Hispanics, Native Americans and Alaskan Natives. In addition, males have higher incidence rates for tuberculosis than females.

The place of occurrence of a disease may be studied at the international, regional, or local level. Tuberculosis occurs with great excess in the nonindustrialized countries. Even within an industrialized country like the United States, substantial regional and local variation in incidence is reported.

Temporal patterns can be examined across years, months, or days, depending upon the time course of the disease in question. For tuberculosis, a progressive decline in incidence over time was observed in the United States until 1984, with a leveling off through 1989 and a rising incidence for the next several years. The change in the temporal pattern of this disease suggested that the introduction of a new factor around 1984, probably HIV, altered the occurrence of tuberculosis.

The concept of an **epidemic** as a rapid and dramatic increase in the incidence of a disease was introduced with analogy to the greater than expected occurrence of tuberculosis after 1984. The use of **ecologic (or correlation) studies** was illustrated by a comparison of incidence rates of AIDS and tuberculosis in selected states. In an ecologic study, the overall amount of a risk factor (eg, AIDS) is related to the occurrence of a disease (eg, tuberculosis) across different populations. This type of correlation can be useful for **generating hypotheses,** but not for testing causal relationships. The influence of a background variable that is related both to the presumed risk factor and the outcome of interest can limit the utility of a correlation analysis. Furthermore, the **ecologic fallacy** can lead to a misleading conclusion when the risk factor and disease are related at the population level but not within particular individuals.

Finally, to distinguish genetic from environmental origins, we discussed the use of studies of disease occurrence in relation to migration patterns. As applied to tuberculosis, persons who migrate from high-risk areas (eg, Asia) to low-risk areas (eg, the United States and Western Europe) experience a progressive decline in incidence over time. This pattern strongly indicates that the primary influences on the occurrence of tuberculosis are environmental.

STUDY QUESTIONS

Questions 1–3: For each migration discussed in the numbered statements below, select the lettered option that describes the most likely effect on the incidence rate of disease among offspring. Each option can be used once, more than once, or not at all.

    A. Greater
    B. Smaller
    C. About the same
    D. Cannot be determined from the information provided

1. When compared with the corresponding rate for non-migrants in Japan (low risk), the incidence rate of colon cancer among offspring of Japanese migrants to the United States, where risk is high among the native-born population, is

2. When compared with the corresponding rate for non-migrants in Africa (high risk), the incidence rate of sickle cell disease among offspring of African migrants to the United States, where the overall risk among the native-born population is low, is

3. When compared to the corresponding rate for non-migrants in Northern Europe (high risk), the incidence rate of atherosclerotic coronary artery disease among offspring of Northern European migrants to Southern Europe, where the risk is low among the native-born population, is

Questions 4–7: For each measure discussed in the numbered statements, select the most appropriate value from the following lettered options. Each option can be used once, more than once, or not at all.

    A. 0.02
    B. 0.49
    C. 0.70
    D. 5
    E. 10
    F. Cannot be determined from the information provided

4. In an international correlation study, the mean annual per capita consumption of alcohol (in ounces) is used to predict national oral cancer mortality rates (in cases per 100,000 person-years). The resulting regression equation is

Oral Cancer Mortality Rate = 5 + 0.02 × (Alcohol Consumed)

    The correlation coefficient is 0.70 and the coefficient of determination is 0.49. What is the predicted oral cancer mortality rate (per 100,000 person-years) in the absence of alcohol consumption?

5. Given the equation in question (4), what is the predicted amount of increase in the oral cancer mortality rate (per 100,000 person-years) per ounce of mean annual per capita alcohol consumption?

6. Given the equation in question (4), what proportion of the variability in oral cancer mortality rates can be accounted for by knowing the corresponding mean annual per capita alcohol consumption?

7. Given the equation in question (4), what is the predicted oral cancer death rate for a country with a mean annual per capita alcohol consumption of 250 ounces?

Questions 8–10: For each numbered situation, select the most appropriate lettered option. Each option can be used once, more than once, or not at all.

    A. Birth cohort effect
    B. Ecologic fallacy
    C. Latent period
    D. Endemic occurrence
    E. Epidemic occurrence

8. Mesothelioma tends to occur 30 years or more after asbestos exposure among workers in the shipbuilding industry.

9. Introduction of strict occupational safety guidelines limits asbestos exposure to workers in an industry with previously heavy exposure, and

consequently, only older workers have asbestos exposure.

10. Communities in which individuals were exposed to asbestos through the shipbuilding trade have a persistent, steady elevation in mesothelioma occurrence when compared with other communities without asbestos exposure.

Questions 11–13: Figure 3–17 is a scatterplot of the incidence of gonorrhea and the death rate from cervical cancer in Alabama, California, Colorado, Illinois, Iowa, Louisiana, Massachusetts, Minnesota, New York, Oregon, South Carolina, and Tennessee.

11. This type of study is best described as

    A. Case-control
    B. Ecologic
    C. Cohort
    D. Randomized controlled trial
    E. Case Series

12. The correlation coefficient for these data is closest to

    A. −0.9
    B. −0.9
    C. 0
    D. +0.1
    E. +0.9

13. This analysis does not establish a cause-and-effect relationship between gonorrhea and cervical cancer because

    A. Only 12 states were studied
    B. Insufficient variation in cervical cancer mortality was observed

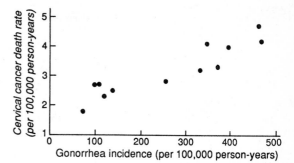

Figure 3–17. Scatterplot of the incidence of gonorrhea in 1989 and age-adjusted death rate from cervical cancer in 1984–88 in selected states of the United States. (Data on gonorrhea from CDC: Summary of notifiable diseases, United States, 1989. MMWR 1990; **38:**1. Data on cervical cancer from Ries LAG et al: *Cancer Statistics Review, 1973–88.* NIH Publication No. 91–2789. National Cancer Institute, 1991.)

    C. There is no comparison group
    D. Another factor related to gonorrhea could be the true cause of cervical cancer
    E. Not all cases of gonorrhea were reported

14. Which of the following diseases is LEAST likely to change in incidence for the offspring of migrants who leave a high-risk country and move to a low-risk country?

    A. Cystic fibrosis
    B. Stroke
    C. Malaria
    D. Unintentional injury
    E. Coronary artery disease

SUGGESTED READING

Comstock GW: Variability of tuberculosis trends in a time of resurgence. Clin Infect Dis 1994;**19:**1015.

Ellner JJ et al: Tuberculosis symposium: Emerging problems and promise. J Infect Dis 1993;**168:**537.

REFERENCES

Clinical Background
CDC: Initial therapy for tuberculosis in the era of multidrug resistance: Recommendations of the Advisory Council for the Elimination of Tuberculosis. MMWR 1993;**42**(RR-7):1.

Hopewell PC: Impact of human immunodeficiency virus infection on the epidemiology, clinical features, management, and control of tuberculosis. Clin Infect Dis 1992;**15:**540.

Iseman MD: Treatment of multidrug-resistant tuberculosis. N Engl J Med 1993;**329:**784.

Jacobs RF: Multiple-drug-resistant tuberculosis. Clin Infect Dis 1994;**19:**1.

Descriptive Epidemiology

Cantwell MF et al: Epidemiology of tuberculosis in the United States, 1985 through 1992. JAMA 1994;**272:**35.

CDC: Estimates of future global tuberculosis morbidity and mortality. MMWR 1993;**42:**961.

CDC: Summary of notifiable diseases, United States, 1993. MMWR 1993;**42:**58.

CDC: Tuberculosis morbidity-United States, 1992. MMWR 1993;**42:**696.

Raviglione MC et al: Global epidemiology of tuberculosis. Morbidity and mortality of a worldwide epidemic. JAMA 1995;**273:**220.

Correlations with Disease Occurrence

CDC: Summary of notifiable diseases, United States, 1993. MMWR 1993;**42:**4.

Dawson-Saunders B, Trapp RG: *Basic and Clinical Biostatistics,* 2nd ed. Appleton & Lange, 1994.

Migration and Disease Occurrence

Medical Research Council Tuberculosis and Chest Diseases Unit: National survey of notifications of tuberculosis in England and Wales in 1983. BMJ 1985;**291:**658.

Medical Surveillance

4

PATIENT PROFILE

A 68-year-old female retired office manager presented with a dry, hacking cough of several months' duration. She reported a history of smoking one pack of cigarettes per day for the past 30 years. To evaluate the patient's cough, her family physician ordered a chest x-ray, which was unremarkable except for an increased density in the hilum (midcentral portion) of the lung fields. A sputum specimen was collected, and abnormally appearing cells were noted upon microscopic evaluation. Since these cells suggested a malignancy, a bronchoscopic examination was performed to allow direct visualization of the large airways. A partially obstructing mass was visible at the distal end of the right main stem bronchus. Brushings from this mass revealed cells consistent with a diagnosis of squamous cell carcinoma. Other diagnostic studies indicated that the cancer had spread to involve the brain and bones. Radiation therapy was administered to all sites of cancer involvement. Nevertheless, the patient's condition rapidly deteriorated, and she died less than 6 months after diagnosis.

INTRODUCTION

In this chapter, attention is focused on one of the most basic functions of epidemiology: *detection of the occurrence of health-related events or exposures in a target population.* The goal of this detection, or **surveillance,** is to identify changes in the distributions of diseases, in order to prevent or control these diseases within a population. The term surveillance literally means "to watch over;" traditionally, medical surveillance activities were developed to monitor the spread of infectious diseases through a population. Today, however, surveillance programs have been applied to a wide variety of other conditions, such as congenital malformations, injuries, occupational health problems, and cancer, as well as other behaviors that affect health. Regardless of the type of outcome under consideration, medical surveillance activities involve the following key features:

(1) Continuous data collection and evaluation.

(2) An identified target population (such as a community, a work force, or a group of patients).
(3) A standard definition of the outcome of interest.
(4) Emphasis upon timeliness of collection and dissemination of information.
(5) Use of data for purposes of investigation or disease control.

The goals of a medical surveillance activity depend upon the state of knowledge about the causes of the condition of interest and the extent to which effective preventive measures are known (Table 4–1). Surveillance activities can provide data about the distribution of a disease by person, place, and time. These patterns of occurrence can help to shed light on possible causes of the disease. For example, if the time and place of disease occurrence are similar for two or more subjects, a shared source of illness, such as an infectious agent, may be involved. Other demographic information about affected individuals, such as age, race, and gender, typically are collected during surveillance and may provide further insight into the modes of disease acquisition. More detailed information on the personal characteristics of affected individuals can be collected through personal interviews.

In the following sections, various aspects of medical surveillance are described. By relating each of these activities to the diagnosis of lung cancer in the Patient Profile, the relationships among different types of surveillance are demonstrated.

SURVEILLANCE OF NEW DIAGNOSES

In the United States, the incidence of cancer is monitored by the National Cancer Institute through a network of population-based registries that collectively comprise the Surveillance, Epidemiology, and End Results (SEER) program. The expression **population-based** means that the target group is the general population defined by place of residence, and the term is used to contrast with other registries, such as hospital-based or medical-practice-based.

The most recently reported SEER data on the incidence of cancer are derived from nine areas, including

Table 4–1. Possible goals of medical surveillance activities.

Identification of patterns of disease occurrence
Detection of disease outbreaks
Development of clues about possible risk factors
Finding of cases for further investigation
Anticipation of health service needs

five entire states (Utah, Iowa, Connecticut, New Mexico, and Hawaii) and four metropolitan regions (Atlanta, Detroit, Seattle, and San Francisco) (Figure 4–1). Although almost 10% of the population of the United States resides within these nine areas combined, this is clearly not a random sample of the nation. The areas were selected largely on the basis of ability to maintain ongoing population-based cancer reporting systems and epidemiologic interest in the population subgroups that reside there. Collectively these registries provide reasonably representative samples of different regions of the country, rural and urban populations, and most major racial and ethnic groups.

The SEER registries use a variety of methods to locate new diagnoses of cancer. The vast majority of diagnoses are identified from hospital admissions through the review of pathology reports and lists of discharge diagnoses. Additional sources of cases include pathology laboratories outside of hospitals, office records of physicians, outpatient treatment facilities, and death certificates. The size of the population at risk of cancer is derived for each geographic area by extrapolation from census estimates.

The 1991 annual age-adjusted incidence rates for the five most common types of cancer among men and

women of all races in the United States are shown in Figure 4–2. Note that the data on breast cancer are confined to women and the data on prostate cancer are confined to men. By convention, the incidence rates for cancer are expressed per 100,000 person-years. The incidence rate for lung cancer means that 58 individuals within a representative sample of 100,000 persons in the United States are expected to develop lung cancer in one year.

The incidence of lung cancer is twice as high among males as among females in the United States. Moreover, as illustrated in Figure 4–3, the incidence of lung cancer is not constant across age groups. This disease is extremely rare in persons under 40 years of age. After age 40, the incidence of lung cancer rises sharply, reaching a peak among persons in their 70s.

The striking relationship between age and incidence of lung cancer (and most other types of cancer) creates a potential complication when comparing the incidence rates of population groups with different age distributions. In other words, simply because of their relative youth, a younger group of individuals will tend to have fewer occurrences of lung cancer than an older group of people. Failure to account for this age discrepancy would result in a distorted comparison of lung cancer incidence rates between the two groups. To allow a comparison of incidence rates that is not influenced by age differences in the underlying populations, one must perform an age-adjustment procedure. The usual approach is referred to as **direct age adjustment** (or direct age standardization), in which *a single standard age structure is applied to the age-specific incidence rates for the groups being com-*

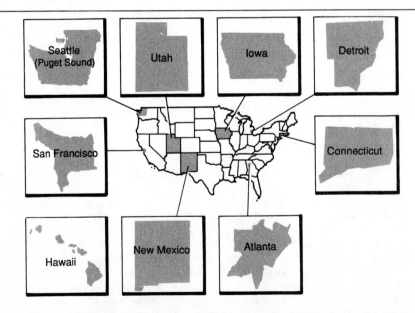

Figure 4–1. Geographic distribution of data collection centers involved in the SEER program. (Modified and reproduced from Ries LAG et al: *SEER Cancer Statistics Review, 1973–91.* National Cancer Institute. NIH Publication No. 94-2789, 1994.)

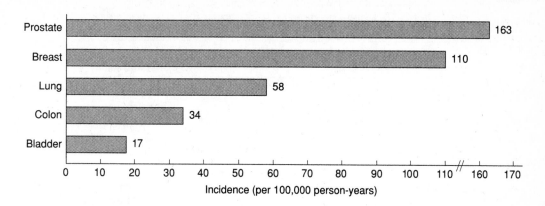

Figure 4–2. Age-adjusted incidence rates for the five leading forms of cancer among men and women of all races in the United States, 1991. The rates for breast cancer are confined to women and the rates for prostate cancer are confined to men. (Data from Ries LAG et al: *SEER Cancer Statistics Review, 1973–91*. National Cancer Institute. NIH Publication No. 94-2789, 1994.)

pared, resulting in summary rates for the groups that are not distorted by differences in age. For direct age adjustment of cancer incidence rates in the United States, the standard age distribution currently in use by the SEER Program is that of the entire population of the country in 1970.

As shown later in this chapter, blacks in the United States have a distribution of ages that is younger than the corresponding age distribution for whites. Since lung cancer tends to occur primarily in older adults, a comparison of overall lung cancer incidence rates for blacks and whites would be misleading, unless an adjustment is made for the underlying racial difference in age distribution. Summary lung cancer incidence rates for whites and blacks can be compared fairly by determining the rate of cancer that would have oc-

curred in each racial group, if they had the same age distribution of the 1970 US population. The choice of the standard age distribution is arbitrary–any distribution can be used as long as it is applied equally to the groups under comparison. We will focus in greater depth on the topic of age adjustment later in this chapter; a discussion of the calculation of adjusted rates can be found in *Basic and Clinical Biostatistics,* Dawson-Saunders and Trapp, 1994).

RATE COMPARISONS

The age-adjusted incidence rates for leading forms of cancer in the United States are shown by race in Table 4–2. From these data, it can be seen that if the

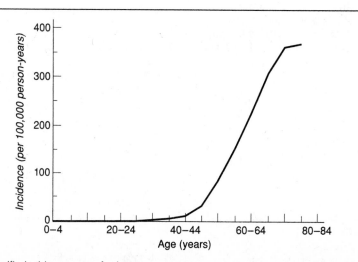

Figure 4–3. Age-specific incidence rates for lung cancer among men and women of all races in the United States, 1987–91. (Data from Ries LAG et al: *SEER Cancer Statistics Review, 1973–91*. National Cancer Institute. NIH Publication No. 94-2789, 1994.)

Table 4–2. The annual age-adjusted incidence rates per 100,000 person-years in whites and blacks for leading forms of cancer in the United States in 1991.[1]

Type of Cancer	Incidence Rate[2]		Black-to-White Rate Ratio
	Blacks	Whites	
Breast[3]	95	114	0.8
Lung	80	58	1.4
Prostate[4]	210	159	1.3
Colon	41	33	1.2
Bladder	10	18	0.6

[1]Data from Ries LAG et al: *SEER Cancer Statistics Review, 1973–91.* National Cancer Institute. NIH Publication No. 94-2789, 1994.
[2]Directly age adjusted to the 1970 population of the United States.
[3]Females only.
[4]Males only.

effect of age is held constant, blacks tend to have higher rates of occurrence of lung, colon, and prostate cancers than do whites. In contrast, breast and bladder cancers tend to occur with greater incidence among whites than blacks.

By dividing the incidence rate among blacks by the incidence rate among whites, a summary measure of disparity in rates of occurrence is obtained. An index of the racial disparity in cancer incidence is the ratio of black-to-white incidence rates, or **rate ratio** (*RR*). If blacks and whites have the same rate of disease occurrence, the rate ratio would have a value of unity (*RR* = 1). When blacks have an elevated incidence compared to whites, the black-to-white rate ratio is greater than one (*RR* > 1). In contrast, when blacks have a lower occurrence rate than whites, the rate ratio is less than one (*RR* < 1). The further the *RR* is away from unity, the greater the disparity in incidence between the races.

The black-to-white rate ratio of 1.4 for lung cancer indicates that the incidence of this cancer in black persons is about 40% greater than it is in whites (Figure 4–4). In contrast, the rate ratio of 0.6 for bladder cancer indicates that the incidence of this cancer in blacks is about 40% lower than it is in whites. These patterns suggest that the factors that influence the development of lung cancer and the factors that influence the development of bladder cancer are distributed differently between the races. These predisposing conditions,

termed **risk factors,** could include genetic susceptibility to the cancers in question, as well as exposure to environmental agents. The most common epidemiologic approaches to evaluating risk factors are discussed in Chapters 8 (Cohort Studies) and 9 (Case-Control Studies). Approaches to the study of genetic susceptibility are presented in Chapter 11.

Variation in incidence across demographic groups can provide important leads about the causation of specific types of cancers. For example, cigarette smoking has been linked to the development of lung and bladder cancers, and among males a larger proportion of blacks than whites smoke. At least among males, therefore, the racial difference in prevalence of cigarette smoking may account for the increased occurrence of lung cancer among blacks. The higher incidence of bladder cancer among whites (especially among males), however, suggests that factors other than cigarette smoking must be involved in the development of this disease.

SURVEILLANCE OF DEATHS

Another index used to measure the population distribution of a disease is the **mortality rate,** which characterizes the rapidity with which deaths from the disease occur over time. The mortality rate is determined by the combined forces of the rate of new diag-

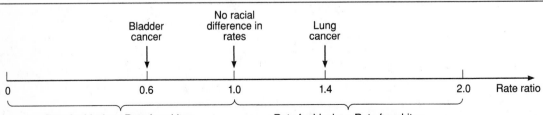

Figure 4–4. Schematic representation of black-to-white incidence rate ratio for cancers of the lung and bladder in the United States.

noses **(incidence rate),** and the likelihood of death following diagnosis **(case fatality).** For diseases such as lung cancer with a high case fatality (ie, a low rate of cure or recovery), mortality rates give a reasonable approximation of incidence rates. As shown in Figure 4–5, the overall age-adjusted mortality rate for lung cancer is about four-fifths as great as the corresponding incidence rate. A malignancy with a more favorable prognosis, such as thyroid cancer, will have a greater disparity between mortality and incidence rates (Figure 4–6). The age-adjusted mortality rate for thyroid cancer is less than one-tenth as large as the corresponding incidence rate, since most persons who develop this disease do not die from it.

Despite the potential disparity between incidence and mortality rates, the distribution of deaths from a disease by person, place, and time still can be useful for surveillance purposes. Pragmatic advantages to the use of mortality information for surveillance purposes are listed below:

(1) Widely collected, virtually complete data; registration of deaths is compulsory in most industrialized countries, and few deaths are not reported.
(2) Standardized nomenclature; the International Classification of Diseases is used to promote uniformity in reporting of causes of death.
(3) Modest cost; recording of deaths is relatively inexpensive.

Mortality statistics thus serve as a convenient tool for epidemiologic surveillance, particularly when incidence data are not available. For example, as already noted, the SEER program covers less than 10% of the population of the United States, but death registration is compulsory throughout the nation. Accordingly, mortality statistics can provide a more complete picture of the geographic distribution of cancer than can be determined from incidence data alone. A map of age-adjusted mortality rates for lung cancer for males and females of all races in the United States illustrates this point (Figure 4–7).

The process of collecting information on deaths in the United States begins with completion of a death certificate. Background demographic data (eg, age, birthdate, birthplace, race, sex, marital status, place of residence, occupation, and education), usually are recorded by the funeral director. A physician is required to certify the conditions responsible, in whole or in part, for the patient's death. For registration purposes, a distinction is made between:

(1) Immediate cause of death.
(2) Conditions that led to the immediate cause of death.
(3) **Underlying cause of death.**

Only the underlying cause of death is tabulated in official statistics. The underlying cause is defined as: (1) the disease or injury which initiated the train of morbid events leading directly to death, or (2) the circumstances of the accident or violence that resulted in the fatal injury. For each of the causes of death listed on the certificate, the physician records the length of time between onset and death. Other required information includes the following: whether an autopsy was performed, the place of death, and the manner of death (ie, natural, unintentional injury, homicide, suicide, or unknown).

Overall, only about 10% of death certificates indicate that an autopsy was performed on the deceased individual (the decedent). The causes of death with the highest percentages of subsequent autopsies are homicides (97%), suicides (56%), and unintentional injuries (49%). An autopsy is performed for fewer than 4% of the patients who die from any one of the following causes: cancer, stroke, chronic obstructive pulmonary disease, or diabetes mellitus. Medical examiners and coroners are responsible for investigating sudden or unanticipated deaths—such as those resulting from homicide, suicide, or unintentional injuries—as well as deaths arising unexpectedly from natural causes. The investigation includes collecting information on the circumstances surrounding the death, and where appropriate, measurement of the decedent's al-

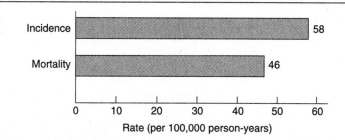

Figure 4–5. Age-adjusted incidence and mortality rates for lung cancer among men and women of all races in the United States, 1991. (Data from Ries LAG et al: *SEER Cancer Statistics Review, 1973–91.* National Cancer Institute. NIH Publication No. 94-2789, 1994.)

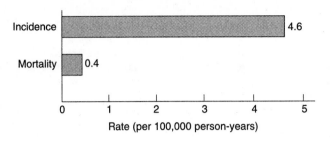

Figure 4–6. Age-adjusted incidence and mortality rates for thyroid cancer among men and women of all races in the United States, 1991. (Data from Ries LAG et al: *SEER Cancer Statistics Review, 1973–91.* National Cancer Institute. NIH Publication No. 94-2789, 1994.)

cohol and drug levels. The information reported by medical examiners and coroners usually is not available at the time of initial certification of death, and therefore, is added later as an amendment.

Death certificates are filed with a local registrar, who checks for completeness of the information provided and then forwards the certificates to the state vital records office. The aggregated certificates are coded, numbered, and stored at the state level, and cer-

tificates for nonresidents are forwarded to their state of residence. The composite death information from each state is transferred to the National Center for Health Statistics for compilation into a national data base. The process of collecting information on deaths in the United States is summarized in Figure 4–8.

As noted previously, there are a number of advantages to the use of death registrations for medical surveillance purposes. At the same time, it must be

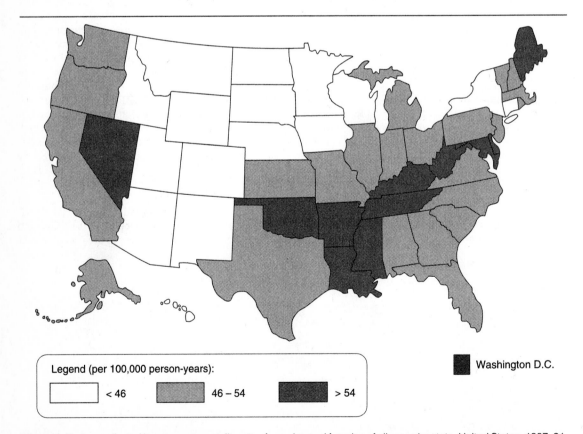

Figure 4–7. Age-adjusted lung cancer mortality rates for males and females of all races by state, United States, 1987–91. (Data from Ries LAG et al: *SEER Cancer Statistics Review, 1973–91.* National Cancer Institute. NIH Publication No. 94-2789, 1994.)

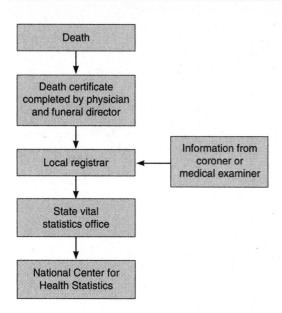

Figure 4–8. Flow diagram for processing of information about deaths in the United States.

recognized that there are several limitations to the information obtained in this manner:

(1) Most physicians receive little formal instruction about how to fill out death certificates. As a result, the reported medical information often is incomplete or inaccurate.

(2) In many situations, the certifying physician may have little particular knowledge of the decedent, leading to further errors in reporting or omissions of important conditions.

(3) The use of only one underlying cause of death in official tabulations can lead to a very incomplete picture of the mortality contributions of various conditions. For example, only 1 of every 10 times that hypertension is reported on a death certificate is it listed as the underlying cause of death.

(4) Concern for the confidentiality of the decedent may cause some physicians to omit sensitive diagnoses. There is evidence, for instance, that AIDS has been underreported as an underlying cause of death.

(5) When standard disease classifications are updated periodically, the rules about assigning underlying causes of death can change, resulting in abrupt, artificial changes in the mortality trends for certain diseases.

(6) With the many steps involved in collecting, editing, coding, and processing of death certificates, summary mortality data for a given year are not reported, even in preliminary form, until about two years later.

For any particular application, the appropriateness of using death registrations for medical surveillance purposes is determined by balancing the advantages of universal coverage, convenience, and accessibility against the limitations of inaccurate and incomplete information, as well as delays in availability. Circumstances in which this type of information is likely to prove most useful include:

(1) Monitoring historical trends in the burden of a disease and forecasting future expectations.

(2) Identifying population subgroups with disproportionate burdens of disease.

(3) Generating hypotheses about risk factors for a disease.

(4) Prioritizing the allocation of health care resources.

(5) Monitoring progress toward meeting health status objectives for a population.

AGE ADJUSTMENT

Mortality rates for all causes of death in the United States are shown by age and race in Figure 4–9. For both whites and blacks, mortality rates begin at high levels during the first year of life, fall to low levels during childhood, adolescence, and young adulthood, and then rise rapidly with increasing age. At every age, however, the death rates for blacks exceed those of whites.

It might be surprising, therefore, that the **crude death rate** (total deaths/total person-years) for blacks (851 deaths/100,000 person-years) is lower than the corresponding rate for whites (880 deaths/100,000 person-years). As indicated in Figure 4–10, the black-to-white ratio of crude mortality rates is 0.97, indicating virtually no difference between the races in the rate of deaths. This apparent paradox is explained by differences in the underlying age distributions of blacks and whites. On average, black persons in the United States tend to be younger than whites (Figure 4–11). For example, only 8.2% of blacks in the United States are 65 years or older, compared to 13.7% of whites. Thus, a smaller proportion of the black population experiences the high mortality associated with advanced age. In order to obtain an undistorted summary comparison of mortality for blacks and whites, the age differential between the races must be eliminated.

As noted previously, the usual approach to removing the influence of age from a comparison of summary rates is direct age adjustment. This technique involves the following steps:

(1) Select a standard age structure. By convention, the standard distribution used for age adjustment of mortality rates in the United States is the age distribution of the total population of the country in 1940.

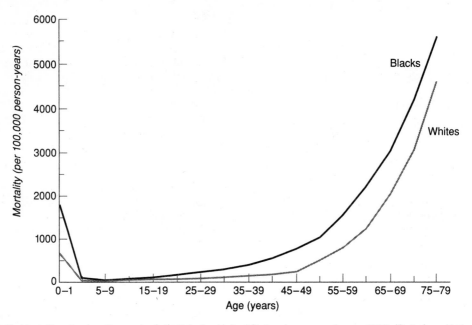

Figure 4–9. Mortality rates for all causes of death in the United States, by age and race, 1992. (Data from National Center for Health Statistics: Advance report of final mortality statistics, 1992. Monthly Vital Statistics Report. **Vol 43,** No. 6 [Suppl], 1994.)

(2) Multiply the age-specific mortality rates for each group being compared by the corresponding age-specific numbers of persons in the standard population. The result is the expected number of deaths for that age group.

(3) Sum the expected numbers of deaths within each age group to yield a total number of expected deaths for each group being compared.

(4) Divide the total number of expected deaths in each group by the total size of the standard population to yield the summary age-adjusted mortality rate.

When this direct age-adjustment procedure is performed on the age-specific death rates for blacks and whites in the United States for 1992, the summary mortality rates shown in Figure 4–12 are obtained. Note that the age-adjusted rates are lower than the corresponding crude rates (Figure 4–10) for both racial groups. Since the 1940 standard population tended to be skewed toward younger ages than either the black or white populations of 1992, the age-adjusted rates are lower than the corresponding crude rates. The change for whites is greater than that for blacks because of a larger differential between the standard (1940) and the more recent (1992) age distribution.

The numerical values of the age-adjusted rates are not particularly meaningful by themselves, since the values will vary according to the standard age distribution used. The utility of the age-adjusted rates is that they allow comparisons across groups, such as the black-to-white rate ratio. It can be seen from Figure 4–12 that the age-adjusted mortality rate for blacks is more than 60% greater than it is for whites (rate ratio = 1.61). Thus, the age-adjusted mortality rate ratio provides a summary measure that is consistent with the increase in black mortality shown in Figure 4–9. Through the use of an adjustment technique, the distorting effect of age has been removed from the contrast of summary mortality rates.

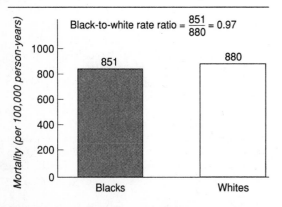

Black-to-white rate ratio = $\frac{851}{880}$ = 0.97

Figure 4–10. Crude mortality rates for blacks and whites in the United States, 1992. (Data from National Center for Health Statistics: Advance report of final mortality statistics, 1992. Monthly Vital Statistics Report. **Vol 43,** No. 6 [Suppl], 1994.)

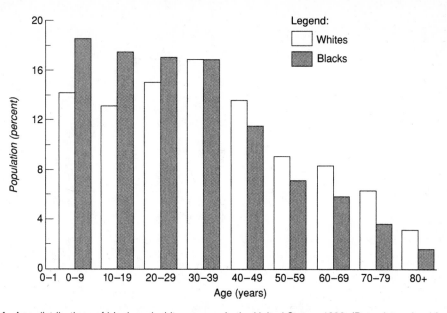

Figure 4–11. Age distributions of black and white persons in the United States, 1992. (Data determined from National Center for Health Statistics: Advance report of final mortality statistics, 1992. Monthly Vital Statistics Report. **Vol 43,** No. 6 [Suppl], 1994.)

MORTALITY PATTERNS

In addition to variation by age and race, mortality in the United Sates also varies by other characteristics. Age-adjusted mortality rates for whites and blacks for calendar years 1975 through 1992 are shown in Figure 4–13. Within each race, the age-adjusted mortality rates tended to decline, although the percentage decline was greater for whites (21%) than for blacks (14%) over this time period. The fall in mortality rates

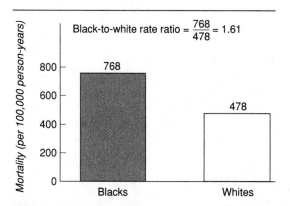

Figure 4–12. Age-adjusted (1940 US population standard) total mortality rates for blacks and whites in the United States, 1992. (Data from National Center for Health Statistics: Advance report of final mortality statistics, 1992. Monthly Vital Statistics Report. **Vol 43,** No. 6 [Suppl], 1994.)

was fairly continuous and progressive among whites. For blacks, however, there was a substantial decline between 1975 and 1979, with increasing rates between 1982 and 1988, followed by progressive declines thereafter.

As shown in Figure 4–14, black males have the highest age-adjusted mortality rate, followed in succession by white males and black females, with the lowest death rates observed among white females. Within both racial groups, males have higher mortality rates than do females. For both genders, blacks have higher mortality rates than do whites.

Table 4–3 lists the annual age-adjusted mortality rates for all persons in the United States according to the 10 leading causes of death. Four of the 5 most common causes of death in this country result from long-term, chronic processes: heart diseases, malignant neoplasms (cancer), cerebrovascular disease (stroke), and chronic obstructive pulmonary diseases.

Age-adjusted mortality rates for the individual causes of death vary by race and gender. Blacks have higher death rates than whites for 8 of the 10 leading causes of death (Figure 4–15). The relative increase in mortality among blacks is greatest for homicide (black-to-white rate ratio = 6.5), followed by HIV infection (RR = 3.7), diabetes mellitus (RR = 2.4), stroke (RR = 1.9), and heart disease (RR = 1.5). Only suicide (RR = 0.6) and chronic obstructive pulmonary diseases (RR = 0.8) are responsible for lower age-adjusted rates of death among blacks than whites.

As depicted in Figure 4–16, males have higher age-adjusted mortality rates for all of the 10 leading causes

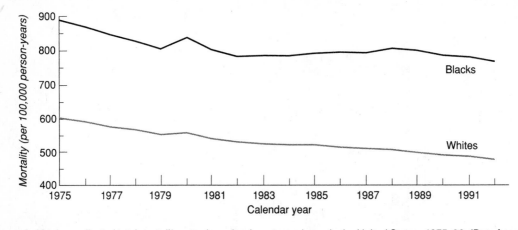

Figure 4–13. Age-adjusted total mortality rates by calendar year and race in the United States, 1975–92. (Data from National Center for Health Statistics: Advance report of final mortality statistics, 1992. Monthly Vital Statistics Report. **Vol 43,** No. 6 [Suppl], 1994.)

of death in the United States. The relative increase in mortality among males is greatest for HIV infection (male-to-female RR = 7.0), followed by suicide (male-to-female RR = 4.3), homicide (RR = 4.0), unintentional injuries (RR = 2.6), heart disease (RR = 1.9), chronic obstructive pulmonary diseases (RR = 1.7), and pneumonia and influenza (RR = 1.7). The ratio of male-to-female death rates is lowest for diabetes mellitus (RR = 1.1) and stroke (RR = 1.2).

Trends in age-adjusted mortality rates for the ten leading causes of death over the time period 1979 through 1988 are displayed schematically in Figure 4–17. Not pictured in this figure is the increase in age-adjusted mortality for HIV disease, since it did not exist as a cause of death in 1979. Dramatic declines in death rates occurred for stroke (−37%), unintentional injuries (−32%), and heart disease (−28%). Concurrent substantial percentage increases in age-adjusted

mortality rates occurred for chronic obstructive pulmonary disease (+36%), diabetes mellitus (+21%), and pneumonia and influenza (+13%). The increase for diabetes mellitus may be attributable, in part, to a change in the instructions for medical certification of deaths that occurred in many states between 1988 and 1989, resulting in a shift toward reporting of diabetes mellitus as the underlying cause of death among decedents who previously would have been assigned to other causes.

Returning to lung cancer, the focus of the Patient Profile, the age-adjusted mortality rate from this disease is the highest for any form of cancer in the United States (Figure 4–18). Lung cancer accounts for more than one-fourth of all deaths from malignant neoplasms in the United States. Between 1973 and 1991 the age-adjusted mortality from lung cancer increased steadily in the United States (Figure 4–19). Overall, the

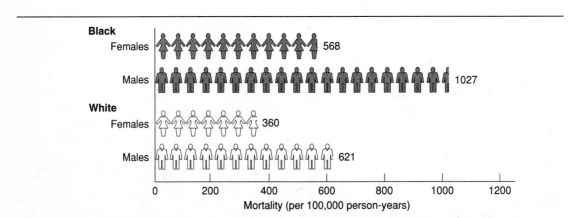

Figure 4–14. Age-adjusted mortality rates for all causes of death by race and gender in the United States, 1992. (Data from National Center for Health Statistics: Advance report of final mortality statistics, 1992. Monthly Vital Statistics Report. **Vol 43,** No. 6 [Suppl], 1994.)

Table 4–3. Age-adjusted mortality rates per 100,000 person-years for the 10 leading causes of death in the United States in 1992.[1]

Rank	Cause of Death	Mortality Rate[2]
1	Diseases of heart	144
2	Malignant neoplasms	133
3	Unintentional injuries	29
4	Cerebrovascular disease	26
5	Chronic obstructive pulmonary diseases	20
6	Pneumonia & influenza	13
7	Human immunodeficiency virus (HIV) infection	13
8	Diabetes mellitus	12
9	Suicide	11
10	Homicide	11

[1] Data from National Center for Health Statistics: Advance report of final mortality statistics, 1992. Monthly Vital Statistics Report. **Vol 43,** No. 6[Suppl], 1994.
[2] Directly adjusted to the 1940 population of the United States.

rate of deaths from this disease increased by over 40% during this time period. Although males account for almost two-thirds of all deaths from lung cancer, the percentage increase in age-adjusted mortality between 1973 and 1991 was much greater for females (140%) than for males (20%). Among males, the age-adjusted death rates for lung cancer reached a plateau from the period 1984 through 1991, whereas the corresponding rates for females continued to climb during those years.

As shown in Figure 4–20, the age-adjusted mortality from lung cancer varies considerably by race and gender in the United States. Among both whites and blacks, there is a considerably greater mortality from this disease among males. Black males have a more than 40% higher lung cancer death rate than white males. In contrast, virtually no racial differential in lung cancer mortality is seen among females.

PREMATURE LOSS OF LIFE

A mortality rate is a convenient and easily understood measure of the burden of a disease on a population. By weighing the impact of all deaths equally, however, a mortality rate does not convey the extent to which persons are dying prematurely. In this context, **premature death** means a death that occurs earlier than would have been expected in the absence of the disease. Clearly, causes of death that tend to occur among young people result in a much greater loss of life expectancy than do causes of death that tend to occur among the elderly. For example, in 1992, persons aged 25 years had an estimated average remaining lifetime of 52 years, compared with only 6 years for persons aged 85 years or older. It may seem paradoxical that persons born more recently were expected to live only to age 77, whereas the older persons were expected to live to age 91 years. Remember, however, that the older persons already had survived to age 85 years, and thus had escaped all of the risk of death between age 25 and 85 years that the younger persons still faced.

A death at age 25 years and a death at age 85 contribute the same amount to a mortality rate. It is clear, however, that the death of a 25-year-old results in a loss of 52 years of life expectancy, compared with a loss of only 6 years of life expectancy for the death of an 85-year-old. In a sense then, the death of the 25-year-old contributes more than eight times the amount of premature loss of life than does the death of the 85-year-old. This is not to say that the life of the 25-year-old is "more important" than that of the 85-year-old. Rather, it simply means that preventing a death has very different consequences for longevity, depending upon the age of the person. To the extent that the benefit of health interventions are assessed by their impact

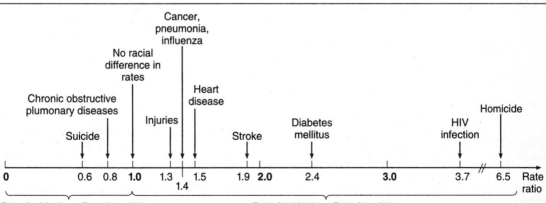

Figure 4–15. Black-to-white ratios of age-adjusted mortality rates for the ten leading causes of death in the United States, 1992. (Data from National Center for Health Statistics: Advance report of final mortality statistics, 1992. Monthly Vital Statistics Report. **Vol 43,** No. 6 [Suppl], 1994.)

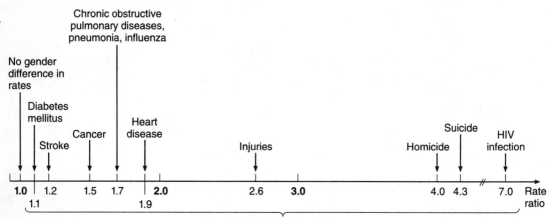

Figure 4–16. Male-to-female ratios of age-adjusted mortality rates for the ten leading causes of death in the United States, 1992. (Data from National Center for Health Statistics: Advance report of final mortality statistics, 1992. Monthly Vital Statistics Report. **Vol 43,** No. 6 [Suppl], 1994.)

on longevity, those that reduce deaths among young persons will appear relatively important.

One approach to estimating the impact of a cause of death on premature loss of life is the **person-years of life lost,** which is calculated in the following manner:

(1) Identify the age at death for each decedent.
(2) Given the decedent's age, estimate the years of life expectancy that were lost because of the death.
(3) Sum the years of life expectancy lost over all decedents.

Selected leading contributors to person-years of life lost in the United States are summarized in Figure 4–21. In 1991, there were 2.2 million deaths which resulted in a total of almost 35 million person-years of life lost. Heart disease, which tends to occur among the elderly, accounted for 33% of all deaths, but only 24% of the person-years of life lost. In contrast, injuries, which tend to occur among the young, accounted for only 4% of all deaths, but almost 9% of person-years of life lost.

The person-years of life lost to selected leading causes of death from cancer are shown in Figure 4–22. The leading contributor is lung cancer, which accounts for more than one-fourth of all of the person-years of life lost to cancer. Breast cancer accounts for 1 out of every 9 person-years of life lost to cancer, and large bowel malignancies account for about 10% of the total.

Another measure of premature loss of life is the **years of potential life lost before age 65 years (YPLL ⊂ 65),** which is calculated in the following manner:

(1) The difference between age 65 years and the age of death is calculated for each decedent.

(2) These differences are summed over all decedents.
(3) This summation is divided by the number of persons under age 65 years in the source population of persons.
(4) The resulting estimate is multiplied by 1000 or 100,000 depending upon the units desired.

The overall YPLL < 65 in the United States during 1991 was 5556 per 100,000 person-years. The YPLL < 65 for selected underlying causes of death are shown in Figure 4–23. The leading contributor to YPLL < 65 is unintentional injuries, which accounts for 17% of the total. As previously noted, unintentional injuries are responsible for only 4% of all deaths. Homicide and HIV infection also account for much larger proportionate shares of total YPLL < 65 (7% and 6%, respectively), than of all deaths (1% each). The comparatively large contributions of unintentional injuries, homicide, and HIV infection to YPLL < 65 result from the young ages at which these fatalities tend to occur.

SURVEILLANCE OF RISK FACTORS

In the preceding section, attention was focused on surveillance of medical events, such as new diagnoses or deaths from specific diseases. Surveillance techniques also can be used to characterize patterns of risk factor distribution by person, place, and time. The Behavioral Risk Factor Surveillance System (BRFSS), which is supported by the Centers for Disease Control and Prevention, collects this type of information. The BRFSS was initiated in 1984 to provide statewide data on lifestyle characteristics that could affect health status. Data are collected by the health departments

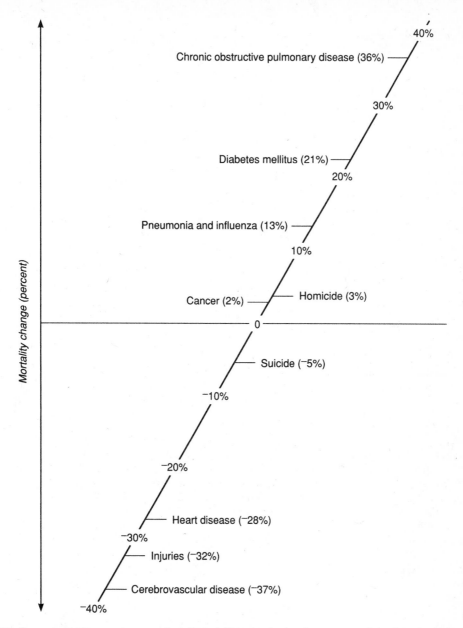

Figure 4–17. Percentage changes in age-adjusted mortality rates for leading causes of death in the United States, 1979–92. (Data from National Center for Health Statistics: Advance report of final mortality statistics, 1992. Monthly Vital Statistics Report. **Vol 43,** No. 6 [Suppl], 1994.)

of most states using a standard protocol. Adult respondents are sampled randomly and briefly interviewed over the telephone.

The most important risk factor for the development of lung cancer is cigarette smoking. Data collected by the BRFSS can be used to describe smoking patterns within the general population. The overall prevalence of cigarette smoking in the United States in 1992, as determined by the BRFSS, was 22%. As shown in Figure 4–24, the estimated prevalence of cigarette use

varied by state of residence, with the highest reported level in Nevada (31%) and the lowest reported level in Utah (16%). The low frequency of cigarette smoking in Utah is attributable to the high proportion of residents who practice Mormonism, a religion that advocates abstinence from tobacco and alcohol. Given the marked differential in cigarette smoking in Utah and Nevada, it is not surprising that the age-adjusted lung cancer mortality in Utah (21.9 cases per 100,000 person-years) was only about one-third as high as that in

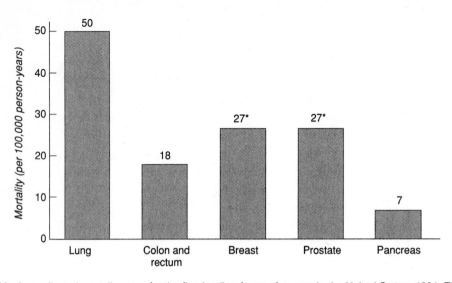

Figure 4–18. Age-adjusted mortality rates for the five leading forms of cancer in the United States, 1991. The rate for breast cancer is confined to women and the rate for prostate cancer is confined to men. (Data from Ries LAG et al: *SEER Cancer Statistics Review, 1973–91.* National Cancer Institute. NIH Publication No. 94-2789, 1994.)

Nevada (60.1 cases per 100,000 person-years) for a recent 5-year time period.

Another system used to collect information on risk factors and health status in the United States is the National Health Interview Survey (NHIS). The NHIS is a continuous nationwide household survey that uses data collected through personal interviews. In 1991, more than 120,000 persons were surveyed by the NHIS. The overall prevalence of current cigarette smoking in the United States during that year, as determined by the NHIS, was 26%. The slight difference in smoking prevalence estimates obtained by the BRFSS and the NHIS may be attributable to differences in sampling schemes, data collection methods, or both.

The NHIS prevalence estimates for cigarette smoking are shown by race and gender in Figure 4–25. These data indicate that cigarette use is most common among black males, followed by white males, white females, and black females, respectively. This pattern is consistent with the race and gender distribution of lung cancer mortality rates previously depicted in Figure 4–20. Although NHIS data indicate that the prevalence of cigarette smoking declined over the decade of the 1980s in all four race-gender groups, cigarette smoking remains the single most preventable cause of

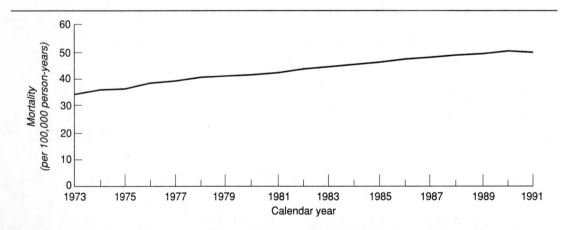

Figure 4–19. Age-adjusted mortality rates for lung cancer by calendar year in the United States, 1973–91. (Data from Ries LAG et al: *SEER Cancer Statistics Review, 1973–91.* National Cancer Institute. NIH Publication No. 94-2789, 1994.)

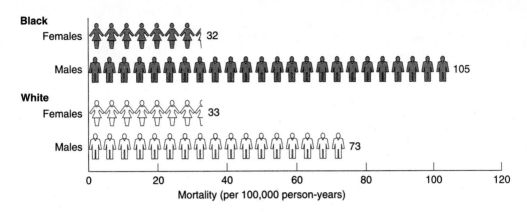

Figure 4–20. Age-adjusted mortality rates for lung cancer by race and gender in the United States, 1991. (Data from Ries LAG et al: *SEER Cancer Statistics Review, 1973–91.* National Cancer Institute. NIH Publication No. 94-2789, 1994.)

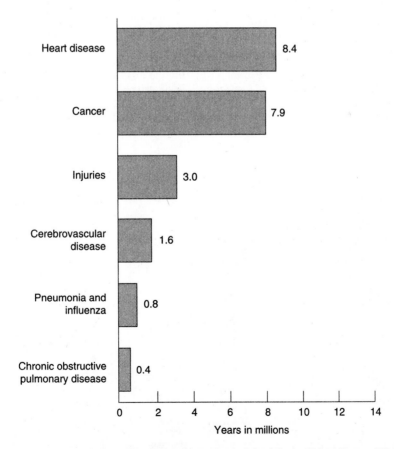

Figure 4–21. Person-years of life lost from selected leading causes of death in the United States, 1991. (Data from Ries LAG et al: *SEER Cancer Statistics Review, 1973–91.* National Cancer Institute. NIH Publication No. 94-2789, 1994.)

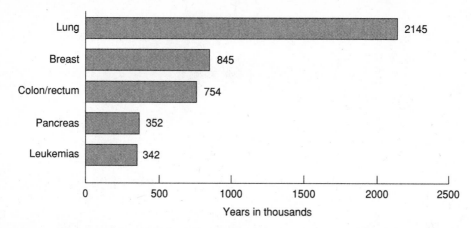

Figure 4–22. Person-years of life lost from selected leading causes of death from cancer in the United States, 1991. (Data from Ries LAG et al: *SEER Cancer Statistics Review, 1973–91.* National Cancer Institute. NIH Publication No. 94-2789, 1994.)

death in the United States. Progress towards meeting the national objective of reducing the prevalence of this behavior can be monitored through risk factor surveillance systems, such as the BRFSS and the NHIS.

SUMMARY

In this chapter, lung cancer was used as a focus for consideration of the role of **surveillance** in epidemiology. Surveillance was defined as the detection of the occurrence of health-related events or exposures in a target population. Successful surveillance activities require continuity over time, standardized methodology, and timeliness of data collection and dissemination.

Surveillance data can be used in different ways, depending upon the type of information collected. Newly diagnosed persons with a disease can yield information on incidence rates; deaths from a disease can be used to describe mortality rates; indices of premature death can be used to assess the impact of a disease on longevity; and prevalence of risk factors can be used to predict future disease occurrence or to assess the status of prevention initiatives.

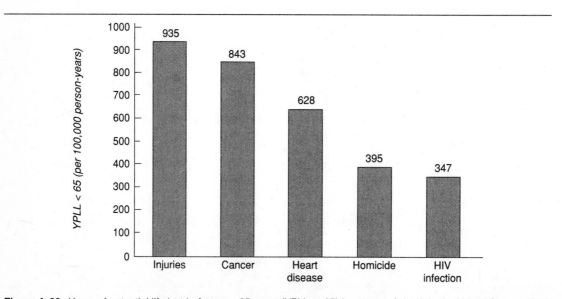

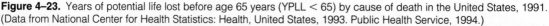

Figure 4–23. Years of potential life lost before age 65 years (YPLL < 65) by cause of death in the United States, 1991. (Data from National Center for Health Statistics: Health, United States, 1993. Public Health Service, 1994.)

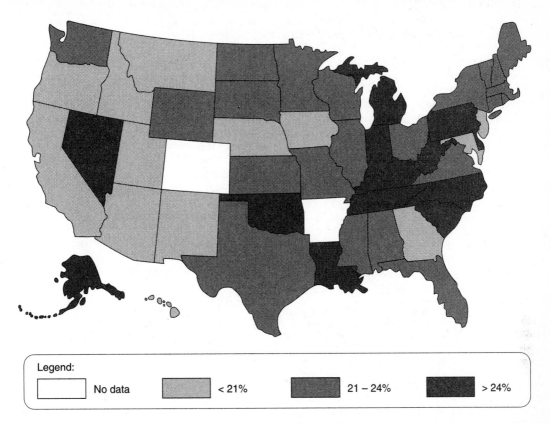

Figure 4–24. Prevalence of cigarette smoking, by state, United States, 1992. Unshaded areas represent states that did not participate in the Behavioral Risk Factor Surveillance System. (Data from CDC: Surveillance for selected tobacco-use behaviors—United States, 1900–94. MMWR 1994;**43:**(SS-3):1.)

Surveillance activities in the United States related to lung cancer include collection of data on newly diagnosed persons (through population-based cancer registries), deaths (through death certificates), and prevalence of cigarette smoking (through population-based personal interview surveys).

The utility of **age adjustment** was demonstrated for the control of differences in underlying age structure, when comparing summary rates of lung cancer incidence or mortality across population subgroups.

Key findings from surveillance related to lung cancer in the United States are listed below.

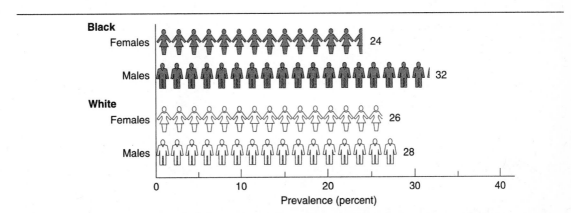

Figure 4–25. Age-adjusted prevalence of cigarette smoking in the United States by race and gender, 1992. (Data from National Center for Health Statistics: Health, United States, 1993. Public Health Service, 1994.)

(1) Lung cancer has the third highest incidence, trailing only breast cancer among women and prostate cancer among men. Malignancies of the lung are the leading cause of death from cancer.

(2) The incidence of lung cancer increases sharply between 30 and 70 years of age.

(3) The overall age-adjusted incidence rate of lung cancer is almost 40% higher in blacks than whites. Contrast of age-adjusted mortality rates reveals a 25% higher rate among blacks.

(4) The age-adjusted mortality rate for lung cancer is about four-fifths of the corresponding incidence rate, indicating a high case fatality. Lung cancer age-adjusted mortality increased by over 40% between 1973 and 1991.

(5) Age-adjusted mortality rates for lung cancer vary widely across states, as do the corresponding prevalences of cigarette smoking.

(6) Lung cancer accounts for about one-fourth of the premature mortality from cancer, and about 6% of total premature loss of life.

(7) The comparatively high age-adjusted mortality rate for lung cancer among black males is paralleled by a comparatively high prevalence of cigarette smoking.

Several features of the Patient Profile illustrate these descriptive patterns of lung cancer distribution: (a) the patient was 68 years of age at presentation, a comparatively high-risk age for lung cancer occurrence, (b) she was a long-term cigarette smoker, thereby substantially increasing her risk of this disease, and (c) the rapidity of her death following diagnosis is consistent with the high case fatality of this disease. With the generally poor treatment results for lung cancer, the greatest promise for controlling the impact of this disease is through preventing the initiation of cigarette smoking and encouraging current smokers to quit.

STUDY QUESTIONS

Questions 1–4: For each numbered condition below, select the most appropriate disease or disorder from the following lettered options. Each option can be used once, more than once, or not at all.

    A. Heart disease
    B. Stroke
    C. Suicide
    D. Hypertension
    E. Colon cancer

1. The condition most likely to be reviewed by a coroner or medical examiner.

2. The condition for which surveillance through death certificates is least likely to be complete.

3. The condition with the greatest male predominance in mortality rates.

4. The condition most likely to be included in data collected by the Surveillance, Epidemiology and End Results Program.

Questions 5–8: For each numbered condition below, select from the following lettered options the most appropriate reason to underestimate the occurrence of the condition when it is evaluated through death certificates. Each option can be used once, more than once, or not at all.

    A. Poor access to diagnostic facilities
    B. Low case fatality
    C. Limited knowledge of patient by certifying physician
    D. Cultural sensitivity of diagnosis
    E. Lack of physician training
    F. Lack of standardized diagnostic coding rules

5. The occurrence of osteoarthritis is underestimated when evaluated through death certificates of former Medicare patients.

6. The existence of prior cardiac disease is underestimated when evaluated through death certificates of persons who died in transit to hospital emergency rooms after experiencing sudden cardiac arrest.

7. The presence of AIDS is underestimated when evaluated through death certificates of persons who died of pneumonia.

8. The occurrence of brain cancer is underestimated when evaluated through death certificates of persons who had resided in remote rural communities.

Questions 9–12: For each numbered condition below, select from the following lettered options the most appropriate trend over time in observed mortality rates. Each option can be used once, more than once, or not at all.

    A. Increasing
    B. Decreasing
    C. About the same
    D. Data are not available

9. Unintentional injuries.

10. Chronic obstructive pulmonary disease.

11. Stroke.

12. Diabetes mellitus.

FURTHER READING

Teutsch SM, Churchill RE: *Principles and Practice of Public Health Surveillance.* Oxford Univ Press, 1994.

Thacker SB, Stroup DF: Future directions for comprehensive public health surveillance and health information systems in the United States. Am J Epidemiol 1994;**140:**383.

REFERENCES

Introduction
Berkelman RL, Buehler JW: Surveillance. In: *Oxford Textbook of Public Health,* 2nd ed. Vol 2. Holland WW, Detels R, Knox G (editors). Oxford Univ Press, 1991.

Surveillance of New Diagnoses
Ries LAG et al: *SEER Cancer Statistics Review,* 1973–91. National Cancer Institute. NIH Publication No. 94-2789, 1994.

Surveillance of Deaths
Stroup NE et al: Sources of routinely collected data for surveillance. In: *Principles and Practice of Public Health Surveillance.* Teutsch SM, Churchill RE (editors). Oxford Univ Press, 1994.

Age Adjustment
Dawson-Saunders B, Trapp RG: *Basic and Clinical Biostatistics,* 2nd ed. Appleton & Lange, 1994.

Mortality Patterns
National Center for Health Statistics: Advance report of final mortality statistics, 1992. Monthly Vital Statistics Report. Vol **43,** No. 6 (Suppl), 1994.

Premature Loss of Life
CDC: Years of potential life lost before age 65, by race Hispanic origin, and sex–United States, 1986–1988. MMWR 1992;**41**(SS-6):13.

National Center for Health Statistics: Health, United States, 1993. Public Health Service, 1994.

Ries LAG et al: *SEER Cancer Statistics Review, 1973–1991.* National Cancer Insitute. NIH Publication No. 94-2789, 1994.

Surveillance of Risk Factors
CDC: Surveillance for selected tobacco-use behaviors–United States, 1900–1994. MMWR 1994;**43**(SS-3):1.

National Center for Health Statistics: Health, United States, 1993. Public Health Service, 1994.

Disease Outbreaks

5

PATIENT PROFILE

A 23-year-old male student presented at 10:30 PM on January 17 at the college infirmary complaining of a sudden onset of abdominal cramping, nausea, and diarrhea. Although the patient was not in severe distress and had no fever or vomiting, he was weak. A number of other students, all with the same symptoms, visited the college infirmary over the next 20 hours. All patients were treated with bed rest and fluid replacement therapy. They recovered fully within 24 hours of the onset of illness.

INTRODUCTION

The concept of an epidemic as a dramatic rise in the occurrence of a disease was introduced in Chapter 3. When an epidemic occurs suddenly and in a relatively limited geographic area, it is described as a **disease outbreak.** The emergence of a disease outbreak requires immediate action to determine the origin of the problem, and ultimately, to prevent other persons from becoming affected.

In many outbreak situations, distinctive clinical features of the affected individuals may suggest the underlying cause (sometimes termed pathogen). A working hypothesis can lead to prompt identification of the causal agent and implementation of control measures. Ideally, the choice of control strategy is predicated upon knowledge of the source of the causal agent and how it is spread.

In other circumstances, however, the clinical features of affected individuals do not suggest a particular pathogen. An urgent response is required, although the investigator does not yet have a specific working hypothesis about the cause. Consequently, the first phase of investigation involves the collection of basic descriptive information to better characterize the illness and its pattern of occurrence. With this background descriptive data in hand, investigators can generate hypotheses and design specific analytical studies to identify the causal factor of the illness.

The development and maintenance of a disease outbreak typically requires each of the following three characteristics:

(1) The presence of a pathogen in sufficient quantities to affect multiple persons.
(2) An appropriate mode of transmitting the pathogen to susceptible persons.
(3) An adequate pool of susceptible persons who are exposed to the pathogen.

These three features are presented schematically in Figure 5–1.

Some outbreaks are self-limited and terminate without any intervention. In other situations, however, the outbreak will continue unless action is taken to prevent further spread. An effective control strategy should address one or more of the three conditions necessary for an epidemic. Specifically, the following interventions could terminate an outbreak:

(1) Removal or elimination of the source of the pathogen.
(2) Blockage of the transmission process.
(3) Elimination of susceptibility (eg, through vaccination or medication).

Epidemiologists often distinguish between two primary modes of transmission in acute outbreaks of disease: (**1**) Person-to-person spread, and (**2**) Common-source exposure.

As the name implies, person-to-person spread occurs when the causal agent is transmitted from one individual to another. As described in Chapter 3, tuberculosis is propagated in this manner, with the pathogen conveyed from an infectious person to a susceptible individual via airborne particles. The investigation of an outbreak of tuberculosis is likely to reveal an initial (or index) case and a number of subsequent cases that develop among the close contacts of the infectious person. An effective control strategy would involve isolation of the index case until that individual is no longer infectious, treatment of the index case with antibiotics to prevent further transmission, and preventive antibiotic therapy for infected close contacts.

A common-source exposure occurs when the causal agent is transmitted to affected individuals by some shared feature of the environment. For example, contaminated food can be the source of pathogenic bacte-

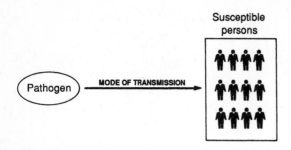

Figure 5–1. Schematic representation of factors required for the development and maintenance of a disease outbreak.

ria for persons who ingest the food. Appropriate control measures for this type of outbreak would involve removal of the contaminated food, as well as review of food preparation practices in order to prevent future outbreaks. Common-source outbreaks are not limited to infectious pathogens. For example, chemical contamination of shared food, air, or water can result in an outbreak of disease.

Outbreaks of disease are fairly common, and not all episodes can be investigated. In deciding whether an investigation is warranted, it is useful to consider the following factors:

(1) Apparent number of persons affected.
(2) Presence of unusual or severe clinical symptoms.
(3) Lack of an obvious explanation for disease occurrence.
(4) Perceived need to implement control measures.
(5) Level of public concern.
(6) Potential for contributing to medical knowledge.

The situation depicted in the Patient Profile did not involve a life-threatening condition, and the symptoms were rather typical of an acute gastrointestinal illness. On the basis of these criteria alone, an investigation of this outbreak would not be justified. On the other hand, a relatively large number of individuals were affected, the cause was uncertain, and members of this college community were concerned about further spread of the epidemic. For these reasons, an investigation of the outbreak was undertaken.

THE EPIDEMIC

This epidemic of apparent gastroenteritis occurred on the campus of a liberal arts college in the northeastern United States. The temporal association of cases led to the working hypothesis that this epidemic

was due to a microbial pathogen from a common source. It was suspected that there was one vehicle for transmission of the disease agent and, since the epidemic quickly peaked in time, that the vehicle was quickly exhausted or removed. The epidemic was investigated by public health authorities.

THE INVESTIGATION

Existing information was gathered quickly, first at the infirmary and then at the college administration office. The index case presented to the infirmary at 10:30 PM on January 17, and by 8 PM on January 18, 47 affected students were examined. A quantitative measure of the extent of an outbreak is the **attack rate** (*AR*). The *AR* is calculated using the following equation:

$$\text{Attack rate (AR)} = \frac{\text{Number of new cases}}{\text{Persons at risk}} \times 100$$

Note that the *AR* is a measure of risk, as defined in Chapter 2. Accordingly, a period of time must be specified in the estimation of an *AR*.

Knowledge that the college enrollment was 1164 allows the *AR* for the gastrointestinal disease outbreak to be calculated. The *AR* for the period from 10:30 PM January 17 to 8:00 PM January 18 was:

$$\text{Attack rate}_{(\text{all students})} = \frac{47}{1164} \times 100 = 4.0\%$$

It readily was apparent, however, that the population at risk could be defined more narrowly because all students who reported to the infirmary lived in dormitories on campus, but only about two-thirds of all enrolled students lived in those dormitories. In other words, the one-third of students who lived outside of dormitories did not appear to be at risk of disease. Since these students were not entered into the numerator of the equation, their inclusion in the denominator makes the calculation potentially misleading. A more precise estimate of the *AR*, based upon the 756 students at risk in the dormitories was:

$$\text{Attack rate}_{(\text{dorm residents})} = \frac{47}{756} \times 100 = 6.2\%$$

By defining the population at risk more precisely, the estimated *AR* increased by more than 50%.

Since the patients' dormitories were recorded on infirmary records, the *ARs* could be calculated by dormitory and by gender (dormitories were separated by gender). These data are presented in Table 5–1. The striking difference in the *ARs* clearly suggested that the residents of two dormitories (1 and 12) were at greater risk than residents of the other 12 dormitories.

Table 5–1. The dormitory of residence of the 47 known cases and the attack rate, as well as the population and gender of the occupants of each dormitory.

Dormitory	Gender	Population at Risk	Number of Cases	Attack Rate (AR %)
1	F	80	19	23.8
2	F	62	2	3.2
3	F	89	0	0
4	F	61	1	1.6
5	F	53	5	9.4
6	M	35	0	0
7	M	63	0	0
8	F	103	4	3.9
9	M	35	1	2.9
10	M	37	0	0
11	F	34	1	2.9
12	M	62	13	21.0
13	M	32	1	3.1
14	M	10	0	0
Total	—	756	47	6.2

A combined *AR* for the two dorms at greater risk can be contrasted with the other 12 as follows:

$$\text{Attack rate}_{(\text{dorms 1, 12})} = \frac{(19 + 13)}{(80 + 62)} \times 100 = 22.5\%$$

The *AR* for the remaining 12 dormitories was:

$$\text{Attack rate}_{(\text{remaining dorms})} = \frac{(47 - 32)}{(756 - 142)} \times 100$$

$$= \frac{15}{614} \times 100 = 2.4\%$$

A ratio of these attack rates may be calculated as follows:

$$\text{Risk ratio} = \frac{AR_{(\text{dorms 1, 12})}}{AR_{(\text{remaining dorms})}} = \frac{22.5\%}{2.4\%} = 9.4$$

This risk ratio means that the *AR* in dormitories 1 and 12 was 9.4 times greater than in the remaining 12 dormitories.

A different ratio could be constructed using only the number of cases. Such a ratio would be 32 cases (dormitories 1 and 12) divided by the 15 cases in the remaining 12 dormitories. This ratio is 32/15, or 2.1. It should be clear, however, that this latter ratio is not an appropriate comparison since it does not take into account the differing sizes of the populations at risk in the dormitories. There were only one-fourth as many students at risk in dormitories 1 and 12, and so one would not expect the same number of cases to occur in these two dormitories as occurred in the other 12. If the residents of dormitories 1 and 12 experienced the same risk as other dormitory residents, then the expected number of cases in dormitories 1 and 12 would be:

Expected cases$_{(\text{dorms 1, 12})}$

$$= \text{Students at risk}_{(\text{dorms 1, 12})} \times AR_{(\text{remaining dorms})}$$

$$= 142 \times \frac{15}{614} = 3.5$$

The frequency data in Table 5–1 also can be used to calculate rates by gender. For males, the *AR* was:

$$AR_{(\text{males})} = \frac{(1 + 13 + 1)}{(35 + 63 + 35 + 37 + 62 + 32 + 10)} \times 100$$

$$= \frac{15}{274} \times 100$$

$$= 5.5\%$$

A similar calculation for females yielded an *AR* of 6.6%. The ratio of attack rates for females-to-males was 1.2, indicating that there was not much gender difference in risk of acquiring this disease.

Visits to some of the campus dormitories by the investigators soon revealed that not all students who became ill had visited the infirmary. Thus, it became important to obtain additional data regarding the nature and extent of the outbreak, which, it was hoped, would be less biased by differences in care-seeking behavior. Questionnaires were prepared and distributed by hand to all students living in seven dormitories chosen to provide a representative sample of the student population. The results from this survey are presented in Table 5–2. A different picture of this epidemic emerged from these results. The overall *AR* now could be calculated as:

$$\text{Attack rate} = \frac{110}{304} \times 100 = 36.2\%$$

Note that the denominator for this *AR* is 304, which was the number of returned questionnaires, and not

Table 5–2. Responses to the questionnaire survey by dormitory.[1]

Dormitory	Population	Questionnaires Returned		Number of Ill Students
		Number	Percent	
5	53	49	92.5	13
6	35	26	74.3	13
7	63	28	44.4	15
8	103	65	63.1	21
9	35	19	54.3	5
12	62	44	71.0	22
Nurses' residence[2]	60	60	100	17
Unidentified[3]	—	13	—	4
Total	411	304	74.0	110

[1]Dormitories 1–4, 10, 11, 13, and 14 were not surveyed.
[2]Nurses' dormitory located off campus.
[3]Dormitory of residence not entered on 13 questionnaires.

411, which was the total number of eligible students. Since nonrespondents could not be classified according to disease status (in the numerator of the AR calculation), their inclusion in the denominator makes the AR calculation invalid. In the initial infirmary data, the ARs for dormitories 6 and 12 were 0 and 21%, respectively. From the survey responses, however, these dormitories did not appear to have different ARs:

$$AR_{(dorm\ 6)} = \frac{13}{26} \times 100 = 50\%$$

$$AR_{(dorm\ 12)} = \frac{22}{44} \times 100 = 50\%$$

In other words, the infirmary records and the questionnaire data gave two very different perspectives on the distribution of the outbreak by place of residence. The explanation for this discrepancy was not immediately apparent, but could have reflected differences in approaches to data collection. The infirmary data were useful in the initial phase of investigation because they were readily available. On the other hand, these data could have been influenced by various factors, such as variation in the severity of illness and care-seeking behavior. The student survey tended to avoid these problems.

The true AR of gastroenteritis on campus was not known. The best estimate was 36.2%, as determined from the student survey, but this AR could have been incorrect since only 74% of the survey questionnaires were returned (see Table 5–2). If the illness experience of the nonrespondents differed appreciably from the three-fourths of students who responded, then the estimated AR could have been incorrect. It is possible, eg, that students who were not affected by the illness were less motivated to respond to the survey. Under these circumstances, the calculated AR of 36.2% would be higher than the true AR for all students. The extent to which the estimated and true AR differ reflects **bias,** or lack of validity. Another potential source of bias could have arisen in the selection of the

dormitories to be surveyed. To the extent that these dormitories were systematically different from the remaining nonsurveyed dormitories, then bias could have been introduced into the estimation of the true AR. Furthermore, if students misreported their illness experience, either intentionally or nonintentionally, then a distorted pattern of the outbreak could have emerged.

The concept of bias will be discussed at length in Chapter 10. Suffice it to say that it is desirable to minimize the amount of bias in any study. In order to reduce the potential for bias in the present context, the amount of missing information must be minimized. Since the investigators could not force students to respond, it would be unrealistic to expect complete participation. Nevertheless, various strategies could be used to increase the response level, eg, the use of reminders and peer support. The pattern of response rates shown in Table 5–2 was clearly nonrandom, with particularly low response levels in dormitories 7, 8, and 9. Focused efforts to increase participation among residents of those dormitories might have helped to increase confidence in the validity of findings.

Several factors could explain why the ARs estimated from infirmary records were low. Some students may have experienced mild illness that did not require medical attention, and others may have sought care elsewhere. Also, it was discovered that dormitories 1 and 12, which initially appeared to have the highest ARs, were located adjacent to the infirmary, and access to this facility was more convenient for residents of these dormitories.

The survey data indicated a much higher AR and more widespread nature of the disease than originally suspected; in fact, more than one-third of all students appeared to be involved. In addition, the abrupt onset of disease and clustering of cases in time suggested a common-source exposure. Data collected during the survey indicated that no large gatherings of students, such as parties or sports events, had recently occurred. Attention then was directed at meals, since most students ate at the college cafeteria. Included in the survey were questions concerning the source of meals eaten on January 16 and 17. Information from the survey is summarized in Table 5–3. Data are presented in a format that is typical for food histories. *ARs* are presented for those who ate and those who did not eat each meal. For example, 152 students ate breakfast on January 16, and of these, 52 reported that they became ill. Thus, the *AR* was (52/152) x 100 = 34.2%. *ARs* were calculated in a similar manner for all meals on these days.

The relationship between eating a particular meal and developing illness was assessed by contrasting *ARs* in those who ate the meal and those who did not. Not surprisingly, most *ARs* were approximately 36%, with little difference between those who did or did not eat a particular meal. The exception was found for the January 17 lunch meal. A ratio of *ARs* (risk ratio) for eaters and noneaters of this meal was calculated as follows:

$$RR_{(1/17\ lunch)} = \frac{AR_{(1/17\ lunch\ eaters)}}{AR_{(1/17\ lunch\ noneaters)}} = \frac{42.2\%}{5.8\%} = 7.3$$

This risk ratio indicates that those who ate this meal were more than seven times as likely to become ill as those who did not eat this meal. Similar risk ratios were calculated for the other meals and were close to 1.0. For example, the risk ratio for dinner on January 17 was 37.5/32.6 = 1.2.

Having identified the meal at which the students most probably were exposed and knowing each student's time of onset of symptoms, it was possible to calculate the **incubation period,** in this case the time between eating the meal and the onset of symptoms, for 101 ill students. The distribution of these incubation periods is shown in Table 5–4 and presented graphically in Figures 5–2 and 5–3. In Figure 5–2, the number of cases that occurred is shown by time in hours between exposure and onset of illness. In Figure 5–3, the cumulative percentage distribution of cases is presented by incubation period. *The median incubation period is the time by which 50% of the cases have occurred.* The median incubation period in Figure 5–3 is 10 hours. A follow-up survey was directed at obtaining information about the noon meal of January 17. Data from the follow-up study are presented in Table 5–5.

In order to identify the food(s) responsible for the outbreak, dietary histories were analyzed. The ques-

tionnaires provided information about particular foods that 251 students ate at the noon meal on Friday, January 17. If students were uncertain about whether they ate the food in question, they were not included in the analysis of that particular food. As a consequence, the total of those who ate and those who did not eat each specific item did not equal 251 for all items.

The ratios of *ARs* yielded values greater than 1.0 for certain items, indicating that the risk of illness was greater among students who ate that item than among those who did not eat the item. For other items the values were less than 1.0, indicating that risk of illness was lower among those who ate the item in question. For example, the risk ratio was 0.7 for fish chowder, 1.0 for fruit salad, and 8.0 for lamb stew pie. It was clear from these data that the risk ratio for illness was considerably higher for those who ate lamb stew pie than for those who did not. This information suggested that lamb stew pie was the most likely source of exposure to the pathogen. Further investigation of the preparation of the lamb stew pie indicated that it was prepared the previous day (January 16), refrigerated, and warmed on the morning it was served.

Although no specific laboratory studies were performed, the etiologic agent that caused this outbreak could be inferred from available information. The illness was marked by gastrointestinal symptoms of limited duration, usually without fever or vomiting; the median incubation period was 10 hours; and a meat dish was presumed to be the most likely source of the pathogen. Based upon these observations, the etiologic agent probably was *Clostridium perfringens.* When ingested from inadequately cooked foods, particularly stews, meats, or gravies, type A strains of this bacterium produce a toxin that causes gastrointestinal symptoms. The incubation period, which may range from 8–22 hours, is typically 10–12 hours. The absence of fever differentiated this particular gastrointestinal illness from shigellosis or salmonellosis, and the absence of vomiting distinguished this illness from food poisoning by staphylococcal bacteria or chemical agents.

Since *C perfringens* food poisoning does not involve person-to-person transmission, it is not necessary to isolate affected patients. Supportive treatment should include oral administration of fluids and elec-

Table 5–3. Analysis of meal-specific exposure histories of the respondents to the questionnaire.

	Students Who ATE Specific Meal				Students Who DID NOT EAT Specific Meal			
	Ill	Well	Total	AR (%)	Ill	Well	Total	AR (%)
January 16								
Breakfast	52	100	152	34.2	51	94	145	35.2
Lunch	89	150	239	37.2	20	44	64	31.3
Dinner	87	150	237	36.7	23	44	67	34.3
January 17								
Breakfast	56	105	161	34.8	42	89	131	32.1
Lunch	106	145	251	42.2	3	49	52	5.8
Dinner	78	130	208	37.5	31	64	95	32.6

Table 5–4. Distribution of incubation periods.

Incubation Period (Hours)	Number of Students	Cumulative Number of Students
≤8	22	22
9	11	33
10	18	51
11	8	59
≥12	42	101

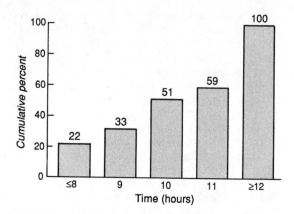

Figure 5–3. Cumulative percentage distribution of cases by time from eating suspect meal to development of symptoms.

trolytes, or intravenous therapy in severe cases. Antibiotic treatment is not required. Taking measures to reduce bacterial proliferation in food sources can prevent outbreaks of *C perfringens* food poisoning. Thorough cooking of meats and stews at an adequate temperature is essential. Dividing stews into small cooking portions helps to ensure uniform heating and decreases the need to store and reheat leftovers.

FOOD-BORNE DISEASE

The episode just described is an example of an outbreak of food-borne disease. When such outbreaks are investigated in the United States, the data typically are collected by state or local health agencies and reported to a national surveillance system coordinated by the Centers for Disease Control and Prevention (CDC). Over a recent 15-year period, almost 7500 food-borne outbreaks were reported. This number probably represents the tip of an iceberg of a much larger number of actual outbreaks, since many episodes are either unrecognized or unreported. Outbreaks in which the clinical manifestations of illness are unusual or severe, or in which an unusual strain of pathogen is detected, are more likely to receive attention and investigation.

Data from the CDC suggest that the historically predominant types of food-borne diseases, such as staphylococcal intoxication and *C perfringens* infec-

tion, now account for a declining proportion of reported outbreaks. Examples of pathogenic agents that appear to be increasing over time are *Salmonella* species, *Campylobacter jejuni*, *Escherichia coli* serotype O157:H7, *Listeria monocytogenes,* and Norwalk virus.

The changing epidemiology of food-borne disease likely reflects trends in the types of foods that are consumed and the origins of those foods, as well as how they are handled and distributed. Over the past two decades in the United States, the consumption of whole milk and red meat has declined, while the intake of poultry, fresh vegetables, and fruits has increased. The domestic growing seasons for fresh fruits and vegetables have been supplemented by importing these commodities from tropical countries. Food-borne outbreaks with a variety of *Salmonella* species have been traced to imported fruits and vegetables, and many other outbreaks probably go undetected because the imports are widely distributed.

Another trend that has affected the epidemiology of food-borne disease is the rising consumption of food in commercial establishments. Pathogens, such as Norwalk virus, can be spread from an infected food handler to a consumer through contaminated food. Training in hygiene and sanitation often is minimal in this industry because the food handlers are low-paid and poorly educated, with rapid turnover in employment. For many of these individuals, sick leave may not be available, so they may work while ill with infectious diseases.

Yet another factor that has influenced the epidemiology of food-borne disease is the growing presence of large-volume food-production facilities. With a trend toward mass-produced foods that are distributed to consumers in remote locations, food-borne diseases may affect large numbers of persons in a variety of locations. Consequently, the classic hallmarks of food-borne disease outbreaks—high attack rates, short in-

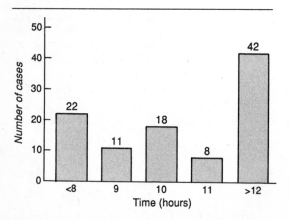

Figure 5–2. Distribution of number of cases by time from eating suspect meal to development of symptoms.

Table 5–5. Food-specific histories of students who ate lunch at the college cafeteria on January 17.

Food or Beverage	Students Who Ate Specific Food or Beverage				Students Who Did Not Eat Specific Food or Beverage			
	Ill	Well	Total	AR (%)	Ill	Well	Total	AR (%)
Fish chowder	16	36	52	30.8	87	103	190	45.8
Lamb stew pie	95	56	151	62.9	7	82	89	7.9
Tuna noodle casserole	12	57	69	17.4	92	80	172	53.5
Pineapple Jell-O salad	58	54	112	51.8	39	69	108	36.1
Fruit salad	32	39	71	45.1	63	82	145	43.4
Cabbage salad	4	5	9	44.4	95	126	221	43.0
Plain Jell-O with vanilla sauce	19	29	48	39.6	80	102	182	44.0
Plain Jell-O without vanilla sauce	62	77	139	44.6	39	56	95	41.1
Milk	91	127	218	41.7	12	13	25	48.0
Coffee	10	31	41	24.4	89	103	192	46.4
Tea	23	19	42	54.8	78	114	192	40.6

cubation periods, clustering of affected persons in time and space—may not occur, making the outbreak difficult to detect. Once an outbreak is suspected, however, the search for the underlying cause typically follows the basic approach outlined in the preceding section.

EMERGING INFECTIOUS DISEASES

Outbreaks of disease sometimes can be linked to the emergence of a new pathogen. The term **emerging infectious disease** is applied to *an infection that has newly appeared in a population or has existed but is rapidly increasing in incidence or geographical range.* One of the more dramatic examples in recent history is disease caused by the human immunodeficiency virus (HIV). There are, however, many other examples, including Lyme disease, hantavirus pulmonary syndrome, and hemolytic uremic syndrome.

Although evolutionary processes can give rise to new infectious agents, most emerging infections probably result from previously existing but obscure pathogens. A number of factors can promote the emergence of these pre-existing pathogens:

(1) Ecologic changes.
(2) Shifts in human populations.
(3) International travel and commerce.
(4) Changes in technological or industrial practices.
(5) Microbial adaptation.
(6) Lapses in the public health system.

Ecologic changes can contribute to emerging infections by placing people into close contact with pathogens not previously encountered by some or all human populations. In addition, ecologic changes can result in conditions that increase the size of a microbial population. The role of ecologic changes in the emergence of an infectious disease is well illustrated by Lyme disease, a systemic illness with characteristic skin rash, joint pain, and in advanced stages, neurologic and cardiac manifestations. This condition is caused by the spirochete, *Borrelia burgdorferi,* which

was first isolated and identified in 1982. This spirochete is borne by a particular deer tick. The first outbreak of Lyme disease was detected in the Connecticut town after which the disease is named. The emergence of Lyme disease in New England probably occurred as a consequence of reforestation of land that had been cleared previously for agricultural purposes. As the forests returned, the deer population grew, allowing in turn, the expansion of the tick population and transmission of the spirochete to humans through tick bites.

Not all ecologic changes that contribute to emerging infections are caused by human activity. Natural changes in ecology also can give rise to emerging infections, as illustrated by the Hantavirus Pulmonary Syndrome (HPS). Hantavirus is named for a river in South Korea where the virus was originally discovered. It is suspected that outbreaks caused by Hantaan virus have occurred in Asia for many centuries, and it was responsible for the condition known as Korean hemorrhagic fever, which affected thousands of soldiers involved in the Korean war during the 1950s. Until 1993, however, hantavirus was not known to cause disease in the United States or to cause an adult respiratory distress syndrome. Beginning with an influenza-like illness, HPS progresses rapidly to respiratory failure, with a high case fatality.

The first outbreak of HPS was detected in the Four Corners region of the southwestern United States during 1993. A new strain of hantavirus was identified, and the reservoir for this pathogen was shown to be the deer mouse, *Peromyscus maniculatus.* The population of this deer mouse in the Four Corners region rose 10-fold between 1992 and 1993, as a result of the end of a 6-year drought. The mouse's predators had decreased during the drought, and with an ample food supply after the drought, the mouse population exploded, expanding the reservoir for the hantavirus and increasing the likelihood of contact with humans.

Emerging infections can be traced to human societal changes, such as migration from relatively isolated rural settings into crowded urban environments. It is speculated, eg, that HIV infection may have originated in rural areas of Africa, but only became epidemic with migration of infected persons into cities. HIV also illustrates the role that human behavior can play in the emergence of a disease. Certain high-risk sexual practices and injecting drug use contributed to the spread of this infection.

For centuries, international travel has been a means by which pathogens are introduced into previously unexposed populations. There are many examples, including the importation of yellow fever from Africa to the Americas during the 16th and 17th centuries. Another historical illustration is the spread of cholera during the 19th century from India to the Middle East and then to Europe. The opportunities for global spread of infections have multiplied in recent years, however, for several reasons. First, the volume of international travel has expanded, increasing the number of person-to-person contacts. Second, the speed of international travel by airplane makes it more likely that infected individuals will be contagious upon arrival at their destinations. When modes of transit were considerably slower than today, there was greater opportunity for an infection to run its course before an infected traveller reached a destination. Third, as noted in the previous section, the growing globalization of food and other markets increases the number of opportunities to convey pathogens from one country to another.

The recent epidemic of cholera in Latin America, where the disease previously had not occurred during the 20th century, illustrates the role of international commerce. Based upon molecular typing of the agent, it is thought that the pathogen, *Vibrio cholerae,* was introduced into Peruvian coastal waters from Asia, perhaps, through the ballast water of a freighter from China. Once introduced, cholera spread to affect more than 500,000 Latin Americans.

Technologic changes now allow food and other products to be produced in mass quantities and distributed widely, thereby enhancing the spread of emerging infections. A recent multistate outbreak of *Escherichia coli* O157:H7 infections illustrates this phenomenon. In 1993, a physician in the State of Washington first noted and reported the hemolytic uremic syndrome in a cluster of children who had presented to local emergency rooms with bloody diarrhea. Investigation by state health officials and officials from three other Western states identified more than 500 affected persons. Their illnesses were linked to the consumption of hamburgers at a particular chain of fast-food restaurants. Cultures of stool from affected persons revealed *E coli* O157:H7, an organism that lives in the intestines of healthy cattle, can contaminate meat during slaughter, and is a pathogen to humans. This organism was isolated from 11 lots of hamburger, collectively accounting for over a million ground beef patties. The affected hamburger was traced back to five slaughterhouses in the United States and one in Canada that were the likely sources of the contaminated meat.

Evolutionary changes in microbes also can give rise to emerging infections. Antibiotic resistance is one such mechanism of adaptation. The problem of multidrug-resistant tuberculosis was described in Chapter 3. Other current examples of pathogens for which antibiotic resistance may impede disease control efforts include penicillin-resistant *Streptococcus pneumoniae* and nosocomial enterococci resistant to vancomycin. In addition to antibiotic resistance, evolutionary changes to established pathogens can limit their control in other ways. Many viruses mutate rapidly, yielding new strains of pathogens with surface antigens that differ from those of existing strains; this phenomenon is known as **antigenic drift**. Reinfection with the new viral strain can arise since its antigens are not recognized by the immune system of the host. In rare instances, a new variant of a pathogen may even result in an entirely new clinical syndrome. The manifestations of streptococcal toxic shock syndrome and necrotizing fasciitis recently linked with group A streptococcal infection may represent this type of phenomenon.

The failure of public health measures also can give rise to emerging infections. For instance, a nonfunctioning water filtration plant in Milwaukee, Wisconsin resulted in contamination of the municipal water supply with *Cryptosporidium* in 1993. This pathogen is a protozoan that infects epithelial cells of the gastrointestinal, biliary, and respiratory tracts of humans and other animals. In humans, the primary manifestations of illness are diarrhea and cramping abdominal pain. Among immunodeficient persons, including those with AIDS, infection can follow a fulminant course, even leading to death. The outbreak in Milwaukee produced illness in more than 400,000 individuals, 4400 of whom required hospitalization.

Emerging infections serve to remind us that the conquest of infectious disease is far from achieved. Despite great successes, such as the worldwide eradication of smallpox, human populations are still exposed to a huge burden of suffering from infectious diseases. The Centers for Disease Control and Prevention (CDC) has developed a strategy to address emerging infectious diseases.

This strategy involves four major components: (1) surveillance, (2) applied research, (3) prevention and control, and (4) infrastructure. Surveillance is intended to enhance the early recognition and prompt evaluation of these outbreaks. Applied research focuses on the development, implementation, and distribution of new diagnostic methods and new vaccines. Prevention and control is designed to promote the collection and dissemination of information about infections. The final strategic component, collectively described as infrastructure, is intended to ensure that appropriate human and laboratory resources are available to support nationwide surveillance and to implement comprehensive prevention and control programs when necessary.

SUMMARY

The investigation of **disease outbreaks** (sudden and geographically limited epidemics) is an essential role of epidemiology. The primary goals of an outbreak investigation are the identification of the causal agent (the pathogen) and the prevention of further cases. The propagation of a disease outbreak requires a pathogen, a viable mode of transmission, and an adequate pool of susceptible persons. Elimination of one or more of these three components will terminate the outbreak. Two basic modes of transmission are **person-to-person** spread and **common-source** exposure. Infectious illnesses can be transmitted by either mode, whereas noninfectious environmental pathogens usually produce disease outbreaks through a common-source transmission.

Not all disease outbreaks warrant investigation. The decision to investigate an outbreak typically is based upon the severity of illness, the number of affected persons, uncertainty about the pathogen, and the perceived need to control further spread of the disease. Investigations usually are conducted by local, state, or federal public health officials.

In this chapter, the principles and methods of outbreak investigation are illustrated by the evaluation of an episode of food poisoning on a college campus. This outbreak came to attention because almost 50 students sought medical care for acute gastrointestinal symptoms in a period of less than 24 hours.

A measure of the risk of developing an illness over a specified period of time is the **attack rate** (*AR*). Based upon infirmary records, the *AR* among all students was estimated to be 4%, but among those residing in dormitories, the estimated *AR* was 6%. The *AR* did not differ by gender, but students residing at two dormitories had higher *ARs* than residents of the other 12 dormitories.

In order to collect more detailed, and perhaps more complete, information than could be obtained from infirmary records, investigators conducted a survey of residents based on a representative sample of dormitories. The survey results indicated a much higher *AR* for dormitory residents (36%) than had been estimated from infirmary records (6%). The possibility of **bias** (systematic error) in both estimates must be considered. Nevertheless, the results of the survey suggested that (a) the outbreak was widespread among dormitory residents and (b) the prior definition of high-risk dormitories based upon infirmary records might be inaccurate.

Comparison of *ARs* for persons who ate and did not eat specific foods indicated a strong association between eating a particular food and risk of the gastrointestinal illness. The distribution of times from ingestion to the onset of symptoms (incubation period) revealed a median interval of about 10 hours. A follow-up survey revealed that lamb stew pie was the most suspect common-source exposure for this outbreak.

Although cultures of the foods and specimens from affected individuals were not obtained, the nature of the symptoms, the median incubation period, and the presumed source of exposure implicated *C perfringens* as the pathogen. Knowledge of the factors that contribute to the proliferation and transmission of this bacteria were used to control the outbreak; such knowledge could be used to prevent similar episodes in the future.

The traditional epidemiology of food-borne outbreaks—high attack rates, short incubation periods, and clustering of affected individuals in time and place—is changing for a number of reasons. The composition of the typical diet has shifted, with decreased consumption of red meat and increased consumption of poultry, fresh fruits, and vegetables. Consequently, exposure to pathogens associated with the latter products is rising. The increased consumption of food from commercial establishments also has resulted in greater opportunity for transmission of infections from food handlers to consumers. The rise of facilities that produce food in massive quantities, combined with the use of distribution systems that deliver foods to geographically remote markets, tend to diminish any clustering in time and space of persons who are infected with pathogens borne by these foods.

Emerging infections can be defined as those that are appearing for the first time in a population, or those that have existed in a population but are rapidly increasing in incidence or geographic range. A number of factors contribute to the emergence of certain infections:

(1) Man-made or natural changes in the environment (eg, accounting for Lyme disease and HPS).
(2) Demographic shifts in populations (eg, accounting for the spread of HIV).
(3) Increased international travel and commerce (eg, accounting for the spread of cholera in Latin America in the 1980s).
(4) Technologic and industrial changes (eg, accounting for the rise of hemolytic uremic syndrome in the Northwest in 1993).
(5) Adaptation of microbes (eg, accounting for antibiotic resistant organisms).
(6) Lapses in the public health system (eg, accounting for infections due to waterborne *Cryptosporidium*).

The emergence of infectious diseases presents a continuing challenge for the recognition, evaluation, and control of disease outbreaks in the United States and elsewhere.

STUDY QUESTIONS

Directions: For each numbered question, select the single best answer from lettered options.

Questions 1–2. During an 8-hour work shift at a corporate headquarters building, 30 employees (20 females and ten males) visited the company's physician with complaints of nausea, vomiting, headaches, and dizziness. All affected individuals responded to supportive treatment and were sent home. In order to search for possible causes of the outbreak, the physician performed an investigation.

1. If 600 persons worked in the building, then the attack rate was
   A. 3%
   B. 5%
   C. 10%
   D. 20%
   E. 30%

2. If 400 females and 200 males worked in the building, the male-to-female risk ratio was
   A. 0.3
   B. 0.5
   C. 1.0
   D. 2.0
   E. 3.0

Questions 3–5. The distribution of cases and population at risk is shown by floor of the building in Table 5–6.

3. The floor with the highest risk of disease was
   A. A
   B. B
   C. C
   D. D
   E. E

4. The risk for workers on the high-risk floor was how many times greater than the average risk among all workers?
   A. 1
   B. 2
   C. 3
   D. 4
   E. 5

5. If the average risk among all workers was applied to the number of workers on the high-risk floor, the expected number of cases on that floor would have been
   A. 1
   B. 2

C. 3
D. 4
E. 5

Questions 6–8. A survey of all workers was conducted to determine whether other persons were affected beyond those who sought care at the physician's office. All 600 employees were surveyed, and 400 questionnaires were completed and returned. A total of 80 persons reported symptoms consistent with the syndrome observed among workers who sought medical attention.

6. The response rate to the questionnaire was
   A. 5.0%
   B. 7.5%
   C. 20.0%
   D. 37.5%
   E. 67.0%

7. Based on the survey data, the attack rate was
   A. 5.0%
   B. 7.5%
   C. 20.0%
   D. 37.5%
   E. 67.0%

8. The percentage of affected individuals who sought medical care was
   A. 5.0%
   B. 7.5%
   C. 20.0%
   D. 37.5%
   E. 67.0%

Questions 9–10. Based upon responses to the survey, the exposure most strongly associated with the development of illness was drinking from a water cooler on the entrance level of the building. The cumulative percentage distribution of times from first drinking that day from the water cooler to the development of symptoms is shown in Figure 5–4.

Table 5–6. Distribution of cases and population at risk by floor of the office building.

Floor	Number of Cases	Persons at Risk
A	4	20
B	7	155
C	6	135
D	8	180
E	5	110
Total	30	600

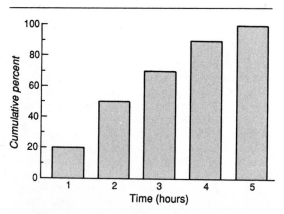

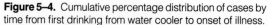

Figure 5–4. Cumulative percentage distribution of cases by time from first drinking from water cooler to onset of illness.

9. From this graph, the median incubation period in hours was
   A. 1
   B. 2
   C. 3
   D. 4
   E. 5

10. Factors that suggest a common-source exposure include all of the following EXCEPT
    A. Tight clustering of cases in time of onset
    B. No more than average risk among office mates of cases
    C. Lack of similar illnesses among family members of cases
    D. Lack of further cases when the water cooler was removed
    E. Large number of affected persons

FURTHER READING

Goodman RA, Buehler JW, Koplan JP: The epidemiologic field investigation: Science and judgment in public health practice. Am J Epidemiol 1990:**132**:9.

Lederberg J et al: *Emerging Infections: Microbial Threats to Health in the United States.* National Academy Press, 1992.

REFERENCES

Introduction
Gregg MB, Parsonnet J: The principles of an epidemic field investigation. In: *Oxford Textbook of Public Health,* 2nd ed, Vol 2. Holland WW, Detels R, Knox G (editors). Oxford Univ Press, 1991.

Kelsey JL, Thompson WD, Evans AS: Epidemic investigation. In: *Methods in Observational Epidemiology.* Oxford Univ Press, 1986.

Food-Borne Disease
Bean NH, Griffin PM: Foodborne disease outbreaks in the United States, 1973–1987: Pathogens, vehicles and trends. J Food Prot 1990:**53**:804.

Hedberg CW, MacDonald KL, Osterholm MT: Changing epidemiology of food-borne disease: A Minnesota perspective. Clin Infect Dis 1994;**18**:671.

Emerging Infectious Diseases
CDC: Addressing emerging infectious disease threats: A prevention strategy for the United States. MMWR 1994;**43**(RR-5):1.

Epstein PR: Emerging diseases and ecosystem instability: New threats to public health. Am J Public Health 1995;**85**:168.

Levins R et al: The emergence of new diseases. Am Scient 1994;**82**:52.

Morse SB: Factors in the emergence of infectious diseases. Emerg Infect Dis 1995;**1**:7.

Diagnostic Testing

PATIENT PROFILE

A 54-year-old high school teacher visited her family practitioner for an annual checkup. She reported no illnesses during the preceding year, felt well, and had no complaints. The hot flashes she had experienced a year ago had resolved without treatment. The physician performed a physical examination, comprising breast, pelvic (including a Papanicolaou smear), and rectal examinations; all were unremarkable. The physician recommended that the patient have a mammogram, which was scheduled for 1 week later.

The results of the mammogram were not normal, and the radiologist suggested that a breast biopsy be performed. The family practitioner notified the patient of the abnormal mammogram and referred her to a surgeon, who concurred that physical examination of the breast was normal. Based upon the mammographic abnormality, however, the surgeon and the radiologist agreed that fine needle aspiration (FNA) of the abnormal breast under radiologic guidance was indicated. Evaluation of the FNA specimen by a pathologist revealed cancer cells, and the patient was scheduled for further surgery the following week.

CLINICAL REASONING

The practice of clinical medicine is the artful application of science. A seemingly straightforward chain of decisions by the physicians in the Patient Profile ultimately led to the diagnosis of breast cancer and subsequent treatment. In practice, however, the process of clinical reasoning can be extremely complex. Each decision made by the clinicians in the Patient Profile included the possibility that information was incorrect. Sir William Osler eloquently described the difficulties of clinical decision-making in 1921:

> The problems of disease are more complicated and difficult than any others with which the trained mind has to grapple . . . Variability is the law of life. As no two faces are the same, so no two bodies are alike, and no two individuals react alike and behave alike under the abnormal conditions which we know as disease. This is the fundamental difficulty in the education of the physician, and

one which he (or she) may never grasp . . . Probability is the guide of life.

The clinical decision-making process is based on probability. For example, in the Patient Profile the clinician knew that a 54-year-old woman with a normal breast examination had a low probability of having breast cancer (~0.3%). An abnormal screening mammogram increased the likelihood of breast cancer to perhaps 13%. The radiologist may have predicted a slightly lower or higher probability of breast cancer, based upon the particular mammographic findings. A positive FNA test increased the probability of breast cancer to about 64%. Again, based upon the particulars of this patient's FNA specimen, such as the appearance of the nucleus or the nuclear/cytoplasmic ratio, the estimate of the probability of breast cancer after the FNA may have been slightly more or less than 64%. Furthermore, different pathologists may reach different conclusions when interpreting the same microscopic specimen, ie, some pathologists may state that cancer cells are definitely present, while others may report that the specimen is suspicious for cancer.

Figure 6–1 is a diagrammatic representation of the diagnostic process that ultimately led to a diagnosis of breast cancer in the Patient Profile. The likelihood of a particular disease at any point in time is given on the horizontal axis. At the far left, the probability of disease is 0, and at the far right, the probability of disease is 100%. Based upon each new meaningful piece of information, the likelihood of disease moves toward 0 or 100%. In the Patient Profile, the probability of breast cancer for the patient increased from near 0 to almost 67% during the diagnostic workup. *The purpose of a diagnostic test is to move the estimated probability of disease toward either end of the probability scale,* thereby providing information that will alter subsequent diagnostic or treatment plans. When the estimated probability of a disease is close to 0, the disease can be ruled out. When the estimated likelihood of a disease is close to 100%, the disease is confirmed.

Although diagnostic procedures, such as x-rays or biopsies, often are considered laboratory tests, almost all approaches to gathering clinical information can be regarded as tests. A patient's responses to questions during history-taking or the presence or absence of physical findings influences the clinician's estimation

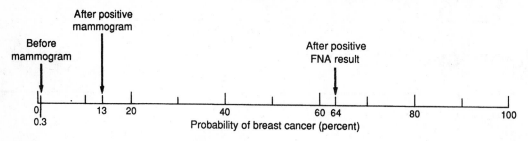
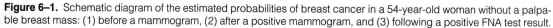

Figure 6–1. Schematic diagram of the estimated probabilities of breast cancer in a 54-year-old woman without a palpable breast mass: (1) before a mammogram, (2) after a positive mammogram, and (3) following a positive FNA test result.

of the probability of a particular disease. In the Patient Profile, if the patient's sister and mother had been diagnosed previously with breast cancer, then the patient's likelihood of having breast cancer prior to any tests could have been as high as 1%. If a palpable breast lump had been present on physical examination, then the likelihood of cancer could have been estimated to be 20–40% prior to the mammogram. Experienced diagnosticians typically form hypotheses early in a patient encounter and then direct the history and physical examination in an effort to refine the estimated probabilities of a relatively small number of diseases.

Tests may be performed for many reasons. In the preceding discussion, attention was focused on determining the probability that a disease was present. Tests also may be used to assess the severity of an illness, predict disease outcome, or monitor response to therapy. Regardless of the purpose of a test, it is important to remember that the test is used to estimate probability of an outcome.

SENSITIVITY AND SPECIFICITY

In a perfect world, medical tests would always be correct. For example, women could undergo a diagnostic test that would unequivocally determine whether breast cancer was present, and the test would have no side effects. A positive test result would indicate that cancer was present, and a negative test result would indicate that the disease was absent. In reality, however, every test is fallible.

Consider a test that has only positive or negative results. After the test is performed, one of four possible scenarios will occur, as demonstrated in Figure 6–2. For the purposes of this discussion, "true" disease status is determined by the most definitive diagnostic method, referred to as a "gold standard." For example, the gold standard for breast cancer diagnosis might be histopathologic confirmation of cancer in a surgical specimen. In cell *a* of Figure 6–2, the disease of interest is present and the test result is positive, or true-positive. In cell *d*, the disease is absent and the test is

negative, or true-negative. In both of these cells, the test result agrees with the actual disease status. Cell *b* represents individuals without disease who have a positive test result. Since these test results incorrectly suggest that disease is present, they are considered to be false-positives. Individuals in cell *c* have the disease but have negative test results. These results are designated false-negatives because they incorrectly suggest that disease is absent.

Any diagnostic test can be evaluated in this manner. The first step in the evaluation of a test is how to determine the "true" disease status. For the FNA test, we could compare results obtained from FNA to the results obtained if every woman subsequently underwent a surgical excisional biopsy procedure. This procedure, the gold standard, is considered to represent the true disease status.

Just such a comparison of FNA results against excisional biopsy was made in 114 consecutive women with normal physical examinations and abnormal mammograms; patients received a FNA followed by a surgical excisional biopsy of the same breast (Bibbo et al, 1988). The results of the comparison are given in Figure 6–3.

Sensitivity and **specificity** are terms used to describe the performance of the FNA test relative to the surgical excisional biopsy. *The sensitivity of a test is*

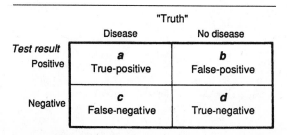
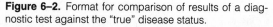

Figure 6–2. Format for comparison of results of a diagnostic test against the "true" disease status.

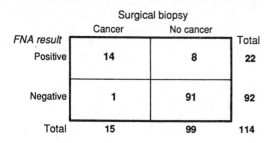

Figure 6–3. Comparison of FNA test results with findings from surgical excisional biopsies in women without palpable breast masses. (Data reproduced, with permission, from Bibbo M et al: Stereotaxic fine needle aspiration cytology of clinically occult malignant and premalignant breast lesions. Acta Cytol 1988;**32**:193.)

defined as the percentage of persons with the disease of interest who have positive test results. Sensitivity is calculated as follows:

$$\text{Sensitivity} = \frac{\text{True-positives}}{\text{True-positives} + \text{False-negatives}} \times 100$$

$$= \frac{a}{a + c} \times 100$$

Substituting data from Figure 6–3, the sensitivity of the FNA test is:

$$\text{Sensitivity} = \frac{\text{True-positives}}{\text{True-positives} + \text{False-negatives}} \times 100$$

$$= \frac{14}{14 + 1} \times 100 = 93\%$$

The greater the sensitivity of a test, the more likely that the test will detect persons with the disease of interest. For the FNA test, 93% of all the patients with breast cancer had positive test results. Tests with great sensitivity are useful clinically to rule out a disease. That is, a negative result would virtually exclude the possibility that the patient has the disease of interest.

Specificity is defined as the percentage of persons without the disease of interest who have negative test results. Specificity is calculated as follows:

$$\text{Specificity} = \frac{\text{True-negatives}}{\text{True-negatives} + \text{False-positives}} \times 100$$

$$= \frac{d}{d + b} \times 100$$

Substituting data from Figure 6–3, the specificity of the FNA test is:

$$\text{Specificity} = \frac{\text{True-negatives}}{\text{True-negatives} + \text{False-positives}} \times 100$$

$$= \frac{91}{91 + 8} \times 100 = 92\%$$

The greater the specificity, the more likely that persons without the disease of interest will be excluded by the test. Very specific tests often are used to confirm the presence of a disease. If the test is highly specific, a positive test result would strongly implicate the disease of interest.

POSITIVE AND NEGATIVE PREDICTIVE VALUE

Sensitivity and specificity are descriptors of the accuracy of a test. Two measures that directly address the estimation of probability of disease are the **positive predictive value (PV⁺)** and the **negative predictive value (PV⁻).** *The PV⁺ is defined as the percentage of persons with positive test results who actually have the disease of interest.* The PV⁺ therefore, allows one to estimate how likely it is that the disease of interest is present if the test is positive. Referring again to Figure 6–2, the PV⁺ is calculated as follows:

$$\text{PV}^+ = \frac{\text{True-positives}}{\text{True-positives} + \text{False-positives}} \times 100$$

$$= \frac{a}{a + b} \times 100$$

The PV⁺ is the percentage of persons with positive test results who have the disease. The calculation of the PV⁺ for the FNA test described in Figure 6–3 is:

$$\text{PV}^+ = \frac{\text{True-positives}}{\text{True-positives} + \text{False-positives}} \times 100$$

$$= \frac{14}{14 + 8} \times 100 = 64\%$$

The average probability of breast cancer among women in this sample prior to the FNA test was 15 affected women out of 114 total women, or 13%. After the FNA test, the probability of breast cancer for a woman with a positive test result increased to 64%.

The PV⁻ is the probability of breast cancer being absent if the FNA is negative. The general formula for the calculation of PV⁻ is:

$$\text{PV}^- = \frac{\text{True-negatives}}{\text{True-negatives} + \text{False-negatives}} \times 100$$

$$= \frac{d}{d + c} \times 100$$

For the FNA test data in Figure 6–3, the PV⁻ is:

$$\text{PV}^- = \frac{\text{True-negatives}}{\text{True-negatives} + \text{False-negatives}} \times 100$$

$$= \frac{91}{91 + 1} \times 100 = 99\%$$

Before the FNA was performed, the average likelihood of not having breast cancer among women in this sample was 99 unaffected women out of 114 total women, or 87%. After a negative FNA result, the probability of not having breast cancer increased to 99%.

Now that the post-FNA probability of disease has been calculated for either a positive or negative test result, one can consider the usefulness of the FNA test for a patient with a nonpalpable breast lesion. A positive test result increased the probability of breast cancer from 13% to 64%. Whether the probability of breast cancer is 13% or 64%, further workup or treatment is indicated. Both before and after a positive FNA result, the clinician would conclude that the likelihood of breast cancer was too great to forgo a test such as a surgical biopsy, which would provide the most definitive diagnosis.

A negative test result, however, would reduce the probability that breast cancer is present to 1% (100% − PV⁻ = 1%). One could choose to defer surgical biopsy and repeat mammographic examinations in several months on women with abnormal mammograms but normal FNAs, accepting a 1 in 100 risk of delayed treatment of an existing cancer. A more aggressive approach would be to perform a surgical biopsy on every woman with an abnormal mammogram. The basis of this decision would be that a probability of breast cancer of 1% is too high *not* to

proceed with a surgical biopsy. The advantage of performing an FNA on patients with abnormal mammograms is that the vast majority of these women could be spared the increased morbidity and expense associated with a surgical biopsy.

In addition to recognizing that all tests are fallible, it is important to appreciate that the usefulness of a test changes as the clinical situation changes. Specifically, the pretest probability of disease in an individual, or the prevalence of disease in a population, greatly influences the predictive value. The concept of variable test performance can be illustrated by comparing the use of FNA in women with mammographically detected breast lesions but without palpable breast masses to the use of FNA in women with breast masses found on physical examination (Figure 6–4).

Notice that the prevalence of breast cancer in these two groups, which is the same as the average pretest probability of disease for individual patients in the corresponding groups, was higher among the women with palpable masses (38%) than among the women without palpable masses (13%). Although the FNA test had identical specificity and sensitivity in these two clinical situations, the PV⁺ of the test was 64% for women without palpable masses but 88% for women with palpable masses. The PV⁺ increased as the pretest probability of disease increased. Therefore, it was easier to

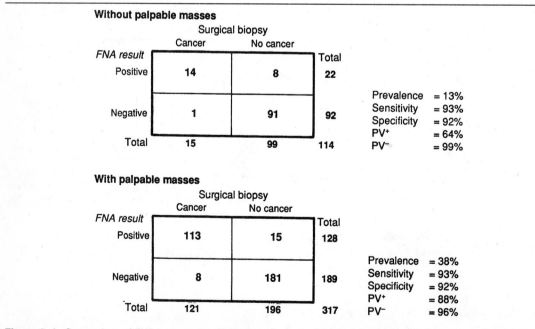

Figure 6–4. Comparison of FNA test results with findings from surgical excisional biopsies in women without palpable breast masses and in women with palpable breast masses. (Data on women without palpable breast masses reproduced, with permission, from Bibbo M et al: Stereotaxic fine needle aspiration cytology of clinically occult malignant and premalignant breast lesions. Acta Cytol 1988;**32**:193. Data on women with palpable breast masses reproduced, with permission, from Smith C et al: Fine-needle aspiration cytology in the diagnosis of primary breast cancer. Surgery 1988;**103**:178.)

confirm the presence of breast cancer in a women with increased baseline likelihood of disease.

The PV^- was 99% when FNA was used among women without palpable masses but decreased to 96% when used for women with palpable masses. The PV^- decreased as the pretest probability of disease increased; this is logical since a disease becomes easier to exclude as the probability of disease decreases before the test is performed. The differences in predictive value between these two populations is due only to the difference in the pretest probability of disease, which, in this case, is based upon whether a palpable mass was present.

Does the difference in predictive values described in Figure 6–4 have clinical implications? As discussed previously, among women with nonpalpable lesions, a negative FNA result ($PV^- = 99\%$) could reduce the probability of disease to 1%, and therefore obviate the need for a surgical biopsy. In the group with palpable masses, after a negative FNA result, the probability of breast cancer still would be 4%, which might warrant further testing, eg, a biopsy. If neither a positive nor a negative test result would change subsequent management, one would question the use of the FNA among women with palpable lumps.

CUTOFF POINTS

In this chapter the use of the FNA was analyzed as a detection method for breast cancer, assuming that the test's report would indicate either "cancer present" or "cancer absent." The dichotomous classification of clinical findings as positive or negative is commonplace and useful. Examples of dichotomous results are a positive or negative history of pain in a breast, the presence or absence of a palpable breast mass on physical examination, and a normal or abnormal alkaline phosphatase level (a serum marker of metastatic spread of breast cancer to bones or liver).

In reality, however, test results often occur along a continuum and, thus, do not indicate only a positive or negative outcome. Breast pain, eg, can be negative, intermittent, or continuous. A breast mass may be measured in centimeters, and the size of the tumor varies among patients. A serum alkaline phosphatase level may range along a continuous scale. In general, the more extreme the value of a continuous test result, the greater the likelihood that the result reflects a laboratory error or an abnormality in the patient.

The results of the FNA test often are classified as follows:

(1) Insufficient material to adequately assess presence or absence of malignant cells.
(2) Benign (no malignant cells present).
(3) Suspicious (atypical cells present but not definitely malignant).
(4) Malignant cells present.

The choice of whether to consider each of these four possible results as positive or negative influences the assessment of test performance. In both the clinical series of patients with breast abnormalities presented above (see Figure 6–4), the patients with inadequate specimens were considered to have negative test results. Another important decision concerning the FNA is whether to classify women with suspicious or atypical results as positive or negative. The ramifications of this decision were explored in an evaluation of the test among women with palpable breast masses. That evaluation of the FNA, shown in Figure 6–5, employs two different assumptions: (1) suspicious FNA results were considered to be positive, and (2) suspicious FNA results were considered to be negative. Note that the sensitivity of the FNA decreased and the specificity increased when women with suspicious FNA findings were considered to have negative test results.

This is an example of changing the **cutoff point,** which is the point at which one considers the test to change from negative to positive. In Figure 6–5 where suspicious FNA results were thought to be positive, the cutoff point was considered to be between normal FNAs and suspicious FNAs. Where suspicious FNA results were considered to be negative, a cutoff point between a suspicious FNA and a malignant FNA was chosen. *Moving the cutoff point changes the test's sensitivity, specificity, positive and negative predictive values, and hence, the way in which the test is used.*

As illustrated in Figure 6–5, a negative FNA result would reduce the probability of breast cancer, but with a 4% chance of breast cancer, a biopsy may still be warranted. A positive FNA result would increase the likelihood of cancer to 88%, but still would not absolutely confirm the diagnosis. Alternatively, by setting the cutoff point between the suspicious and malignant categories, the positive PV of the test becomes 100%. This could be useful clinically, since women with a positive FNA would require no further diagnostic tests prior to definitive surgical treatment (usually partial or complete removal of the affected breast). Indeed, the positive FNA has been characterized by many clinicians as a test that precludes the need for surgical excisional biopsy, thereby saving the patient an additional procedure and reducing the cost of treatment.

SCREENING TESTS

In the Patient Profile, a mammogram was recommended to the patient as a **screening test** for breast cancer. The purpose of a mammogram is to detect breast cancer earlier in the course of the disease than would otherwise occur if the test were not performed. Figure 6–6 is a schematic representation of the course of disease over time, and illustrates the possibility of

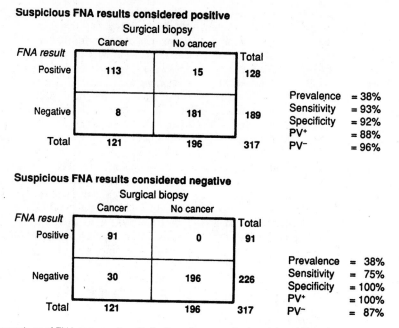

Suspicious FNA results considered positive

Surgical biopsy

FNA result	Cancer	No cancer	Total	
Positive	113	15	128	Prevalence = 38%
Negative	8	181	189	Sensitivity = 93%
				Specificity = 92%
				PV+ = 88%
Total	121	196	317	PV− = 96%

Suspicious FNA results considered negative

Surgical biopsy

FNA result	Cancer	No cancer	Total	
Positive	91	0	91	Prevalence = 38%
Negative	30	196	226	Sensitivity = 75%
				Specificity = 100%
				PV+ = 100%
Total	121	196	317	PV− = 87%

Figure 6–5. Comparison of FNA test results with findings from surgical excisional biopsies among women with palpable breast masses. (Data reproduced, with permission, Smith C et al: Fine-needle aspiration cytology in the diagnosis of primary breast cancer. Surgery 1988;**103**:178.)

detecting disease earlier using a screening test, thereby allowing for more effective treatment and prolonged survival. Inherent in this schematic diagram are two important concepts: (1) individuals with a disease can be identified by a screening test before the time of routine diagnosis (eg, when symptoms occur), and (2) treatment at the time of detection by screening, as opposed to the time of routine diagnosis, results in an improved chance of survival.

Breast cancer is a prototypical example of a progressive disease. As with most neoplasms, a breast cancer is believed to begin as a single malignant cell, which grows rapidly and forms a proliferating tumor. Over time, breast cancer cells can spread through the lymphatic system to the axillary lymph nodes and eventually to other parts of the body via the lymphatic system, the vascular system, or both. The earlier in the course of the disease that breast cancer is discovered,

the less likely that the cancer will spread to lymph nodes and other sites.

It has been known for many years that length of survival from time of diagnosis of breast cancer is related to the size of the tumor and the extent of spread to adjacent and remote sites. When mammography was first introduced, it was obvious that cancerous lesions in the breast—even those that could not be felt by even the most skilled clinician—could be detected. Researchers postulated that by screening asymptomatic women with mammography, breast cancer could be detected at an earlier stage, and, therefore, affected women as a group would experience increased survival. This logic seems infallible, but two important biases—**lead-time bias** and **length-biased sampling**—must be considered when evaluating any screening program.

As illustrated in Figure 6–7, *lead-time bias is an increase in survival as measured from disease detection*

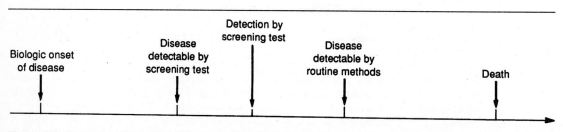

Figure 6–6. The natural history of a disease over time, including the preclinical stage when a screening test can detect the disease.

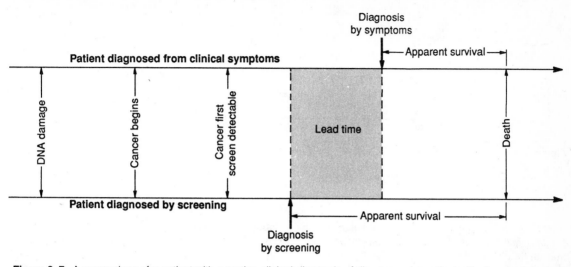

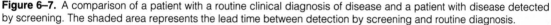

Figure 6–7. A comparison of a patient with a routine clinical diagnosis of disease and a patient with disease detected by screening. The shaded area represents the lead time between detection by screening and routine diagnosis.

until death, without lengthening of life. Notice in Figure 6–7 that the person detected with screening and the person detected without screening die at exactly the same time, but the time from diagnosis until death is greater for the screened patient because the cancer was recognized earlier. The time from early diagnosis by screening to routine diagnosis is defined as the lead time.

Length-biased sampling occurs when disease detected by a screening program is less aggressive than disease detected without screening. On average, breast cancers detected in a screening program may be less aggressive than cancers that are diagnosed when symptoms appear. This occurs because less aggressive cancers typically grow at a slower pace than more aggressive malignancies, and therefore the length of time that a cancer is detectable by screening is greater for slow-growing neoplasms. If one were to measure length of survival, individuals with breast cancers detected by screening would appear to live longer because the cancers in these patients grow at a slower pace than the cancers in routinely diagnosed patients.

To overcome lead-time bias and length-biased sampling, and therefore, to assess the true benefit of a screening program, it is useful to measure disease-specific mortality rates within an entire population. Individuals who are either randomly assigned to a screening program or who receive no screening are followed to determine whether they die from the disease of interest. Such a study was performed in the 1960s by the Health Insurance Plan (HIP) of New York. In the HIP study, women were randomly assigned to receive routine care or to undergo a screening program comprised of yearly mammographic and breast examinations.

The results of that study on the usefulness of mammography as a screening tool appear in Figure 6–8. In the evaluation of any screening test, it is important to

identify false-negative results. In the HIP study, in the screened group asymptomatic women with a positive result were referred for biopsy. At the time, there was no definitive or "gold-standard" test like FNA that could be performed on healthy women after a mammogram to determine whether cancers had been missed. An approximation of the number of false-negative screening tests (47 in this example) was derived by determining the number of cancers that arose between yearly screening examinations; these were designated "interval cancers." If a symptomatic cancer occurred after a screening mammogram but prior to the next mammogram, it was presumed that the first mammogram was falsely negative.

In Figure 6–8, notice that mammography had an excellent specificity (98%), yet the false-positive tests still outnumbered the true-positive tests by over 7 to 1 ($PV^+ = 12\%$). This means that among women with positive mammograms who were referred for surgical biopsy to obtain a definitive diagnosis, more than seven biopsies were negative for every breast cancer that was found. This high false-positive rate is related to the low prevalence of breast cancer in the general population. A low PV^+ is fairly typical for a screening test designed to detect a disease that is relatively infrequent in the general population at any point in time. It is important, therefore, to consider the possible anxiety, expense, and morbidity associated with false-positive results when screening initiatives are introduced into the general population.

The purpose of the HIP study was to determine if repeated use of mammography could reduce breast cancer mortality. The use of a concurrent control group allowed investigators to assess the relationship between mammographic screening and mortality from breast cancer. A random assignment of women to either

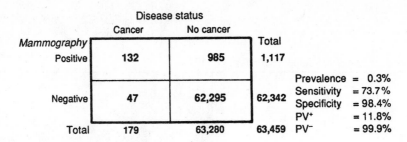

Figure 6–8. Results of mammographic screening in the Health Insurance Plan (HIP) of New York study. (Data reproduced, with permission, from Shapiro S et al: *Periodic Screening for Breast Cancer: The Health Insurance Plan Project and its Sequelae,* 1963–1986. Johns Hopkins, 1988.)

screening or routine care tended to balance the screened and unscreened groups with respect to factors that might affect subsequent breast cancer mortality (see discussion of randomization in Chapter 7). Evaluation of age-specific breast cancer mortality rates, rather than length of survival, diminished the possible distorting effect of lead-time bias. After the initial screening, slow-growing tumors presumably were removed from the screened women, and the effectiveness of subsequent annual mammograms in reducing breast cancer mortality was less likely to reflect length-biased sampling. The HIP researchers concluded that mammography reduced breast cancer mortality among the screened population by 30% when compared to the control group of women who were receiving routine care. The results of this landmark study, combined with findings from investigations of similar design in other countries, established the effectiveness of mammographic screening.

A list of criteria for a successful screening program is presented in Table 6–1. A mammographic screening program for breast cancer can be assessed using these criteria. Breast cancer is an important public health problem in the United States; at some time during her lifetime, one out of every nine women will be diagnosed with breast cancer. Early detection allows less extensive surgical treatment and reduces morbidity and mortality from this disease. Since breast cancer incidence increases steadily with age, a high-risk population can be defined as any group of women who are over 50 years of age. Although screening recommen-

dations for women under age 50 remain controversial, it is widely recommended that women aged 50 or older have a mammogram once a year. Although the test does cause some discomfort, most women find the procedure acceptable. There is an extremely small risk of breast cancer associated with the radiation received during mammography. This increased risk is negligible, however, when compared to an average woman's baseline risk of the disease. Finally, mammography is a relatively sensitive and specific test.

SUMMARY

In this chapter, the principles of evaluating and interpreting diagnostic tests were introduced, using the diagnosis of breast cancer as an example. The process of reaching a diagnosis can be represented as a weighing of probabilities. When a particular diagnosis is excluded or ruled out, the probability that the disease is present is close to 0. When a particular diagnosis is confirmed, the probability that the disease is present is close to 100%. The challenge for the clinician is to collect information that will allow successive improvements in probability, until a disease is either confirmed or excluded.

All clinical information is subject to error. Accounting for the various errors that can arise in diagnostic testing allows the physician to select tests and interpret the results of those tests appropriately. One type of error is referred to as a **false-negative** result be-

Table 6–1. Criteria for a successful screening program.

Basis for Criteria	Criteria
Effect of morbidity and mortality on population	Morbidity or mortality of the disease must be a sufficient concern to public health. A high-risk population must exist. Effective early intervention must be known to reduce morbidity or mortality.
Screening test	The screening test should be sensitive and specific. The screening test must be acceptable to the target population. Minimal risk should be associated with the screening test. Diagnostic workup for a positive test result must have acceptable morbidity, given the number of false-positive results.

cause the test fails to detect a disease when it is present. A test is said to be **sensitive** when the percentage of false-negative errors is low. A second type of error is referred to as a **false-positive** result because the test indicates that a disease is present when in fact it is not. A test with a low percentage of false-positive results is said to be **specific.**

Sensitivity and specificity are characteristics of a diagnostic test. It is useful to consider two other measures, **positive predictive value** (PV$^+$) and **negative predictive value** (PV$^-$), which are used to interpret the results of a diagnostic test. PV$^+$ is the percentage of persons with a positive test result who truly have the disease of interest. PV$^-$ is the percentage of persons with a negative test result who truly do not have the disease of interest. Both positive and negative predictive values are heavily influenced by either the pretest probability that the patient has the disease of interest, or by the prevalence of the disease in the particular population that is tested.

In some situations, a test result has only one of two possible outcomes: positive or negative. In other circumstances, however, multiple levels of outcome or even a continuous range of values can occur. For multilevel or continuous outcome test results, a dividing line or **cutoff point** can be chosen to separate findings considered to be positive or negative. The choice of a cutoff value affects the sensitivity and specificity of a test, and consequently the positive and negative predictive values as well. Raising the threshold for considering a result to be positive typically will lead to a gain in specificity (fewer false-positives) but a loss of sensitivity (more false-negatives or missed cases). On the other hand, lowering the threshold for considering a result to be positive typically will reduce the level of false-negatives (raise sensitivity) and increase the likelihood of false-positives (lower specificity).

The use of tests to detect a disease at an earlier time than it would be diagnosed through routine methods is referred to as **screening.** The evaluation of a screening test must take into account two types of distorting effects: **lead-time bias** and **length-biased sampling.** Lead-time bias can occur in a comparison of survival time, since cases detected by screening are discovered to have the disease earlier in the clinical course and, therefore, may appear to survive longer, even though the time of death is the same as if no screening had occurred. Lead-time bias may be minimized by evaluating mortality rates—rather than duration of survival—as the outcome. Length-biased sampling can occur when the screening test preferentially detects slowly progressive disease that is less likely to cause death or may result in a delayed death. Length-biased sampling can be reduced by repeated screening efforts, since slowly progressive forms of disease can be removed by the initial screening and, thus, should not be overrepresented in later screenings.

A successful screening program requires focus on a disease with appreciable health impact, for which early diagnosis and effective treatment can reduce the risk for significant morbidity and mortality. In addition, it is essential to define a high-risk population for whom (a) the test is acceptable and (b) the test can be administered with minimal risk. The false-negative, and particularly the false-positive, errors of the screening test should be relatively small, and the expense and morbidity of further evaluation of false-positives must be acceptable. When evaluated using these criteria, screening mammography is judged to be a very useful technique, at least for women over age 50.

STUDY QUESTIONS

Questions 1–4: For each measure described below, select the most appropriate numerical value from the following lettered options. Each option can be used once, more than once, or not at all.

A. 0.10	**E.** 0.56
B. 0.16	**F.** 0.70
C. 0.30	**G.** 0.90
D. 0.44	**H.** 0.96

1. What is the sensitivity of the prostate specific antigen (PSA) test for detecting prostate cancer in a clinic population of 1000 men aged 60 or older, with a prevalence of prostate cancer of 10%, among whom 70 of the prostate cancer patients have positive (abnormal) test results and 90 of the patients without prostate cancer have positive test results?

2. What is the specificity of the test described in question (1)?

3. What is the positive predictive value of the test described in question (1)?

4. What is the negative predictive value of the test described in question (1)?

Questions 5–8: For each of the numbered items below, select the most appropriate measure from the following lettered options. Each option can be used once, more than once, or not at all.

A. Sensitivity
B. Specificity
C. Positive predictive value
D. Negative predictive value
E. False-positives
F. False-negatives

5. Among 100 patients with Alzheimer's disease, 15 subjects score within the normal range on a battery of tests of cognitive performance.

6. Among 500 persons with positive screening tests for antibodies to the human immunodeficiency virus (HIV), 492 are infected with the virus.

7. Among 1000 women without breast cancer, screening mammograms are normal for 920 women.

8. Among 750 patients with normal screening test results for serum cholesterol, 50 actually have elevated serum cholesterols.

Questions 9–12: For each numbered item below, select the most appropriate limitation for applying results from a screening test. Each lettered option can be used once, more than once, or not at all.

A. Low sensitivity
B. Low specificity
C. Lead-time bias
D. Length-biased sampling
E. Low prevalence

9. Sigmoidoscopic screening preferentially tends to detect slow-growing colonic cancers that are less likely to become fatal, vs faster-growing, aggressive, undetected cancers.

10. Chest radiographs tend to lead to earlier recognition of lung cancers, with no impact on delaying the eventual time of death.

11. A screening test for developmental disabilities in children fails to detect a substantial proportion of children with such disabilities.

12. When applied in the general population, a screening test that is normal among 99% of unaffected persons and abnormal among 97% of affected persons nevertheless yields a low positive predictive value.

Questions 13–14: A comparison of clinically diagnosed versus autopsy-confirmed myocardial infarctions was performed among 1000 consecutive deceased patients, as shown in Figure 6–9.

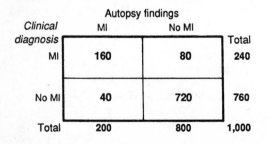

Clinical diagnosis	Autopsy findings		
	MI	No MI	Total
MI	160	80	240
No MI	40	720	760
Total	200	800	1,000

Figure 6–9. Comparison of clinical diagnosis of myocardial infarction (MI) with autopsy findings in 1000 consecutive patients who underwent surgery.

13. From these data, the prevalence of myocardial infarction at autopsy was closest to

A. 20%
B. 67%
C. 80%
D. 90%
E. 95%

14. The sensitivity of the clinical diagnosis was closest to

A. 20%
B. 67%
C. 80%
D. 90%
E. 95%

Question 15: A comparison of clinically diagnosed versus autopsy-confirmed gastric and peptic ulcers was performed in 10,000 consecutive deceased patients, as shown in Figure 6–10.

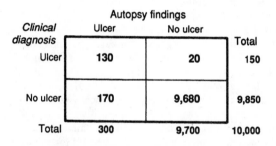

Clinical diagnosis	Autopsy findings		
	Ulcer	No ulcer	Total
Ulcer	130	20	150
No ulcer	170	9,680	9,850
Total	300	9,700	10,000

Figure 6–10. Comparison of clinical diagnosis of gastric and peptic ulcer with autopsy findings in 10,000 consecutive patients who underwent surgery.

15. From these data, the prevalence of autopsy-confirmed gastric and peptic ulcer was closest to

A. 3%
B. 43%
C. 87%
D. 98%
E. 100%

FURTHER READING

Anderson RE, Hill RB, Key CR: The sensitivity and specificity of clinical diagnostics during five decades. JAMA 1989;**261**:1610.

REFERENCES

Bibbo M et al: Stereotaxic fine needle aspiration cytology of clinically occult malignant and premalignant breast lesions. Acta Cytol 1988;**32**:193.

Osler W: Medical education. In: *Counsels and Ideals,* 2nd ed. Houghton Mifflin, 1921.

Shapiro S et al: Breast cancers detected—Sensitivity and specificity of screening. In: *Periodic Screening For Breast Cancer: The Health Insurance Plan Project and Its Sequelae,* 1963–1986. Johns Hopkins, 1988.

Smith C et al: Fine-needle aspiration cytology in the diagnosis of primary breast cancer. Surgery 1988;**103:** 178.

Clinical Trials

7

PATIENT PROFILE

An active 13-year-old middle school student complains to her parents of increasing thirst, frequency of urination, and fatigue that has persisted for a week. The following morning, the girl and her parents visit their family pediatrician. During the history, the physician notes the above-mentioned symptoms, as well as a decrease in the girl's academic performance over the previous week. She is drinking more than 3 liters a day, and urinating approximately 8 times during a 24 hour period; at least one of those times requires her to awaken from sleep. On physical examination, she is found to be afebrile, with a pulse of 110, which is slightly elevated for the patient, a normal blood pressure lying and sitting, and a normal respiratory rate. The pediatrician notes that the girl's weight has dropped 2 kilograms since a visit 3 months earlier. The remainder of the physical examination is unremarkable.

In the office, the pediatrician performs a urinalysis, which reveals a normal microscopic exam; the dipstick exam of the urine is negative for blood, white blood cells, and bilirubin, but is 4+ positive for glucose and 1+ positive for ketones. To the parents, the pediatrician mentions a concern that the girl may have diabetes mellitus. A complete blood count and blood chemistries are sent to a local laboratory, and the doctor arranges for the patient and her parents to see a pediatric endocrinologist within the hour.

In the endocrinologist's office, the results of the blood tests confirm that the girl has a markedly elevated blood glucose (565 mg/dl) and a slightly elevated blood urea nitrogen (24 mg/dl). Her serum bicarbonate is normal. The endocrinologist discusses the diagnosis of type I diabetes mellitus with the patient and her parents and asks them to speak with a nurse educator in the office to begin to learn about diabetes mellitus, the self administration of insulin, dietary control, and glucose monitoring.

CLINICAL BACKGROUND

In the United States, the prevalence of diabetes mellitus is estimated to be between 2–4%. The two basic types of diabetes mellitus are contrasted in Table 7–1. Type I diabetes is characterized by a markedly decreased or absent production of insulin, possibly due to an autoimmune destruction of the pancreatic beta cells. Without insulin to facilitate the entry of glucose into cells, plasma glucose levels rise. When the plasma glucose exceeds a level that can be reabsorbed by the kidney (approximately 180 mg/dl), the glucosuria obligates an osmotic diuresis. The concentration of glucose in the urine requires that excessive water be eliminated in the urine. An excess of energy is also lost in the urine in the form of glucose.

The resulting loss of water and calories leads to the cardinal signs of diabetes: increased urination, thirst, and appetite, as well as weight loss and dehydration. Prior to the discovery of insulin, patients diagnosed with type I diabetes mellitus died of their disease within weeks. After the purification of insulin from animals, subcutaneous injections of insulin allowed patients with type I diabetes mellitus to survive. Today, type I diabetic patients inject synthetically manufactured human insulin. The development of machines that measure plasma glucose from a small sample of blood obtained by finger stick now enables patients to monitor their blood glucose levels at home.

Although the discovery of insulin and the development of glucose monitoring virtually eliminated acute deaths due to insulin deficiency, persons with type I diabetes continued to suffer the long-term complications of the disease—premature atherosclerotic cardiovascular and peripheral vascular disease resulting in heart attacks, stroke, and amputations; retinopathy, ie, damage to the arterial vessels that can lead to blindness; and nephropathy, ie, damage to the micro-vasculature of the kidney ultimately leading to kidney failure.

During the 1980s, the cause of these long-term complications was debated within the medical community. One group argued that if blood glucose levels were controlled more tightly, a corresponding decrease in the long-term complications of diabetes would result. Others postulated that other physiologic abnormalities associated with diabetic disease contribute to the long-term vascular complications. This debate is of critical importance to our patient, a teenager with newly diagnosed diabetes. Conventional, twice-a-day injections of regular insulin in combination with a

Table 7–1. Comparison of type I and type II diabetes.

	Type I	Type II
Synonym	Insulin dependent diabetes mellitus (IDDM), juvenile onset	Non-insulin dependent diabetes mellitus (NIDDM), adult onset
Age of onset	Usually <30	Usually >40
Ketosis	Common	Uncommon
Body weight	Non-obese	Obese (50–90% of patients)
Endogenous insulin secretion	Severe deficiency	Moderate deficiency
Insulin resistance	Occasional	Almost always
HLA* association	DR3, DR4	None
Identical twins	<50% concordance	Almost 100% concordance
Islet cell antibodies	Frequent	Absent
Treatment with insulin	Always necessary	Usually not required

* HLA = Human leukocyte antigen

longer-acting insulin would control her glucose well enough to avoid complications associated with very high blood glucose levels. However, more "intensive" therapy with four injections of insulin per day and more frequent monitoring of blood glucose levels would more closely approximate secretion of insulin by the normal pancreas, and theoretically might reduce the risk of long-term vascular complications. At the same time, more intensive therapy also could result in more frequent episodes of low blood glucose levels (hypoglycemia), which rarely can result in coma. The pediatric endocrinologist might also be concerned that frequent episodes of hypoglycemia would interfere with the normal growth of an adolescent.

While there are theoretical reasons why a physician would want to maintain normal blood glucose levels in our patient, there are also hazards associated with the intensive therapy described above. To determine the safety and efficacy of new therapies, researchers must conduct a clinical trial. *A randomized, controlled clinical trial is a study design in which one treatment is compared directly with another treatment to determine which of the two options would be of greatest benefit.*

INTRODUCTION TO CLINICAL TRIALS

In the Patient Profile, the clinician is faced with a treatment decision: whether to use one of two regimens for blood glucose control. Hippocrates' axiom— "First, do no harm"—is a time-honored warning to clinicians contemplating medical intervention. "One must attend in medical practice not primarily to plausible theories," Hippocrates wrote, "but to experience combined with reason." In other words, a treatment plan should seem reasonable in theory but should also be tested experientially. More than 2000 years ago, Hippocrates noted that the benefits of a treatment should be judged according to the treatment's effects on patients.

In modern medical practice, a randomized, controlled clinical trial of one therapy versus another is the accepted standard by which the usefulness of a treatment is determined. To practice modern medicine and select appropriate therapy, one must understand the design and conduct of clinical trials.

This important method of evaluating treatments utilizes two types of knowledge, both alluded to by Hippocrates: reason and experience. "Reasonable" treatment is that which is suggested by a knowledge of basic biomedical science. For the clinical situation presented in the Patient Profile, a knowledge of the pathophysiology of diabetes mellitus and the long-term complications of this disease would indicate the need for tight control of blood glucose levels and the avoidance of any possible long-term complications of diabetes. As stated by Hippocrates, however, the clinician cannot base therapeutic decisions on theory alone, but must submit the dictates of reason to the test of experience.

Clinicians employ two types of experience to assess a treatment regimen—their own personal experience and the written or orally conveyed experience of their colleagues. Written experience may take the form of a report of a single case, a series of cases, or a comparison of one treatment versus another. *The direct comparison of two or more treatment modalities in human groups is referred to as a clinical trial.* The development of the clinical trial is a product of the application of modern scientific method to clinical medicine. The purpose of the clinical trial is to provide clinicians with information that will help them prescribe appropriate, timely treatment for their patients.

Experiments on human populations have inherent difficulties not found in the laboratory. The laboratory scientist can carefully control the conditions under which an experiment is conducted. For instance, genetically identical male mice 30 days old may be divided into two groups, kept in the same environment, and given identical diets except for a single micronutrient to ascertain the effect of that nutrient on the development of disease. Except for the rare instance of identical twins, however, human beings are variable in their genetic constitutions and their environments. Control of a human subject's environment or compliance with a treatment regimen cannot be controlled, as it can in conducting animal experiments. Furthermore, human patients and researchers have direct personal interests in the outcomes of trials. To acknowledge and account for the complexities of the human subject is the challenge of conducting a clinical trial.

STATEMENT OF THE RESEARCH QUESTIONS

As in a laboratory experiment, the first step in performing a clinical trial is to formulate the major research question. This question, usually referred to as an hypothesis, is refined to determine important study parameters, eg, the types of interventions to be compared, the nature of the outcomes to be assessed, the number of subjects in each treatment group, and the eligibility requirements for enrollment.

The parameter that is measured to answer the most important question of the clinical trial is the **primary end point.** When determining the primary end point, clinical researchers must consider the following questions:

(1) Which end points are most important clinically?
(2) Which end points can be measured in a reasonable manner?
(3) What practical constraints exist, such as population size, financial resources of the research study, and ability to follow patients on a long-term basis?

Researchers in the United States and Canada designed a clinical trial to address the following question: *Is intensive therapy, including more frequent insulin injections and blood glucose monitoring, "superior" to standard therapy for diabetes mellitus?*

To assess treatment efficacy, more than one end point can be measured. Types of end points include measures of quality of life, length of survival, percentage of patients surviving, complication rate, and intermediate end points that are predictive of survival or quality of life (Table 7–2). In assessing "superiority" for the treatment of diabetes mellitus, possible outcome measures include the following:

(1) The percentage of patients surviving at a specified time following the initiation of treatment.
(2) A patient's ability to maintain an active lifestyle.

(3) The risk of having a major complication from treatment.
(4) The risk of experiencing one of the vascular events associated with diabetes mellitus.
(5) Measurement of hemoglobin A1-C (HgbA1C), which is an indicator of the degree to which blood insulin levels have risen over the previous month.
(6) Blood glucose levels.

Examples of two of these questions restated symbolically as hypotheses follow:

$$H_0 : \pi_0 = \pi_1$$

where H_0 is the so-called **null hypothesis** and π_0 and π_1 are the percentages of persons in the standard therapy or intensive therapy groups, respectively, who develop diabetic retinopathy during the 5-year period following entry into the study.

$$H_0 : \mu_0 = \mu_1$$

where μ_0 and μ_1 are the mean HgbA1C levels at 1 year following entry into the trial for persons in the standard therapy or intensive therapy groups, respectively.

Note that these hypotheses are stated in the null form—ie, *there is no difference between the treatment groups regarding the specified end point.* The purpose of the clinical trial is to test whether the observed outcomes are consistent with these null hypotheses. If the observed data are not consistent with the null hypothesis, then the null hypothesis (H_0) is rejected in favor of an **alternative hypothesis** (H_A) such as the following:

$$H_A : \pi_0 \neq \pi_1$$

where π_0 and π_1 again are the respective percentages of persons developing diabetic retinopathy during the 5-year period following entry into the study in the standard therapy and intensive therapy groups. This alternative hypothesis states that the two treatments will differ with respect to the development of diabetic retinopathy. Similarly, an alternative hypothesis for the HgbA1C outcome could be stated as follows:

$$H_A : \mu_0 \neq \mu_1$$

Table 7–2. Types and examples of end points used in clinical trials.

Type of End Point	Example
Quality of life	Ability to perform usual daily tasks
Survival	Percentage of patients alive 1 year after entering trial
Complications	Percentage of patients who develop serious allergic reactions
Intermediate measures	Percentage of patients who have recurrence of symptoms

where μ_0 and μ_1 again are the respective mean HgbA1c for the standard therapy and intensive therapy groups. In other words, this alternative hypothesis states that the two treatments will differ with respect to mean HgbA1c levels achieved in patients after treatment.

The most important end-points for any therapy of a potentially fatal disease would be survival, or survival accounting for quality of life. However, researchers in this trial of therapy for diabetes chose diabetic retinopathy as the primary end point of the study. The researchers chose this particular end point for several reasons:

(1) Death from diabetes often occurs decades after the onset of the disease. Since a large number of patients in the trial would have no evidence of complications of diabetes, the trial could not have been completed in a timely manner if death were the primary end point.

(2) Retinopathy is a serious complication of diabetes. Vascular damage in one organ correlates with vascular damage at other sites of the body. Since vascular disease is a predominant physiologic process resulting in morbidity and mortality from the disease, the researchers felt that it was a reasonable choice as a primary end-point.

(3) The eye provides a unique view by non-invasive methods of damage to the vascular system. Furthermore, the measurement of the progression of retinopathy could be standardized and evaluated by taking photographs of each patient's retina at various points in time; moreover, researchers could evaluate the amount of retinal damage as documented in the photos without learning the treatment group to which each patient had been randomized.

(4) Retinopathy, an intermediate end point, is thought to be predictive of two important final end points: survival and quality of life.

SAMPLE SIZE DETERMINATION

The number of subjects to be enrolled in a clinical trial—ie, the sample size—must be determined at the same time as the primary research end point. At the conclusion of any experiment, data are analyzed and a statistical decision is made to reject or accept the null hypothesis. This decision is based upon probabilities and, unfortunately, may be correct or incorrect. The relationship between the possible results of the diabetes trial and the "truth" is shown in Figure 7–1. For the purposes of this discussion, "truth" can be thought of as the results of the intervention, if applied correctly to the entire universe of patients with the clinical condition under study. A clinical trial can be considered a sample of the "truth." Using a sample of a population, one hopes to make valid inferences about the entire

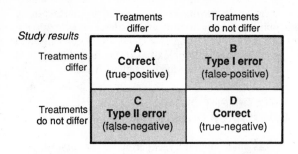

Figure 7–1. Comparison of study results and "truth."

population, but since one can evaluate only a sample, the risk of mistaken conclusions exists.

In cells A and D of Figure 7–1, the results of the study agree with the "truth." In cells B and C, however, the study results do not agree with the "truth"—ie, errors are made. These two types of error differ in their origin and implications.

If the study finds a difference in treatments, when in actuality there is no difference (cell B), then a type I error is present. Under this circumstance, the *study results are falsely positive.* In the trial of diabetes therapy, a type I error would have occurred if the investigators had concluded that there is a difference between treatments in the proportion of patients who developed retinopathy, when in "truth" there is no difference in those two proportions. *If the study fails to find a difference in treatments when in actuality there is a difference (cell C), a type II error is said to have occurred.* Under this circumstance, *the study results are falsely negative.* In the trial of diabetes therapy, a type II error would have occurred if the investigators had concluded that there is no difference between treatments in the proportion of subjects determined to have progressive retinopathy, when in fact one of the treatment regimens is associated with a reduced risk of retinopathy.

Falsely positive or falsely negative studies can occur because of faulty methodology, chance occurrences, or both. While methodologic error can be minimized by careful attention to study design, errors due to chance can never be completely eliminated. Such errors, however, can be estimated. The notation used to denote the likelihood of a type I error—that the observed difference between groups is not a true difference but is due instead to chance—is the **alpha level.** Conversely, the notation used to describe the likelihood of a type II error—that the study did not find a difference when there actually is one—is called the **beta level.** Researchers specify the alpha and beta levels when planning a study. The alpha level is specified commonly as 0.05, which means that the investigator is willing to accept a 5% risk of committing a type I error (falsely concluding that the groups differ when in reality they do not). The investigator must also specify beforehand the beta level, or risk of committing a type II error. Often a level of 0.20 for beta is considered adequate—in other words, a 1 in 5 chance of missing a true difference between the groups is allowed. The **statistical power,** or ability of a study to detect a true difference between groups, is $(1 - \beta)$. Statistical power for a study with a beta level of 0.20 would be 0.80, or 80%. Such a study would have an 80% chance of detecting a specified difference in outcome between the treatment groups.

Once the alpha and beta levels have been specified, the research team must specify another extremely important study parameter before determining sample size—the magnitude of the difference in outcome between treatment groups that the study will be designed to detect. This difference between the treatments under comparison is of great importance and should be selected on the basis of clinical information. In deciding on the level of outcome difference worthy of detection, the investigator might consider one or more of the following questions:

(1) What difference in outcome would be important to clinicians treating this type of patient?
(2) What difference would be meaningful to a patient who may suffer the consequences of the disease?
(3) What difference in outcome would justify use of the more effective treatment in spite of greater expense or greater side effects?

Formulas for the determination of sample size and illustrative calculations are provided in Appendix B. Suffice it to say here that all three factors just mentioned (acceptable levels of type I and type II errors and the expected magnitude of difference in outcome between groups) are inversely related to the required sample size (Table 7–3). That is, if one can tolerate only a 1% chance of committing a type I error rather than accepting a 5% error level, then the sample size must be increased. Similarly, a decrease in the acceptable level of type II error (enhanced statistical power) is accompanied by a need to study more subjects.

As the expected magnitude of difference in outcome (eg, proportion of subjects developing retinopathy) between treatment groups decreases, a larger sample size is required to detect the difference. In contrast, as the variability of the outcome (eg, the standard deviation of HgbA1c) diminishes, fewer subjects are required to

Table 7–3. Factors that affect sample size requirements.

Factor	Effect on Sample Size Required
↓Acceptable type I error	↑
↓Acceptable type II error	↑
↓Variability of outcome measures	↓
↓Expected differences in outcome and between groups	↑

demonstrate a difference in outcome between the groups.

RANDOMIZATION

A central tenet of the clinical trial is that patients should be assigned to treatment groups by a method that maximizes the probability that the two groups will be similar in background characteristics that may influence either the response to therapy or the primary outcome measure. For the modern clinical trial, the assignment to treatments is done by **randomization.** *With randomization, the determination of treatment group assignment is based upon probability alone and is not influenced by the physician's or patient's preference.*

The assignment for each patient is independent of the assignment for all other patients. That is to say, the treatment assignment of each patient is not influenced by the assignment of any other patient. When there are two possible treatment assignments with equal sample sizes (as in the diabetes trial), then each patient has a 50% chance of being assigned to either treatment. Such an assignment could be decided by a coin toss: eg, if the coin comes up heads, the patient is assigned to standard therapy; if the coin comes up tails, the patient is assigned to intensive therapy. Of course, tossing a coin is a rather inelegant way to assign patients to treatment groups, so many investigators use more sophisticated devices, such as tables of random numbers or computer-generated random assignments. The basic design of a randomized controlled clinical trial is illustrated in Figure 7–2, using the diabetes trial study as an example.

As recently as 50 years ago, the primary means of evaluating the benefit of a new treatment was to treat a series of patients with the new method and then compare the outcome with that observed in the past for a group of patients who received the standard therapy. The patients who received the standard therapy are called **nonconcurrent** or **historical controls.** Consider how such a study might have been performed to address the diabetes treatment question. If researchers wanted to test the hypothesis concerning the clinical efficacy of intensive therapy (experimental treatment) versus standard (or control treatment), a group of patients would be given intensive therapy and the proportion of patients who develop retinopathy in a specified period of time would then be compared to the proportion of patients who develop retinopathy among a group of patients treated at an earlier time with standard insulin therapy (Figure 7–3). There are several inherent problems with this approach:

(1) The diagnostic criteria for progression of retinopathy may change over time.
(2) The techniques used to measure retinopathy may change over the time period of the study.

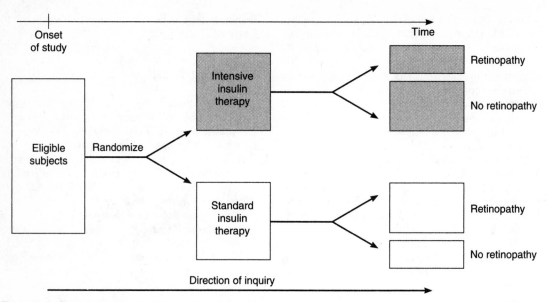

Figure 7–2. Schematic diagram of the design of a randomized controlled clinical trial comparing standard with intensive insulin therapy for the treatment of diabetes mellitus. Shaded areas correspond to patients randomized to intensive insulin therapy.

(3) Additional treatment modalities, such as advances in knowledge regarding dietary control, could become available over time and for ethical reasons would have to be employed on the patients during the second part of the study.

(4) Most importantly, the patients who presented with diabetes during the time when patients were being treated with standard insulin therapy may not have been similar in prognostic characteristics (sex, age, socioeconomic status) to the group who present during the intensive treatment period.

If concurrent controls are necessary to compare treatment groups, a basic question arises: *How should patients be assigned to each treatment group?*

One could have physicians or patients choose which treatment a patient will be given. This technique,

however, is seriously flawed. Although health care providers strive to be objective decision-makers, they are empathetic to the needs of their patients and often have opinions concerning the efficacy of a treatment prior to the results of clinical trials. Patients—who of course have a direct personal interest in any treatment result—would very likely choose a treatment based on their assessment or expectation of its efficacy.

In order to avoid unfair comparisons that may result from these preferences of patients and physicians, the assignment to treatment group should therefore be determined by chance, independently of the wishes of clinicians and patients. *The purpose of randomization is to achieve "equality" of baseline characteristics of treatment groups, so that the comparison of treatments is considered fair.* To assess the equality of the treatment groups, demographic and prognostic factors may be compared between groups. If patients have been

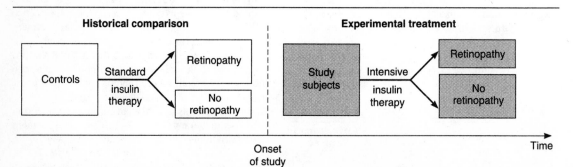

Figure 7–3. Schematic diagram of the comparison of intensive insulin therapy for diabetes mellitus against the historical experience of standard insulin therapy for previous patients with diabetes mellitus. Shaded areas correspond to patients receiving intensive insulin therapy.

randomly allocated, it is expected that the groups will be similar in demographic and prognostic features.

Table 7–4 is an example from the diabetes trial of the comparison of treatment groups after randomization. Note that there were two groups or cohorts of patients who were studied in this trial. The primary prevention group was defined by their complete lack of retinopathy at entry into the trial. The secondary prevention group included patients who already had signs of diabetic retinopathy at time of entry into the trial. The separation of the trial participants into groups is a technique known as **stratification.** The researchers chose to stratify by the presence or absence of retinopathy because they felt that this variable was of great importance in assessing the effect of treatment. By stratifying, the researchers assured that they would have randomized within each of these two important but different groups.

As can be seen in Table 7–4, the two treatment groups are remarkably similar with regard to age, gender, duration of disease, insulin dose, glycosylated hemoglobin, mean blood glucose, and in other characteristics known to be risk factors for vascular disease for subjects in both the primary and secondary prevention groups.

If one wants to ensure that similar numbers of patients with certain important prognostic characteristics are included in each treatment group, those characteristics can be accounted for in the randomization process. Suppose researchers wanted to guarantee that at the end of the diabetes study there would be equal percentages of males and females in each treatment group. The order in which the two treatments were assigned to groups of four patients of the same gender could be random; the first four male patients would be assigned to either standard or intensive therapy and the next four males would be assigned to the other group. Females would be assigned in the same manner. At the end of the study there would be an equal number of male and female patients in each treatment group. Assignment of patients in this manner is termed **block randomization.** *The purpose of randomization in blocks of patients is to protect against imbalanced treatment assignment (due to "luck of the draw") with respect to prognostically important patient subgroups.*

THE PLACEBO EFFECT AND BLINDING

In the year 1801, Haygarth reported the results of what may have been the first **placebo-controlled trial.** A popular treatment for many diseases at that time was to apply metal rods, known as Perkins tractors, to the body and thus relieve symptoms through a supposed electromagnetic influence of the metal. Haygarth treated five patients with imitation wooden tractors and found that four gained relief. The following day, he used the metal tractors on the same five patients and obtained identical results: relief in four of the five subjects. In describing the results of his experiment, Haygarth quoted James Lind, who is credited with performing the first clinical trial: "An important lesson in physic is here to be learnt, viz., the wonderful and powerful influence of the passions of the mind upon the state and disorders of the body. This is too often overlooked in the cure of diseases . . ."

The influence of treatment of any kind on patients' perceptions of their illness cannot be forgotten when designing a clinical trial. This concept is of greatest importance when the outcome measure is subjective. The patient's desires may also influence decisions made by clinicians subsequent to the initial randomization in a clinical trial. An additional factor that could potentially lead to differential treatment of groups within a trial is the clinician's decision process during a clinical trial. For example, will a clinician who has certain beliefs concerning a treatment's efficacy be likely to discontinue a therapy believed to be inferior in favor of the alternative therapy?

To account for the placebo effect and to reduce the introduction of bias due to patients' and clinicians' conceptions, studies may be conducted in a **blinded** fashion (Table 7–5). *"Blinding" means that the treatment assignment is not known to certain persons.* In a **single-blinded study,** the treatment assignment is un-

Table 7–4. Distribution of baseline characteristics of patients enrolled in the diabetes therapy trial.[1]

Characteristic	Standard Therapy (N = 378)	Intensive Therapy (N = 348)
Age (yr)	26 ± 8[2]	27 ± 7
Adolescents, 13–18 yrs (%)	19	16
Male sex (%)	54	49
White race (%)	96	96
Duration of IDDM (yr)	2.6 ± 1.4	2.6 ± 1.4
Insulin dose (U/kg of body weight/day)	0.62 ± 0.26	0.62 ± 0.25
Glycosylated hemoglobin (%)	8.8 ± 1.7	8.8 ± 1.6
Mean blood glucose (mg/dl)	229 ± 80	234 ± 86
Body weight (% of ideal)	103 ± 14	103 ± 13

[1]Adapted and reproduced, with permission, from The Diabetes Control and Complications Trial Research Group: The effect of intensive treatment of diabetes on the development and progression of long-term complications in insulin-dependent diabetes mellitus. N Engl J Med 1993;**329**:977.

[2]Plus-minus values are means ± standard deviation.

known to the patients; in a **double-blinded study,** the treatment assignment is unknown either to the patients or to their physicians. In a double-blinded study, the treatment assignment is revealed to the patient and physician only if there are serious or unexpected side effects—or when the study is completed.

In the diabetes therapy trial, neither patients nor their physicians were blinded to their treatment group. This was not possible since the patients and physicians are intimately involved in regulation of insulin dose on either arm of the trial. The researchers did "blind" the physicians who evaluated the photographs of the retina when assessing subjects for retinopathy. This was done to eliminate the possibility of **observer bias.**

Although blinding of both the patients and the treating physicians is desirable, there are trials, such as the diabetes trial, that cannot be conducted in a blinded fashion because the treatments are so obviously different that it is not feasible to keep the assignment secret. Whenever possible, however, blinding should be employed, since lack of blinding could influence perceptions of outcome and reduce the confidence in study results.

ETHICAL ISSUES CONCERNING CLINICAL TRIALS

The investigator who contemplates entering a patient into a randomized clinical trial is faced with several ethical dilemmas. First, is the randomized clinical trial method ethically acceptable? One of the most important ethical tenets in medicine is that the patient's welfare is of primary concern, and a caregiver should prescribe the optimal treatment for a patient. One could argue that even if a clinician has only a hunch or feeling that one treatment is superior, the patient should be offered that treatment. Randomization between two treatments, therefore, might be considered to be unethical. Given the seriousness and possible side effects of medical interventions, however, the axiom "first, do no harm" must always be borne in mind. The history of medicine is replete with examples of treatments now known to be either of no benefit or actually harmful. The clinical trial is considered to be the best method available to determine the benefits and potential harm of treatment regimens.

If one accepts that the clinical trial method is appropriate, then one must decide how to perform trials as ethically as possible. Following is a list of guidelines for medical professionals who are conducting clinical trials:

(1) None of the treatment options included in a randomized trial should be known to be inferior to another based on previous randomized studies, and if a standard treatment regimen exists, it should be used as the control.

(2) The trial should address a question that is of clinical importance and seek to answer the question in a way that will be useful for future patients.

(3) Patients should be told that they are part of a clinical experiment and should be informed in understandable language about all treatment options, the risks and benefits, and the nature of randomization. The patient who then agrees to participate is said to have given **informed consent,** which implies that the patient freely chooses to be included in the trial.

(4) The investigators undertaking the trial should be able to recruit in a timely manner the number of patients needed to meet the required sample size.

EVALUATION OF CLINICAL TRIALS

Relatively few physicians design clinical trials, and a limited number enter patients into clinical trials—but all clinicians read published accounts of clinical trials and use the results to guide the treatment of patients. A checklist of questions to help the physician interpret and evaluate these trials appears in Table 7–6.

Design Issues

The null hypothesis—and what would constitute a meaningful difference in outcome—should be stated in the methods section of a reported clinical trial. In the diabetes therapy trial, the primary outcome and the difference that was considered meaningful were clearly stated prior to beginning the trial. Trials should be designed to test one specific hypothesis or only a few hypotheses, and these should be evident to the reader.

The characteristics of the study population are especially important when assessing the relevance of a particular trial to an individual practitioner's patients. In the diabetes therapy trial, the eligibility and exclusion criteria are clearly stated, as summarized in Table 7–7. Summary data about gender, age, and medical histories of the participants appear in Table 7–4. The combination of the entry criteria and the demographic characteristics of the study's entrants provides the reader with an adequate description of the study group. With this information, the reader is better able to judge whether the results of this study are applicable to a par-

Table 7–5. Summary of various types of blinding to assignment of treatment in clinical trials.

Blinding	Knowledge of Treatment Assignment	
	Patient	Investigator
None	Yes	Yes
Single	No	Yes
Double	No	No

Table 7–6. Checklist for evaluating clinical trials.

1. **What was the null hypothesis?**
   a. What was the outcome of interest?
   b. What was thought to be a meaningful difference in outcome?
2. **Which group was being tested?**
   a. How was the study population for the trial selected? (1) Exclusion criteria (2) Random versus volunteer
   b. What were the group's demographic and health characteristics?
3. **How many subjects were entered in the study?**
   a. Was the size decided prior to the onset of the study?
4. **How were the experimental and control groups selected?**
   a. Were they selected in a way to ensure equal distribution of known risk factors?
5. **Were the treatment regimens described adequately?**
   a. If appropriate, was there a nontreated group?
   b. If the control is "standard therapy," was the treatment reasonable?
6. **Was this a blinded study?**
   a. Did the patients know which treatment they received?
   b. Did the physicians know which treatment patients received?
   c. Did the persons measuring outcome know if patients were in the control or experimental group?
7. **What were the results?**
   a. Were the treatment groups similar with regard to known prognostic factors?
   b. Were side effects recorded and reported?
   c. Who was included in the final results?
   d. Who was lost to follow-up? Did they differ from those who completed the study?
   e. During analysis, were patients kept in their originally assigned groups?
   f. Were enough of the data presented so that the conclusions can be justified?
   g. Were known risk factors accounted for in the analysis?
   h. Were confidence intervals reported?
   i. If the results were negative, was statistical power addressed?
8. **Were the results biologically plausible and consistent with previous literature?**
   a. If not, was this addressed?

ticular patient. Often, patients are excluded from a trial for pragmatic reasons, such as inability to comply with treatment or lack of fluency in the language of the investigators. These exclusions, however, may limit the ability to generalize study findings to other patient groups.

Once randomized to a particular treatment regimen, a patient may adhere to that regimen (comply) or may elect not to follow the prescribed regimen. Possible reasons for noncompliance are listed in Table 7–8. The investigator cannot force participants to comply, since such coercion would violate the rights of subjects to participate of their own free choice.

There are several possible ways, however, to increase compliance in a clinical trial (Table 7–9). The investigator may be able to select subjects who can be expected to be compliant. Motivation to participate is likely to be enhanced if the patients perceive themselves to be at high risk of an adverse health consequence. In the diabetes trial, eg, all enrolled subjects

had an illness that put them at risk for the long-term vascular complications of diabetes. Also, participants are apt to be motivated to comply if the offered treatments may reduce the need for painful or debilitating therapy. In the diabetes trial, for instance, patients may have hoped that more intensive therapy, or participation in a clinical trial with stringent guidelines for treatment, would help to reduce the long-term complications of disease.

In nonurgent situations, the investigator may be able to assess probable compliance before randomization is performed. To monitor compliance, eg, the investigator may ask eligible participants to take either an active or an inert medication. This pretest interval is referred to as a "run-in" test period. Individuals who show a likelihood of compliance are randomized to the treatments of interest, and those likely to be noncompliant are excluded from the trial. Other strategies to increase compliance include providing incentives for participation or maintaining frequent contact with sub-

Table 7–7. Summary of enrollment criteria for subjects in the primary prevention group of the diabetes therapy trial.

Patient Characteristic	Enrolled Subjects
Age	13–39 years
Diagnosis	insulin dependent diabetes mellitus
Duration of disease	1–5 years
Past medical conditions	Absence of hypertension, hypercholesterolemia, and diabetic complications or medical conditions
Complications of diabetes	No retinopathy, urinary albumin excretion of <40 mg per 24 hours

Adapted and reproduced, with permission, from The Diabetes Control and Complications Trial Research Group: The effect of intensive treatment of diabetes on the development and progression of long-term complications in insulin-dependent diabetes mellitus. N Engl J Med 1993;**329**:977.

Table 7–8. Possible reasons for noncompliance in a randomized clinical trial.

1. Misunderstanding of instructions.
2. Inconvenience of participation.
3. Side effects of treatment.
4. Cost of participation.
5. Forgetfulness.
6. Disappointment with results.
7. Preference for another treatment.

jects. Compliance also is likely to be enhanced by keeping the duration of the intervention as brief as possible.

Regardless of how carefully a clinical trial is designed, it is likely that some subjects will not adhere to the treatment regimen. The extent to which participants actually comply can be assessed by various approaches. Personal reports by subjects and family members provide a simple but questionably reliable basis to determine compliance. In drug studies, a traditional approach to assessing compliance is to count the number of unused pills at regular intervals. However, because pills can disappear for reasons other than ingestion by the subject, pill counts provide suggestive but not definitive evidence of compliance. The most conclusive evidence of compliance with a drug regimen is likely to be obtained by measurement of the drug (or a metabolite) in the subject's blood or urine. Even this type of biologic assay, however, has limited utility, with the most obvious constraints being cost, inconvenience to subjects, and the difficulty of collecting specimens from some individuals. Moreover, long-term compliance typically cannot be assessed by measurements of such specimens, since the presence of most drugs is detectable in blood or urine for no more than a few days. The diabetes trial was fortunate to be able to measure glycosylated hemoglobin, a long-term measure of glucose control, as a secondary endpoint. Although the measurement of glycosylated hemoglobin is not a direct measure of compliance, it provided an independent measure of effect of the two treatment groups that was expected to differ if the treatments did differentially affect subjects' plasma glucose levels.

Despite the difficulties inherent in assessing compliance, it is important to estimate the extent to which subjects adhere to the assigned regimens. The ability of a study to identify a true effect of treatment (statistical power) may be diminished if a substantial proportion of the participants do not comply with the assigned treatment. That is, the observed difference in outcomes between the study groups may be reduced because of noncompliance. Accordingly, it may be necessary to include a larger initial sample size to compensate for the loss of discriminatory power. As will be emphasized later in this chapter, it is important to include all randomized patients in the main analysis of a clinical trial. Therefore, every effort should be made to determine the outcomes of both compliant and noncompliant subjects.

Analysis of Results

Loss of some patients to follow-up is likely to occur in any clinical trial. The more patients who are lost and the less that is known about them, the less confidence one can place in the results of the trial. In the analysis of results from a clinical trial, *patients should be left in the treatment group originally assigned by the study (intention to treat) even if they received one of the other treatments after the original treatment regimen failed.* In the diabetes therapy study, eg, 95 women assigned to the standard therapy group received more intensive therapy during a pregnancy. In another smaller subgroup of patients, researchers discontinued intensive therapy and resumed standard therapy. These patients remained in the standard therapy group during analyses, however. This may seem counterintuitive, since these patients actually received some of both treatment regimens. The purpose of this trial, however, was to help clinicians determine the best treatment at the time of initial presentation for entry into the trial. Subsequent treatment decisions may include the alternative treatment, but those subsequent decisions have no bearing on the original clinical question posed by the trial and thus are not pertinent to group assignment. Design of the diabetes therapy trial with consideration of intention to treat is illustrated schematically in Figure 7–4.

All participants who are randomized should be included in the analysis of a clinical trial. Selective removal of subjects from the comparison of outcomes, even if it seems justified for pragmatic reasons, may lead to erroneous conclusions. Consider, eg, the question of whether to include noncompliers in the analysis. Since these individuals did not receive the assigned treatments as intended, it may seem illogical to leave them in the analysis. It has been shown, however, that noncompliers tend to have worse outcomes

Table 7–9. Strategies to enhance compliance with treatment assignment in randomized clinical trials.

1. Select motivated persons.
2. Pretest ability and willingness of participants to comply.
3. Provide simple and lucid instructions to subjects.
4. Offer incentives to comply (eg, no charge for therapeutic intervention and associated examinations).
5. Provide positive reinforcements to subjects for adherence to treatment regimen.
6. Maintain frequent contact with participants and remind them about importance of adherence to the regimen.
7. Measure adherence through pill counts or sampling of biologic specimens.
8. Limit duration of intervention.

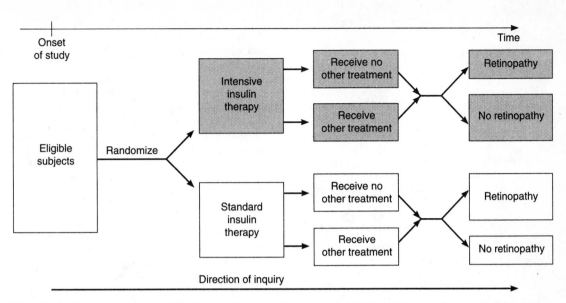

Figure 7–4. Schematic diagram of the design of a randomized controlled clinical trial comparing standard insulin therapy with intensive insulin therapy for the treatment of diabetes mellitus with analysis by intention to treat. Shaded areas correspond to patients randomized to intensive insulin therapy.

than compliers, regardless of their treatment assignment. If the treatment assignment affects the level of compliance, then failure to account for compliance in the analysis can produce a misleading result.

Removal of noncompliers from the analysis may also limit the ability to generalize study findings to clinical practice. In recommending treatment to a particular patient, the physician must consider the possibility that the treatment will not be completed as intended. The essential question of a clinical trial is whether or not a treatment should be offered at a particular point in time. The relevant information on treatment benefit, therefore, is the outcome among all patients who were offered the treatment, rather than just those who completed it.

A well-reported clinical trial should contain enough of the primary data to enable the reader (1) to compare the main outcome measure between the treatment groups and (2) to perform basic statistical tests to determine whether it is reasonable to exclude chance variation as a cause of observed differences between the compared groups. For the clinical trial, it is useful to review three very common types of comparisons: the comparison of two risks, the comparison of time to an event (survival analysis), and the comparison of two means.

Many outcomes from a clinical trial are yes/no outcomes, (eg, death or no death, cure or no cure, recurrence or no recurrence) and therefore can be displayed in simple tabular format. Whether a patient developed retinopathy in the primary prevention group in the diabetes therapy trial is presented in Table 7–10.

The incidence rate of developing retinopathy in each arm of the primary treatment group was determined by dividing the number of subjects who developed retinopathy by the number of person-years of follow-up. **Person-years** are calculated by summing up the years that each subject is in the study prior to the development of retinopathy. This allows for including all subjects in the results of a study, regardless of how long each subject was enrolled. This issue is common to the clinical trial, since recruitment of subjects into a trial often occurs over several years. The incidence rate (IR) of retinopathy in the standard therapy group was calculated to be 4.7 per 100 patient-years of follow-up, and 1.2 per 100 patient-years of follow-up for the intensive therapy group. There are several ways to compare these two rates.

One way to compare the rates is to calculate the percentage of retinopathy incidence that would be avoided if intensive therapy were used instead of standard therapy. This percentage is known as the **percentage rate reduction,** and is calculated as follows:

Table 7–10. Results of the diabetes therapy trial concerning the risk of developing retinopathy.

Retinopathy	Treatment		Total
	Standard Therapy	Intensive Therapy	
Yes	91	23	114
No	287	325	612
Total	378	348	726

Adapted and reproduced, with permission, from The Diabetes Control and Complications Trial Reearch Group: The effect of intensive treatment of diabetes on the development and progression of long-term complications in insulin-dependent diabetes mellitus. N Engl J Med 1993;**329**:977.

Percentage Rate Reduction = $\dfrac{IR_{(standard)} - IR_{(experimental)}}{IR_{(standard)}}$ $\times 100$

If the percentage rate reduction = 0, there is no reduction in incidence rate attributable to the new therapy, and the treatments are judged to be equivalent. The further the percentage rate reduction is from zero, the greater the difference is between the two groups. For the diabetes trial, the percentage of retinopathy that could have been prevented by patients using intensive therapy rather than standard therapy is calculated:

$$\text{Percentage Rate Reduction} = \frac{4.7 - 1.2}{4.7} \times 100$$

$$= 74\%$$

That is, almost three-fourths of the retinopathy that occurred in the standard therapy group could have been avoided if those patients had been treated with intensive therapy. The value of 74% is known as a **point estimate** because it is the single value along the scale from 0–100% that is most consistent with the results of the trial.

A useful method to gauge the precision of any point estimate is to calculate the 95% confidence intervals for the estimate. If the clinical trial were repeated many times, the values falling between the upper and lower bounds of the 95% confidence interval would include the true point estimate value 95% of the time. If the 95% confidence interval of the percentage risk reduction includes 0, the data are consistent with the null hypothesis, and the difference between the groups is not statistically significant at an alpha level of 0.05. If the 95% confidence interval does not include 0, the difference is statistically different at an alpha level of 0.05.

The approximate 95% confidence interval (CI) for the percentage rate reduction in the diabetes therapy trial calculated above is 60–83%. Since the interval does not include 0, this decreased rate is considered statistically significant at an alpha level of 0.05. This means that, given the observed data, if the trial were repeated often, 95% of the time the percentage rate reduction would fall between 60% and 83%. The 95% confidence interval for the percentage rate reduction for retinopathy is illustrated schematically in Figure 7–5.

Another method of comparing two rates is by forming a ratio of the rates, the so-called **rate ratio (RR)**. For other situations, where risks rather than rates of events are estimated, the risks of endpoints can be measured for the experimental and control groups, then contrasted by dividing the experimental group risk of adverse events by the control group risk; this is the risk ratio or **relative risk**. If the $RR = 1.0$, the rate (or risk) of the outcome of interest in the two treatment groups is exactly equal. The further the ratio is from 1.0, the greater the difference in rate (or risk) between the two groups. For this trial, the rate of retinopathy in the intensive therapy group compared with the standard therapy group would be calculated as follows:

$$\text{Rate Ratio} = \frac{\dfrac{1.2 \text{ cases}}{100 \text{ patient-years}}}{\dfrac{4.7 \text{ cases}}{100 \text{ patient-years}}} = 0.26$$

That is, the rate of developing retinopathy in the intensive treatment group is about one-quarter that of the standard therapy group. The value of 0.26 is another example of a point estimate, because it is the single value along the rate ratio scale most consistent with the observed data. Similar to the percentage rate reduction, one can also calculate 95% confidence limits for the RR point estimate. If the 95% confidence interval

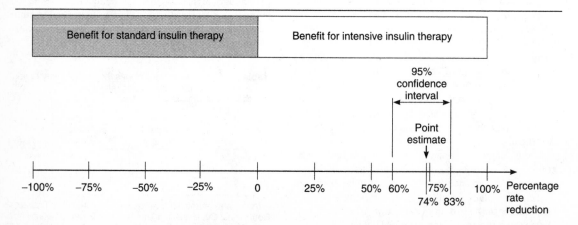

Figure 7–5. The point estimate and corresponding approximate 95% confidence interval for the percentage rate reduction in the diabetes therapy trial.

includes the null value of 1.0, there is no statistical difference between rates in the two groups, and the null hypothesis would be accepted. If the 95% confidence interval does not include 1.0, the difference in rates between the two groups would be considered statistically significant at the 5% level. The point estimate and 95% confidence interval for the rate ratio of retinopathy in the diabetes therapy trial is illustrated schematically in Figure 7–6. Note that the point estimate of the *RR* does not lie at the midpoint of the 95% confidence interval. The asymmetry of the confidence interval occurs because the distribution of possible values of the *RR* is skewed toward the right (ie, all the values corresponding to a benefit for conventional therapy are compressed into the range of zero to 1, whereas the values corresponding to a benefit for intensive therapy are spread from 1 to positive infinity).

The *RR* is a simple, easily understood method to evaluate results of clinical trials. For time-to-event data, however, survival analysis has several advantages over the *RR*. The survival curve, as described in Chapter 2, is a graphic presentation of time-to-event data. Since it graphically depicts events as they occur over time, the survival curve provides information on the rapidity with which events occur. Furthermore, the survival curve can make use of data from patients who are followed for varying lengths of time. For the diabetes trial, the cumulative risk of retinopathy was plotted over time (Figure 7–7). While this figure is not a display of survival (life versus death), it does represent "survival" without the occurrence of the event of interest, in this case retinopathy. A patient who is followed for only 3 years provides useful information on risk of developing retinopathy for that period of time but would provide no information pertinent to a comparison beyond 3 years. Survival analysis also allows one to estimate median survival duration (eg, time-to-retinopathy-development) as well as the percentage of survivors (eg, persons without retinopathy) at any time along the curve.

Time-since-first-treatment is depicted along the horizontal axis, and the percentage of patients without retinopathy is displayed on the vertical axis. At the time of initial treatment (years = 0), 0% of the patients in each group have developed retinopathy. As time from treatment progresses, the percentage of patients who are diagnosed with retinopathy increases, though more rapidly in the control group. At the end of 9 years of follow-up, 14% of the patients treated with intensive therapy have been diagnosed with retinopathy, compared with 55% of the standard therapy subjects.

The survival curves could be used to estimate the relative risk of being diagnosed with retinopathy at any point in time. For example, the intensive to conventional group relative risk of retinopathy at 5 years is as follows:

$$\text{Relative Risk} = \frac{6}{15} = 0.4$$

This relative risk indicates that the intensive therapy subjects have about 60% less risk than conventional therapy subjects of developing retinopathy within five years. Alternatively, the median time-to-development-of-retinopathy for the two groups can be estimated and contrasted. The median time is the point at which half of an initial study group remains free of the occurrence of interest. In this example, the estimated median time to development of retinopathy for the standard therapy group is 8.5 years. The median time to retinopathy for the intensive therapy group has not been reached after 9 years of follow-up. That is, the patients treated with the intensive therapy are developing retinopathy at a slower rate than are the standard therapy subjects.

Several tests of significance can be used to compare survival curves (see Dawson-Saunders and Trapp, 1994). As is demonstrated by the diabetes trial data, although this type of analysis is called survival analysis, it is not limited to the analysis of deaths. Any event that

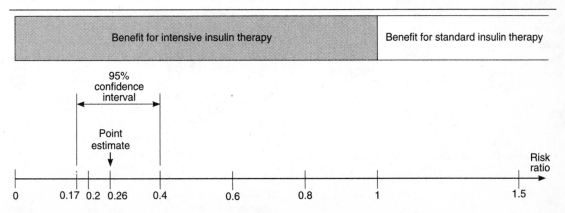

Figure 7–6. The point estimate and corresponding approximate 95% confidence interval for the rate ratio of retinopathy in the diabetes therapy trial.

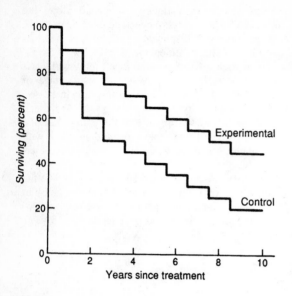

Figure 7–7. Cumulative incidence of a sustained change in retinopathy in patients with IDDM who receive intensive insulin or standard insulin therapy. (Adapted and reproduced, with permission, from the Diabetes Control and Complications Trial Research Group: The effect of intensive treatment of diabetes on the development and progression of long-term complications in insulin-dependent diabetes mellitus. N Eng J Med 1993; **329:**981.)

occurs over time (time-to-disease-recurrence, time-to-return-to-work, etc) can be compared in this fashion.

Another comparison frequently used in clinical trials is the comparison of means. In the diabetes trial, eg, blood glucose was measured at the onset of the study and at regular intervals thereafter. In Table 7–4, one of the baseline characteristics compared between the standard therapy and intensive therapy groups is the mean blood glucose. One could choose to distribute patients into several discrete categories of blood glucose (eg, <140, 140–179, 180–239, 240 or greater), but that would involve a loss of useful information about the actual observed glucose measurements. Instead, the mean or average blood glucose can be compared. The null and alternative hypotheses for this comparison would be stated as follows:

$$H_0 : \mu_1 = \mu_2$$
$$H_A : \mu_1 \neq \mu_2$$

A test of the equality of two means can be accomplished by performing a *t* test as follows:

$$t = \frac{\bar{x}_1 - \bar{x}_2}{\left(s_p \sqrt{\dfrac{1}{n_1} + \dfrac{1}{n_2}} \right)}$$

where $\bar{x}_1$ and $\bar{x}_2$ are the observed mean blood glucose levels of the standard and intensive treatment groups, respectively; s_p is an estimate of the pooled variance of the two means; and n_1 and n_2 are the sample sizes for each group. To illustrate the use of a t test, the observed mean blood glucose levels in patients treated with intensive and conventional therapy can be compared as follows:

$$t = \frac{231 - 155}{\left(44.8 \sqrt{\dfrac{1}{378} + \dfrac{1}{348}} \right)} = 22.8$$

A *t*-statistic of 22.8 for this sample size corresponds to a *P*-value of <.0005. In other words, there is less than a .05% chance that a difference in means as large as that observed with these sample sizes could have occurred by sampling variability alone. Accordingly, the null hypothesis of no difference between the means is rejected.

If a study concludes that no difference exists between treatment regimens, the amount of difference the authors thought was important should be specified, as well as the likelihood that the study did not find a difference due to chance alone. The likelihood that a negative result is due to chance is the beta error; 1 minus the beta error $(1 - \beta)$ is the statistical power (see Sample Size Determination).

The reader should interpret the results of a single trial in the context of other clinical trials and other information. If a single trial calls into question previous clinical research or contradicts what is theoretically expected, then additional trials or basic research may be required to help understand the results of the clinical trial.

SUMMARY

The randomized controlled clinical trial is the most widely accepted approach to compare the benefits of alternative treatments. The advantages and disadvantages of this research method, as compared with alternative study designs, are set forth in Table 7–11. The principal strength of this approach derives from assigning treatments to patients by randomization, thereby tending to balance the study groups with respect to both known and unknown prognostic factors.

Before enrolling patients in a clinical trial, the investigator can determine the baseline and follow-up information that will be required on all subjects. Procedures then can be put in place to enable the researchers to collect data in a fairly complete and accurate manner. The investigator can also allocate subjects to desired dose levels rather than relying upon physician or patient preferences. When blinding of the evaluators or patients is feasible, the assessment of clinical outcomes is less likely to be influenced by knowing which treatment was used.

Randomized controlled clinical trials are subject to certain constraints, however. Restrictive criteria for inclusion of subjects may produce a very homogeneous study population but, at the same time, may restrict one's ability to extrapolate results to patients with other characteristics. Clinical trials—particularly those involving chronic processes—may require years of follow-up to determine the outcome of treatment. A prolonged observation period leads to higher costs, increases the likelihood that patients will be lost to follow-up, and delays the time at which a treatment recommendation can be made. The use of intermediate end points, such as glucose levels or glycosylated hemoglobin in the diabetes trial, can help to limit the length of required follow-up. Nevertheless, a definitive conclusion about treatment benefit often requires years of observation.

Large sample sizes typically are required in clinical trials when the magnitude of difference in responses between study groups is small. Furthermore, large numbers of subjects are likely to be required to demonstrate differences between study groups when there is wide variability in responses to treatment. Increasing the size of the study population not only raises the cost of a trial but may also lead to pragmatic difficulties in locating a sufficiently large pool of eligible patients.

Ethical concerns may arise in a clinical trial if one or more of the treatment options has serious potential side effects. Ethical dilemmas can also arise when early data suggest—but do not establish—a therapeutic advantage for one of the treatments. In this situation, a decision must be made about whether the trial should be continued until a definitive conclusion is reached or should be terminated earlier so that all patients have the opportunity to receive the apparently superior treatment. In order to minimize the possible influence of real or perceived conflicts of interest, it is desirable that an external advisory group review these ethical questions.

An investigator cannot control the behavior of subjects enrolled in a clinical trial. Even after initial informed consent has been given to participate in a clinical trial, a subject has the right to withdraw at any time. Some subjects may elect to remain in the trial but not comply with the assigned regimen.

Noncompliance can reduce the statistical power of a clinical trial and thereby lead to a false-negative conclusion. Accordingly, every effort must be made to achieve maximal compliance with assigned treatment without infringing the patient's right to refuse therapy.

Ultimately, treatment decisions should be based on the best evidence available concerning therapeutic benefit. The standard approach to gathering this evidence is the randomized controlled clinical trial. Although this type of investigation is labor-intensive, time-consuming, and expensive, it can provide the most convincing evidence of the superiority of one treatment over another. Through the use of randomized clinical trials such as the diabetes therapy study, the delivery of patient care can be based upon rigorous scientific information.

STUDY QUESTIONS

Directions: For each question, select the single best answer.

1. A randomized clinical trial was designed to compare two different treatment approaches for asthmatic attacks. The purpose of randomization in this study was to
   A. Obtain treatment groups of similar size
   B. Select a representative sample of patients for study
   C. Increase patient compliance with treatment
   D. Decrease the likelihood that observed differences in clinical outcome are due to chance
   E. Obtain treatment groups with comparable baseline prognoses

2. In a double-blinded clinical trial concerning the treatment of osteoarthritis, half of the patients received a nonsteroidal anti-inflammatory agent and the other half received a pharmacologically inert substance. Two-thirds of the patients in the former group and one-third of the patients in the latter group reported relief of symptoms. The patients' perceptions of improvement on treatment with an inert substance is best described as
   A. Intention to treat
   B. Noncompliance

Table 7–11. Advantages and disadvantages of randomized controlled clinical trials.

Advantages	Disadvantages
Randomization tends to balance prognostic factors across study groups.	Subject exclusions may limit ability to generalize findings to other patients.
Detailed information can be collected on baseline and subsequent characteristics of participants.	A long period of time often is required to reach a conclusion.
Dose levels can be predetermined by the investigator.	A large number of participants may be required.
Blinding of participants can reduce distortion in assessment of outcomes.	Financial costs are typically high.
Assumptions of statistical tests tend to be met.	Ethical concerns may arise.
	Subjects may not comply with treatment assignments.

C. Placebo effect
D. Type II error
E. False-positive result

3. In a randomized clinical trial comparing the effectiveness of a new vaccine for measles to that of a standard vaccine, the evaluating clinicians knew which vaccine each patient received, but the patients themselves were unaware of the treatment assignment. This design is best described as
A. Unblinded
B. Single-blinded
C. Double-blinded
D. Triple-blinded
E. None of the above

4. The purpose of informed consent in a clinical trial for treatment of hypertension is to
A. Increase the patients' knowledge of possible risks and benefits of treatment options
B. Increase the level of patient participation
C. Decrease the likelihood of malpractice suits
D. Decrease the likelihood of a placebo effect
E. Decrease the likelihood of patient blinding to treatment assignment

5. Which of the following actions is most likely to result in an increase in the statistical power of a clinical trial comparing different weight loss programs?
A. Blinding of the clinicians who evaluate weight loss
B. The use of a comparison group that receives only a pharmacologically inert substance
C. Measurement of patient satisfaction with treatment rather than actual reduction in weight
D. Increasing the number of patients studied
E. Restricting the study population to patients with mild obesity

6. A small clinical trial is designed to compare the effectiveness of a new treatment vs a standard chemotherapeutic regimen for lymphoma. No difference in 5-year survival percentages is observed despite the fact that, in truth, the new treatment is superior. The failure to detect a benefit for the new treatment is best described as
A. Observer bias
B. Placebo effect
C. Type I error
D. Type II error
E. Blinding

7. In a clinical trial comparing medical and surgical treatment of duodenal ulcers, 20% of the patients randomized to medical treatment ultimately underwent a surgical procedure and 10% of the pa-

tients initially assigned to surgery later required additional medical management. Analysis of this study according to initial treatment allocation, ignoring subsequent change in therapy, is best described as
A. Blinding
B. Intention to treat
C. Type I error
D. Observer bias
E. Placebo effect

8. In a hospital-based clinical trial of the management of paranoid schizophrenia, relief of symptoms in patients treated with a new drug is compared with symptom relief among patients previously treated with a standard drug. Which of the following is LEAST likely to be a cause of an unfair comparison of the relative benefits of the new and standard drugs?
A. Changes over time in the criteria used to diagnose paranoid schizophrenia
B. Changes over time in the methods used to assess symptom relief
C. Changes over time in the nature of patients referred to the hospital
D. Inability to blind clinical evaluators to treatment status of patients treated with the new drug
E. Lack of use of a separate untreated control group

9. A clinical trial was conducted to evaluate the benefits of an intensive exercise program in reducing subsequent mortality among persons who survive at least 30 days after an initial myocardial infarction. Patients were randomized to receive either usual care (controls) or the exercise program. Among 100 controls, 30 died within the 3-year follow-up period, compared with 50 deaths among the 100 patients on the exercise program. The relative risk of death for the exercise group compared to controls was
A. 0.20
B. 0.30
C. 0.50
D. 0.60
E. 1.67

Table 7–12. Baseline characteristics in a randomized clinical trial of the prevention of osteoporosis.

Characteristic	Level	Experimental	Control
Age (years)	Mean value	67	65
Race	% black	28	24
Body weight	% over ideal	64	42
Calcium supplements	% users	54	60
Exercise	% daily	46	38

10. A randomized clinical trial was undertaken to evaluate the effect of supplemental estrogen in preventing osteoporosis among postmenopausal women. The experimental group of 50 women received a daily pill of low-dose estrogen, and the control group of 50 women received a placebo. The baseline characteristics of the two groups are shown in Table 7–12. Assuming that each characteristic is comparably related to the risk of developing osteoporosis, the factor most likely to contribute to an unfair comparison of experimental and control groups was

A. Age
B. Race
C. Body weight
D. Calcium supplement use
E. Regular exercise

FURTHER READING

Buyse MC: Potential and pitfalls of randomized clinical trials in cancer research. Cancer Surv 1989;**8:**91.

Ratain JS, Hochberg MC: Clinical trials: A guide to understanding methodology and interpreting results. Arth Rheum 1990;**33:**131.

REFERENCES

Andreoli TE et al: *Cecil Essentials of Medicine.* Saunders, 1993.

Bull JP: The historical development of clinical therapeutic trials. J Chron Dis 1959;**10:**218.

Bulpitt CJ: *Randomized Controlled Clinical Trials.* Martinus Nijhoff, 1983.

Dawson-Saunders B, Trapp RG: *Basic and Clinical Biostatistics.* 2nd ed. Appleton & Lange, 1993.

Diabetes Control and Complications Trial Research Group. The effect of intensive treatment of diabetes on the development and progression of long-term complications in insulin-dependent diabetes mellitus. N Engl J Med 1993;**329:**977.

Gehlbach SH: *Interpreting the Medical Literature* 2nd ed. MacMillan, 1988.

Haygarth J: *Of the Imagination as a Cause and as a Cure of Disorders of the Body.* R. Crutwell, 1801.

Spilker B: *Guide to Clinical Interpretation of Data* Raven Press, 1986.

Cohort Studies 8

PATIENT PROFILE

A pediatrician was called to the hospital to attend the delivery of a newborn. The mother, a 28-year-old primigravida, had experienced elevated blood pressure during an otherwise uncomplicated pregnancy. The labor was induced because the pregnancy had continued 2 weeks past the expected date of delivery. During labor, evidence of fetal distress occurred. When the membranes ruptured, the obstetrician noted thick greenish fluid containing meconium. At the time of delivery, the male newborn was limp, cyanotic, with no spontaneous respiratory effort, and a heart rate of only 50 beats/min. When meconium was suctioned from his mouth and nose, the baby did not grimace, cough, or sneeze.

Vigorous efforts at resuscitation were initiated, including bag-and-mask ventilation with 100% oxygen and chest compressions, but the Apgar score at 1 minute of life was 1. The Apgar score (Table 8–1), an index of neonatal asphyxia, can range from 0 (very asphyxiated) to 10 (no asphyxia). Despite continuing resuscitation, the 5-minute Apgar score only improved to 2, with a heart rate of 110 beats/min. The 10-minute Apgar score remained depressed at 3, and the neonate was transferred to the Newborn Intensive Care Unit. With aggressive medical management, the 3100-g neonate continued to improve without evidence of acute neurologic complications. He was discharged from the hospital on the 12th day of life.

CLINICAL BACKGROUND

Perinatal asphyxia can be defined as fetal hypoxia during labor and delivery. Hypoxia in the perinatal period is believed to be a major cause of perinatal deaths, as well as impaired development and neurologic function among survivors. The causes of perinatal asphyxia are not completely understood, but a number of factors have been associated with hypoxia during labor and delivery, including preeclampsia or eclampsia, maternal hypotension, placental insufficiency, and prematurity. The passage of meconium and the presence of this material in the amniotic fluid indicate possible fetal distress.

The pathogenesis of perinatal asphyxia is presented in Figure 8–1. The development of severe metabolic acidosis in the fetus indicates a lack of oxygen. This is because tissues must resort to anaerobic glycolysis for energy production. The degree of hypoxia that a fetus can tolerate before cellular injury occurs is variable and depends on a variety of factors, including previous asphyxia during the pregnancy, metabolic needs versus metabolic reserves, and blood flow to vital organs.

In experimental studies on newborn primates, varying degrees of asphyxia have been induced. These studies have shown that, for brain injury to occur, the fetus must be exposed to marked asphyxia for at least 25 minutes. These studies also indicate that this degree of asphyxia will probably lead to fetal death, rather than survival with neurologic impairment. In general, research has shown the immature nervous system to be more resistant to hypoxic injury than the mature brain.

STUDY DESIGN

In the Patient Profile, the newborn's parents are understandably distraught by the unanticipated complications in their baby's first hours of life. Naturally, they have questions about what the future will bring. Will their son develop normal mental capacity? Will he have physical disabilities? Questions like these from concerned parents often can be answered from the pediatrician's own clinical experience. If, however, a physician has seen only a few such patients, he or she must consult the medical literature to answer parental concerns.

In undertaking such a search, the pediatrician will find a variety of case reports of infants who have had severe perinatal asphyxia and have developed various acute and chronic medical problems. Some of these reports describe dismal outcomes, including death. However, there are also reports of cases of severe asphyxia during delivery, followed in later childhood by normal neurologic development and excellent school performance. Thus, the pediatrician may be uncertain about what to tell parents. Clearly, a broad spectrum of outcomes is possible. What the pediatrician in our example needs to find is a study that offers reliable evidence of the likelihood of each of the various possible outcomes.

Table 8–1. Apgar score for evaluation of neonatal asphyxia.[1,2]

	Score		
Sign	0	1	2
Heart rate (beats/min)	Absent	<100	>100
Respiration	Absent	Slow, irregular	Regular, crying
Muscle tone	Limp	Slow flexion	Active motor
Color	Blue, pale	Body pink, extremities blue	Completely pink
Reflex response to catheter in nostril	None	Grimace	Cough, sneeze

[1]The values for each of the five categories are added to yield a result from 0 to 10.
[2]Adapted from Apgar V, James LS: Am J Dis Child 1962;**104**:419.

The most definitive conclusions could be drawn from a **clinical trial.** This would be a study in which newborns are randomly assigned to different levels of perinatal asphyxia and then followed with measurements of outcome, such as achievement of developmental milestones and school performance. This type of study has actually been performed on laboratory animals, but such a study on human infants would be unethical. An investigator could not intentionally expose humans to potentially harmful conditions simply to learn about the effects on outcome.

Since intentional exposure of human newborns to asphyxia cannot be justified on ethical grounds, the investigator might resort to observing the outcomes of newborns who develop asphyxia under natural circumstances. This type of study is characterized as **observational** because the investigator does not determine the assignment of exposure but rather passively observes events as they unfold. The observational study design that is most similar to the clinical trial is a **cohort study.** In this type of study, as illustrated in Figure 8–2, the investigators identify a population **(cohort)** and determine their initial characteristics (exposure status). A cohort for an asphyxia study might consist of infants born with perinatal asphyxia and babies born without this condition. The researchers then follow the cohort over time and determine the outcome in the exposed and unexposed groups. It is important to remember that in a cohort study, information about the risk factor (exposure) is determined prior to the observation of disease status.

A large cohort study was conducted in the United States on the utility of Apgar scores as predictors of chronic neurologic disability. In this study, investigators evaluated 49,000 infants whose Apgar scores were recorded at 1 and 5 minutes of age. For those infants who did not achieve a score of 8 or higher at 5 minutes, Apgar scores were also recorded at 10, 15, and 20 minutes. All the children were then followed to the age of 7 years. The occurrence of seizures was determined through clinical observations in the newborn nursery; interval histories were recorded at 4, 8, 12, and 18 months of age and yearly thereafter. The presence of cerebral palsy was determined by physical examination at age 7 years. A psychologic and developmental assessment was also performed at age 7. The design of this study appears in Figure 8–3.

This study demonstrated that low Apgar scores are a risk factor for the development of cerebral palsy. However, 55% of the children with cerebral palsy at age 7 had Apgar scores of 7 or higher at 1 minute, and 73% scored 7 or higher at 5 minutes. Of the 99 children who survived and had Apgar scores of 0–3 at 10, 15, or 20 minutes, 12 were found to have cerebral palsy. Eleven of those 12 were also mentally retarded. Ten of those infants had seizures in the first 24 hours of life. Of the children who survived and had Apgar scores of 0–3 at 10 minutes or later, 80% were free of any major handicap at early school age.

This study of a large population of children provides the pediatrician in the Patient Profile with the kind of information needed to discuss the baby's prognosis with his parents. The study represents an experience that no single practitioner could compile, even in a

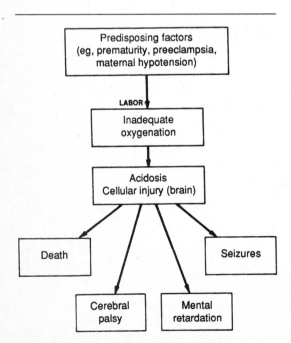

Figure 8–1. Schematic representation of the pathogenesis of perinatal asphyxia.

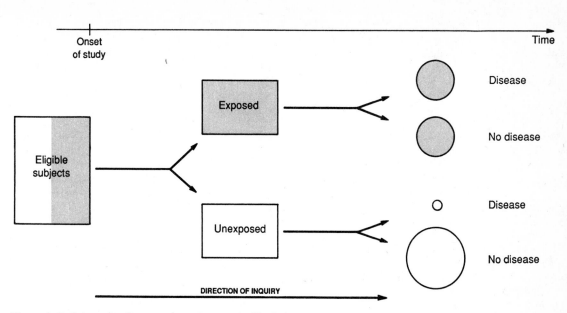

Figure 8–2. Schematic diagram of a cohort study. Shaded areas represent exposed persons, and unshaded areas represent unexposed persons.

lifetime of practice. The pediatrician can now advise the parents that, although their baby does have an increased risk of cerebral palsy and developmental delay, such an outcome occurs in only about 1 of 8 asphyxiated neonates. Since the baby did not have a seizure in the first 24 hours of life, the prognosis may be more favorable. It should be reassuring to the par-

ents to learn that 80% of even the most severely asphyxiated newborns were free of major neurologic handicap at early school age.

Perhaps the contributions of cohort studies can be illustrated best by the Framingham Heart Study, one of the most widely recognized and most influential studies of this type. In that investigation, the status of the

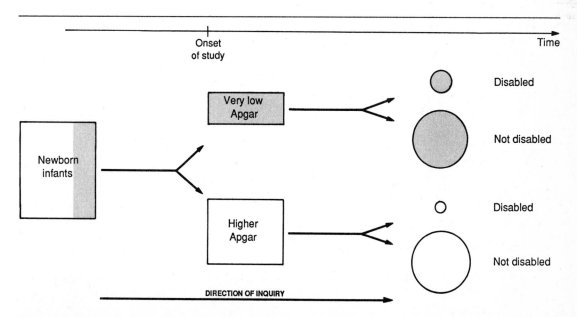

Figure 8–3. Schematic diagram of a cohort study of the relationship between perinatal asphyxia and chronic neurologic disability. Shaded areas represent newborns with very low Apgar scores, and unshaded areas represent children with intermediate or high Apgar scores.

residents of Framingham, Massachusetts, was determined with respect to potential risk factors for cardiovascular disease. Beginning in 1950, a sample of 6500 individuals aged 30–59 years was chosen from a total population of approximately 10,000 people in that age group. Approximately 5100 subjects with no clinical evidence of atherosclerotic cardiovascular disease agreed to participate in the study. Each subject was examined at the beginning of the study and reexamined every 2 years thereafter. For example, the investigators identified subjects with elevated blood pressure, smokers, and subjects with elevated serum cholesterol levels. The population was followed over 35 years to identify subjects who suffered a myocardial infarction, stroke, or other adverse cardiovascular event. This protocol allowed investigators to determine if an individual with hypertension, eg, was more likely to suffer a stroke than someone with normal blood pressure.

More than 250 research reports have been produced by the Framingham Heart Study investigators and their collaborators. The Framingham Heart Study is the source of much of our current knowledge about the risk factors for cardiovascular morbidity and mortality. This cohort has also been used to collect information regarding various other diseases.

The Framingham population was chosen for many reasons, in particular, because it is a stable community with a broad representation of occupations. The Framingham study is limited, however, because its participants are mainly white, middle class individuals.

TIMING OF MEASUREMENTS

A cohort study usually is **prospective,** ie, the risk factor exposure and subsequent health outcomes are observed after the beginning of the study (Figure 8–2). For example, a prospective cohort study of neonatal asphyxia and subsequent mental retardation could be started in 1996. The degree of birth asphyxia could be determined for births occurring through 1997, and the development of mental retardation could be assessed between 1997 and 2002 or later. An alternative name for such a cohort study is a **longitudinal study.**

Occasionally, a cohort study is **retrospective** (or historical), ie, it utilizes information on prior exposure and disease status. As shown in Figure 8–4, a retrospective cohort study of neonatal asphyxia and neurologic disability designed in 1997 might involve a review of the medical records of infants born in a particular hospital in 1986 to determine level of asphyxia, followed by a review of school achievement records over the period 1996–1997 to determine the degree of intellectual functioning. Note that exposure to risk factors and the subsequent development of the health outcome occur prior to the beginning of the retrospective cohort study.

The advantage of the retrospective cohort design is that all the events under study have already occurred, and conclusions can therefore be drawn more rapidly. In addition, the cost of a retrospective cohort study might be substantially lower for the same reason. The

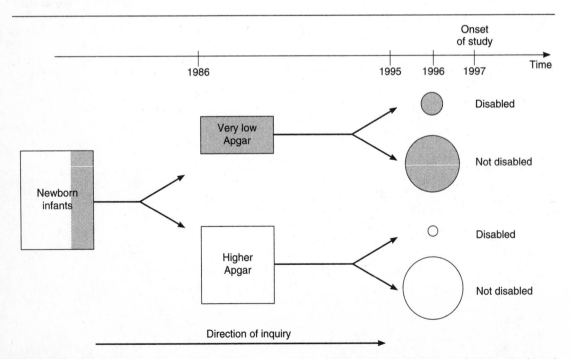

Figure 8–4. Schematic diagram of a retrospective cohort study of the relationship between perinatal asphyxia and chronic neurologic disability. Shaded areas represent newborns with very low Apgar scores, and unshaded areas represent children with intermediate or high Apgar scores.

retrospective approach also may be the only feasible way to study the effects of exposures that no longer occur, eg, discontinued medical treatments. On the other hand, in a retrospective cohort study, one must usually rely upon existing records or subject recall; both are usually less complete and accurate than data collected in a prospective study. Attributes of the prospective and retrospective cohort study designs are compared in Table 8–2.

It should now be clear that a prospective cohort study often takes a long time to complete. Furthermore, in order to have enough subjects to reach a valid conclusion, a cohort study (either prospective or retrospective) usually requires a fairly large number of individuals with the potential to develop the outcome of interest. For example, in the study of perinatal asphyxia, data concerning 49,000 subjects were accumulated over a 7-year period. For this reason, such studies can be expensive to complete. In fact, if the disease outcome under study is rare, the sample size required for a cohort study may be so large that it would be impractical to undertake such a study. On the other hand, if the exposure or risk factor is rare, a well-designed cohort study may offer superior statistical power to evaluate exposure-disease associations, because this type of study allows selective inclusion of exposed persons. In the perinatal asphyxia situation, eg, one could include all newborns with Apgar scores of 0–3 but only a sample of the larger pool of newborns with higher scores.

Following subjects over a long period of time can lead to various problems. Subjects may move away or leave the study for other reasons, including death from other causes than the disease under investigation. If the losses to follow-up are substantial, and the lost subjects differ in outcome from those who remain in the study, the validity of the results can be affected seriously. It is also possible for exposure status to change during the course of the study. Obviously, birth asphyxia occurs only once at the beginning of a lifetime. In other circumstances, however, the exposure under study may be subject to variation over time. For example, a cigarette smoker may quit, or, in an occupational cohort study, employees may change jobs and, therefore, their level of exposure to an occupational hazard may also change. Diagnostic methods for the disease under study may also vary over time.

The advantages and disadvantages of cohort studies are presented in Table 8–3.

SELECTION OF SUBJECTS

Selection of subjects for a cohort study is influenced by various factors, including (a) the type of exposure under investigation, (b) the frequency of the exposure in the population, and (c) the accessibility of subjects and the likelihood of their continuing participation. Both exposed and unexposed groups must be free of the outcome of interest at the start of the study, and they must be similarly-eligible to develop the outcome during the course of the study. If some subjects already have the outcome at the onset of the study, the temporal relationship between the exposure and the disease will be obscured.

The Exposed Group

The type of exposure under investigation is critical for selection of the exposed group. Some exposures during pregnancy are common, such as gestational diabetes or hypertension. For these exposures, a general population of pregnancies could be used to construct the cohort. Other exposures, such as in vitro fertilization, are not common among all pregnant women. In order to use a cohort study design to evaluate whether in vitro fertilization is a risk factor for developmental disability in the offspring, it may be necessary to sample exposed subjects from an infertility clinic rather than from among pregnant women in the general population.

Feasibility issues are also important when selecting the exposed population. The investigator should identify an accessible population that is motivated to participate in the study and unlikely to discontinue participation. The availability of historical information such as medical records may also be a factor in selecting this group. Examples of groups that have been chosen for feasibility reasons include nurses, members of health maintenance organizations, stable communities, and labor union members.

The degree of exposure may differ depending on the goals of the study. For some exposures, subjects are classified into either of two groups: exposed and unexposed. In vitro fertilization is an example of this type of dichotomization. Other studies involve a range of exposure levels, eg, Apgar scores as an indicator of perinatal asphyxia. The investigator may take a graded exposure variable, such as the Apgar score, and transform it into a categorical exposure by dividing subjects into those whose score exceeds a certain designated

Table 8–2. Comparison of the attributes of retrospective and prospective cohort studies.

Attribute	Retrospective Approach	Prospective Approach
Information	Less complete and accurate	More complete and accurate
Discontinued exposures	Useful	Not useful
Emerging, new exposures	Not useful	Useful
Expense	Less costly	More costly
Completion time	Shorter	Longer

Table 8–3. Advantages and disadvantages of cohort studies.

Advantages	Disadvantages
Direct calculation of risk ratio (relative risk)	Time-consuming
May yield information on the incidence of disease	Often requires a large sample size
Clear temporal relationship between exposure and disease	Expensive
Particularly efficient for study of rare exposures	Not efficient for the study of rare diseases
Can yield information on multiple exposures	Losses to follow-up may diminish validity
Can yield information on multiple outcomes of a particular exposure	Changes over time in diagnostic methods may lead to biased results
Minimizes bias	
Strongest observational design for establishing cause-and-effect relationship	

value (eg, Apgar score of 3) and those whose score falls below that value. The value chosen to separate groups is referred to as a **cutoff point** and can be selected in various ways. For example, the cutoff point might be selected on the basis of the underlying distribution of values, such as the point that separates the 10% of subjects with the lowest Apgar scores from the remainder of the population. Alternately, one can use a standard cutoff point believed to have pathophysiologic implications, regardless of the underlying distribution in the population.

Thus, Apgar scores can be classified into dichotomous categories (0–3 versus > 3), into multiple ordered categories (0–3, 4–6, 7–10), or by gradations (continuous). If the exposure can be categorized into multiple levels or gradations, the investigator can determine whether a relationship exists between the dose of the exposure and the response. In the present context, eg, one can ask whether the risk of chronic neurologic disability rises as the Apgar score decreases. If such a trend is observed, the argument that perinatal asphyxia is a cause of chronic neurologic disability is strengthened.

The Unexposed Group

Feasibility issues for the unexposed group are similar to those that apply to the exposed group. The unexposed group must be accessible for entry into the study and for follow-up. When the purpose of a cohort study is to investigate a community, such as in the Framingham Heart Study, that community is the source of the unexposed persons. Since there may be more unexposed people in the community than are needed for the investigation, a representative sample may be taken. In the Framingham Heart Study, several risk factors were of interest, all of which were relatively prevalent in the community. In this situation, a sample of the entire community was drawn and then subdivided into exposure groups, depending upon the risk factor of interest in a particular analysis. In the study of perinatal asphyxia, the unexposed group was defined as the infants with the highest Apgar scores (7–10), indicating the lowest degree of perinatal asphyxia.

For cohort studies that involve the selection of a specific exposed population, selection of an appropriate comparison population may be less clear-cut. For example, if one is studying in vitro fertilization as a risk factor for congenital malformations, the comparison group might be pregnant women who are followed in other obstetric practices. If, however, the comparison pregnancies are not followed with a comparable level of clinical scrutiny, or if the unexposed pregnancies differ from the exposed pregnancies in other ways that might be related to congenital malformations, the study may lead to a false conclusion. The investigator may relate an observed increased risk of congenital malformation to in vitro fertilization when, in fact, the elevated risk is due to some other difference between the exposed and unexposed groups. This type of problem illustrates why a randomized controlled clinical trial may be less susceptible to error than a cohort study. With randomization, factors known to be related to the development of disease—as well as other factors not yet recognized as related to the disease—tend to be balanced between the groups. This justifies confidence that an observed association is, in fact, due to the exposure of interest rather than to some other characteristic.

The underlying principle in selecting the unexposed group is that it should yield a fair comparison with the exposed group. Occasionally, the frequency of outcome occurrence in the exposed population is compared with the outcome frequency in the general population. This is particularly useful when members of the general population are very unlikely to be exposed to the study factor. However, the general population may not be comparable with those in the exposed group. For example, follow-up for disease occurrence may be more (or less) complete than for the exposed study group. This may lead to erroneous conclusions. Furthermore, if the exposed and unexposed groups are chosen from different time periods (a nonconcurrent study), medical care or other factors may differ between the groups in a way that makes the comparison unfair and the results invalid. Suggestions for the selection of exposed and unexposed subjects are presented in Table 8–4.

DATA COLLECTION

The investigator must collect information on both the independent variable (exposure) and the dependent variable (response) during the course of a cohort study.

Table 8–4. Guidelines for selection of exposed and unexposed subjects in cohort studies.

| Guidelines | | |
Unexposed	Exposed	Unexposed and Exposed
Both exposed and unexposed groups should be free of the disease of interest and equally susceptible to development of the disease at the beginning of the study.	The baseline characteristics of exposed persons should not differ systematically from those of unexposed persons, except for the exposure of interest.	Unexposed persons should be sampled from the same (or comparable) source population as the exposed group
Equivalent information (quantity and quality) should be available on exposure and disease status in the exposed and unexposed groups.		Multiple comparison groups of unexposed subjects chosen in different ways may reinforce the validity of findings.
Both groups should be accessible and available for follow-up.		

Exposure

It is essential to define the exposure clearly. Some exposures are acute, one-time episodes, never repeated in a subject's lifetime, eg, asphyxia at birth. Other exposures are long-term, such as cigarette smoking or the use of oral contraceptives. Exposures may also be intermittent, eg, pregnancy-induced hypertension, which may occur during one pregnancy, disappear after delivery, and perhaps reappear during subsequent pregnancies. The types of exposure characteristics that should be considered are presented in Table 8–5.

A subject who originally satisfies the criteria for inclusion in a cohort study should not be excluded subsequently from the analysis because of a change in exposure status during follow-up. This type of exclusion may lead to a biased conclusion. Specifically, it is possible that a change in exposure status may indicate a change in outcome status. For example, in studying the relationship between the use of an anti-nausea medication during pregnancy and subsequent risk of spontaneous abortion, the use of the medication may be discontinued because of early signs of threatened abortion. Excluding this subject from the analysis, therefore, may result in an underestimate of the true link between the medication and the risk of abortion. The potential for changes in exposure status has important implications for the frequency of follow-up. Frequent reassessment of exposure and outcome status may be required if exposure status changes over time.

The source of available information about exposure may constrain the ability of the investigator to define and measure exposure experience. If the information comes from medical records, as is sometimes necessary in a retrospective cohort study, the quality of exposure information may be poor. For example, there are inherent disadvantages in using Apgar scores from medical records. Sometimes the Apgar scoring system is recorded by the medical staff as part of the required paperwork after delivery, without careful timing of the observations and detailed assessment by multiple observers. The medical staff providing patient care may be distracted by other responsibilities. In the previously cited prospective cohort study of neonatal asphyxia, a specially-trained independent observer who was not responsible for patient care recorded the score in a standard manner on a standardized study form at exactly 1, 5, and 10 minutes of life.

In general, objective measures of exposure or biologic markers of exposure are preferred over subjective measures. For example, in a study of maternal use of illicit drugs and pregnancy outcome, one approach to exposure assessment would be to question pregnant women about their use of illicit drugs. Self-reports of illicit drug use, however, are likely to underrepresent actual exposure. Repeated measurements of drug metabolites in urine might provide a more accurate and reliable assessment of exposure.

Clinical Response

Before the start of the study, it is imperative to determine that subjects do not have the outcome (disease) under investigation. This may be especially difficult if the outcome is a disease that develops slowly, has an insidious onset, and is asymptomatic until its late stages. One approach to this problem is to exclude cases that emerge early in the course of the investigation, under the assumption that the biologic onset of disease preceded the beginning of the study.

The degree of surveillance for disease should be similar in the exposed and unexposed groups. The frequency of examination and the duration of follow-up depend on the type of exposure and the outcome under investigation. For some diseases, the time from exposure to development of disease is short. A cohort study of the relationship between exposure to perinatal asphyxia and death within the first week of life, eg, would

Table 8–5. Measurements of exposure used in cohort studies. (*Example:* gestational hypertension.)

Measurements of Exposure	Examples
Intensity	Mean blood pressure level
Duration	Weeks of hypertension
Regularity	Number of affected pregnancies
Variability	Range of measured blood pressures

have a short follow-up period. Other outcomes, such as chronic neurologic disability, may require years to assess. Because the investigators were interested in performance and cognitive ability at early school age, the study of the relationship of perinatal asphyxia to neurologic development required 7 years of follow-up.

Information on outcome status may come from various sources. Some cohort studies rely on information from physician and hospital records. This would be particularly pertinent for a cohort study focusing on a population with good access to health care and standardized record-keeping practices, such as a prepaid health plan. Other cohort studies may combine physician records with periodic examinations by the investigators. The Framingham Heart Study is an example of this type of study. Another approach to collecting information on disease is to have the subjects report whether they develop the outcome of interest. The study may also involve reviews of medical records in a subset of subjects to confirm self-reports.

If the outcome under study is death from any cause, the investigator may use information from death certificates. Death certificates may have limited utility, however, if the study focuses on a specific disease, since cause-of-death information on death certificates may be inaccurate (see Chapter 4). Obviously, in that circumstance the best information would come from autopsy reports. This approach may not be feasible, however, since most people who die are not autopsied.

If diagnostic evaluations are required by the investigator during the study, an appropriate diagnostic test for the disease must be available (see Chapter 6). This approach has limitations because diagnostic tests are not always available or feasible. In order to ensure a fair comparison between the exposed and unexposed groups, the accuracy and reliability of diagnosis must not differ between the groups. Thus, it can be helpful if those who assess outcomes are unaware of the subjects' exposure status. The study of perinatal asphyxia relied on standard neurologic examination and psychologic tests. The examiners had no access to the medical records and, thus, were blind to the Apgar scores of the children. This blinded approach should facilitate an assessment of neurologic outcomes that is comparable for exposed and unexposed children.

It is possible for exposure status to alter the surveillance for disease. An example of this problem could occur in a study of neonatal asphyxia and intellectual development. If a physician is more likely to administer psychologic and developmental tests to an infant who had a difficult birth with low Apgar scores, that child is more apt to be diagnosed as having subtle developmental problems than another child who has not been singled out for close surveillance. This could lead to an overestimate of the relationship between neonatal asphyxia and subsequent developmental disability. This problem, however, can be avoided, as in the cited study, by ensuring that a standard diagnostic protocol is followed, regardless of exposure status.

ANALYSIS

Several different approaches can be used to analyze the results of a cohort study, as described in the following sections.

Risk Ratio

The results of a cohort study can be summarized with the format shown in Table 8–6. In that table, the letters A–D represent numbers of subjects in the four possible combinations of exposure and outcome status (in this instance, death).

A. Exposed persons who later die.
B. Unexposed persons who later die.
C. Exposed persons who do not die.
D. Unexposed persons who do not die.

The total number of subjects in this study is the sum of A + B + C + D. The total number of exposed persons is A + C, and the total number of unexposed persons is B + D.

Among exposed persons, the risk (R) of death is defined as:

$$R_{(exposed)} = \frac{\text{Exposed persons who die}}{\text{All exposed persons}}$$

$$= \frac{A}{A + C}$$

As indicated in Chapter 2, risk can vary between 0 (no exposed persons die) and 1 (all exposed persons die). As in all statements of risk, some time period for the development of the outcome must be specified. For example, the outcome might be the risk of death in the first year of life. Among unexposed persons, the risk of death is defined as:

$$R_{(unexposed)} = \frac{\text{Unexposed persons who die}}{\text{All unexposed persons}}$$

$$= \frac{B}{B + D}$$

As indicated in Chapters 4 and 7, one approach to contrasting the risk in two groups is to create a ratio measure. The **risk ratio** (RR) or relative risk is:

$$RR = \frac{R_{(exposed)}}{R_{(unexposed)}} = \frac{A/(A + C)}{B/(B + D)}$$

Table 8–6. Summary of risk data from a cohort study.

Outcome[1]	Exposed	Unexposed	Total
Death	A	B	A + B
No death	C	D	C + D
Total	A + C	B + D	A + B + C + D

[1]In some studies, the outcome is development of disease rather than death.

If the exposed and unexposed persons have the same risk of death, then the *RR* is 1 (ie, the null value). That is, exposure is not related to the outcome. If the risk among exposed persons is greater than the corresponding risk among unexposed persons, then the *RR* is greater than 1 (ie, hazardous exposure). In contrast, if the risk among exposed persons is smaller than the corresponding risk among unexposed persons, then the *RR* is less than 1 (ie, beneficial exposure).

The calculation of risk ratio can be illustrated from the study of perinatal asphyxia. The data in Table 8–7 relate to infants who weighed more than 2500 g at birth. Exposure is defined as an Apgar score of 0–3 at 10 minutes of life, and the comparison group of less exposed newborns had Apgar scores of 4–6 at 10 minutes. In the actual study, a third group with Apgar scores of 7–10 was included, but the data are not described here in detail.

The risk among exposed newborns is:

$$R_{(exposed)} = \frac{42}{122} = 0.344 = 34.4\%$$

That is, about 1 out of 3 newborns weighing more than 2500 g and having very low Apgar scores at 10 minutes died during the first year of life. The risk among "less exposed" newborns is:

$$R_{(less\ exposed)} = \frac{43}{345} = 0.125 = 12.5\%$$

In other words, 1 in 8 neonates weighing over 2500 g and having intermediate Apgar scores at 10 minutes died during the first year of life.

Without any further calculations, it should be obvious that the neonates with very low 10-minute Apgar scores had a worse prognosis than those with intermediate 10-minute Apgar scores. Quantification of the magnitude of this effect is achieved by calculating the risk ratio:

$$RR = \frac{42}{122} \bigg/ \frac{43}{345} = 2.8$$

The *RR* of 2.8 means that newborns at this birth weight with very low 10-minute Apgar scores are almost 3 times more likely to die in the first year of life

Table 8–7. Relationship between 10-minute Apgar scores and risk of death in the first year of life among children with birth weights of at least 2500 g.[1]

	Apgar Score 0–3	Apgar Score 4–6	Total
Death	42	43	85
No death	80	302	382
Total	122	345	467

[1]Data used, with permission, from Nelson KB, Ellenberg JH: Apgar scores as predictors of chronic neurologic disability. Pediatrics 1981;**68**:36.

than similar-weighing newborns with intermediate 10-minute Apgar scores. The *RR* is a measure of the strength of association between exposure and outcome. The further the *RR* is from the null value of 1, the stronger the association. The strength of association is an important criterion in evaluating whether an observed association is likely to represent a cause-and-effect relationship. The *RR* of 2.8 is consistent with a moderate-to-strong relationship between the exposure (10-minute Apgar score) and outcome (infant death).

As discussed in Chapter 7, a sense of the statistical precision of this estimated risk ratio can be obtained by calculating **confidence intervals** around the point estimate of 2.8. Using the approximation method described in Appendix C, the 95% confidence interval for the data presented in Table 8–7 is (1.9, 4.1). That is, at the 95% level of confidence, the range of *RR* values consistent with the observed data fall between 1.9 and 4.1. Thus, the data indicate a risk of death in infants with very low Apgar scores that ranges between roughly a doubling and a fourfold increase (Figure 8–5). As demonstrated in Chapter 7, the point estimate does not lie in the middle of the *RR* confidence interval. The asymmetry of this interval derives from the skew of the range of values of the risk ratio toward the positive direction (ie, all beneficial effects are compressed into the range 0–1, whereas hazardous effects range from 1 to positive infinity).

Since the null value is excluded from this 95% confidence interval, one can conclude that the findings are **statistically significant.** In other words, these data are not consistent with the null hypothesis of no association between Apgar scores and infant mortality (at the prespecified 95% level of confidence). An association as strong as that observed between Apgar scores and infant mortality, therefore, cannot be explained by chance alone.

As indicated earlier, the argument that the linkage between Apgar score and death in the first year of life is one of cause-and-effect is strengthened if a dose-response relationship can be demonstrated. A third group of newborns, with Apgar scores of 7–10, was therefore included in the study. Comparison of the risk of death in that group against the previous reference group with intermediate Apgar scores of 4–6 yields a risk ratio of 0.15, with an approximate 95% confidence interval of (0.11, 0.21). This result means that newborns with a 10-minute Apgar score of 7–10 have only about one-sixth the risk of death in the first year of life as newborns with Apgar scores of 4–6. This disparity is statistically significant, and the very narrow width of the confidence interval indicates a statistically precise estimate (because it is based upon a large number of observations).

The dose-response relationship between Apgar score and the risk ratio of death in the first year of life for newborns weighing more than 2500 g is shown in Figure 8–6. The reference group against which others were compared in the preceding calculations was the

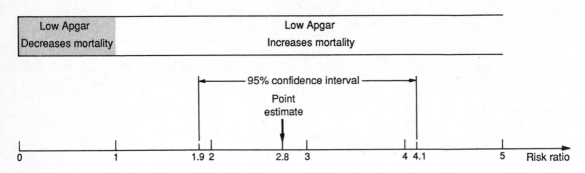

Figure 8–5. Point estimate and 95% confidence interval for risk ratio comparing infant mortality in newborns who weigh more than 2500 g and have 10-minute Apgar scores of 0–3 to infant mortality for similar-weighing newborns with 10-minute Apgar scores of 4–6. (Data used, with permission, from Nelson KB, Ellenberg JH: Apgar scores as predictors of chronic neurologic disability. Pediatrics 1981; **68**:36.)

group with Apgar scores of 4–6 (ie, the risk ratio for this group is defined as 1). A clear trend of decreasing risk ratio with increasing Apgar score is seen, and this trend is unlikely to have occurred by chance alone. Thus, there is strong evidence in these data for a dose-response relationship.

Attributable Risk Percent

The risk of a specified outcome can be compared with measures other than a ratio. For example, one can simply subtract the risk for one group from that for another. This measure is termed the **risk difference,** or excess risk. Some authors use the term "attributable risk" for this measure, but that expression is discouraged here because it may be confused with other expressions. The risk difference (*RD*) is defined as:

$$RD = R_{(exposed)} - R_{(unexposed)}$$

$$= \frac{A}{A + C} - \frac{B}{B + D}$$

Using the previously cited data relating 10-minute Apgar scores (0–3 versus 4–6) to the risk of death in the first year of life, we calculate the risk difference as:

$$RD = \frac{42}{122} - \frac{43}{345} = 0.344 - 0.125 = 0.219$$

That is, the risk of death in the first year of life is increased by 0.219 for newborns who weigh more than 2500 g and have a 10-minute Apgar score of 0–3, compared with similar-weighing newborns with a 10-minute Apgar score of 4–6.

Another measure of interest is the **attributable risk percent** (*ARP*), in which the risk difference is expressed as a percentage of the total risk experienced by the exposed group:

$$ARP = \frac{R_{(exposed)} - R_{(unexposed)}}{R_{(exposed)}} \times 100$$

$$= \frac{A/(A + C) - B/(B + D)}{A/(A + C)} \times 100$$

For the Apgar score-infant mortality data, the attributable risk percent is:

$$ARP = \frac{(0.344 - 0.125)}{0.344} \times 100 = 63.7\%$$

In other words, almost two-thirds of the total risk of infant mortality for newborns who weigh more than 2500 g and have 10-minute Apgar scores of 0–3 is related to an Apgar score below the 4–6 level. The attributable risk percent typically is used as an indicator of the public health impact of exposure. These data suggest that birth asphyxia is a major contributor to—but not the sole cause of—infant mortality among severely asphyxiated children.

Rate Ratio

The analyses presented thus far are based upon comparisons of risk estimates across exposure groups. In a cohort study, the measured outcome may be an incidence (or mortality) rate rather than a risk. The format used to summarize rate data in a cohort study appears in Table 8–8. The rate ratio is derived as follows:

$$Rate\ ratio = \frac{Rate\ of\ outcome\ among\ exposed\ persons}{Rate\ of\ outcome\ among\ unexposed\ persons}$$

$$= \frac{A/PT_{(exposed)}}{B/PT_{(unexposed)}}$$

The magnitude of the rate ratio is interpreted in the same manner as the risk ratio (<1 = protective effect, 1 = no effect, >1 = harmful effect of exposure). The further away from the null value, the stronger the association between exposure and the rate of the outcome.

The data collected in the study of perinatal asphyxia were not presented in a manner that allows calculation of rate ratios.

To illustrate this measure, then, data are drawn from the Chicago Heart Association Detection Project in Industry (Dyer et al, 1992). That investigation involved

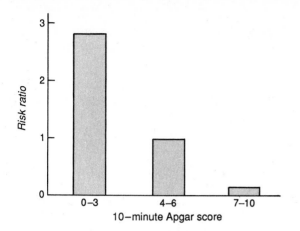

Figure 8–6. Dose-response relationship for the association between 10-minute Apgar scores and risk of death in the first year of life among newborns with a birth weight over 2500 g. (Data used, with permission, from Nelson KB, Ellenberg JH: Apgar scores as predictors of chronic neurologic disability. Pediatrics 1981;**68**:36.)

almost 40,000 men and women at 84 cooperating companies and institutions in the Chicago area. Subjects were enrolled between 1967 and 1973, screened for cardiovascular disease risk factors, and then followed an average of 14–15 years. For white males aged 25–39 at entry, the relationship between baseline serum cholesterol and subsequent rate of coronary heart disease (CHD) is shown in Table 8–9. The rate ratio is:

$$\text{Rate ratio} = \frac{26/36,581}{14/68,239} = 3.5$$

In other words, the CHD mortality rate among white males with borderline high cholesterol levels was about 3.5 times higher than that of white males with lower cholesterol levels. Adjustment for underlying age differences in the study groups reduced the observed rate ratio to 3.1. Comparison of CHD mortality among white males 25–39 with high serum cholesterol levels (>6.2 mmol/L[>240 mg/dL]) to those with normal levels (≤5.1 mmol/L [≤197 mg/dL]) yielded an age-adjusted rate ratio of 5.1. Thus, a dose-response relationship was evident between baseline serum cholesterol level and subsequent CHD mortality.

Table 8–8. Summary format of rate data from a cohort study.

	Exposed Persons	Unexposed Persons	Total
Number of outcomes	A	B	A + B
Person-time (PT)	$PT_{(exposed)}$	$PT_{(unexposed)}$	$PT_{(total)}$

Table 8–9. Relationship between baseline serum cholesterol level and subsequent coronary heart disease mortality rate among white males aged 25–39 at entry into the Chicago Heart Association Study.[1]

	Cholesterol Level		
	5.2–6.2 mmol/L[2]	⊆5.1 mmol/L[3]	Total
Deaths	26	14	40
Person-years	36,581	68,239	104,820

[1]Data from Dyer AR, Stamler J, Shekelle RB: Serum cholesterol and mortality from coronary heart disease in young, middle-aged, and older men and women from three Chicago epidemiologic studies. Ann Epidemiol 1992;**2**:51.
[2]201–240 mg/dL.
[3]≤197 mg/dL.

SUMMARY

In this chapter, the basic approach to the design and analysis of cohort studies is presented, with illustrations drawn primarily from the literature on birth asphyxia. A cohort study is a type of observational investigation in which subjects are classified on the basis of level of exposure to a risk factor and followed to determine subsequent disease outcome. **Prospective** cohort studies are conducted by making all observations on exposure and disease status after the onset of the investigation. A **retrospective** cohort study involves observations on exposure and disease status prior to the onset of the study. The retrospective approach offers several pragmatic advantages but may result in less accurate and complete information on exposure and disease status.

Cohort studies are statistically efficient for the study of rare exposures because the exposed individuals can be selectively included in the study. On the other hand, cohort studies are inefficient for the investigation of slowly developing or rare diseases. The evaluation of chronic diseases through the cohort approach requires a long follow-up period and increases the chances that subjects will be lost from the study. The evaluation of rare diseases with the cohort study approach requires a large sample size and therefore is expensive and labor-intensive.

There are several basic strategies to analyze cohort studies. If data are collected on the risk of developing an outcome during a specified period of time, the summary measure of effect typically is the **risk ratio,** or the risk of the outcome among exposed subjects divided by the risk of the outcome among unexposed individuals. An alternative approach to contrasting risks is the **risk difference,** which is the risk among exposed persons minus the risk among unexposed. If the risk difference is divided by the risk among exposed, a measure termed the **attributable risk percent** is derived. The attributable risk percent is an indicator of the proportion of risk that may be attributable to the exposure per se. When data in a cohort study are based upon the rate of disease outcome, the standard measure of effect is the **rate ratio.** The checklist provided in Table 8–10 may serve as a useful guide in evaluating the design and the analysis of published cohort studies.

The prospective cohort study of perinatal asphyxia cited in this chapter indicates that Apgar scores can serve as a useful predictor of subsequent risk of death and neurologic disability. An inverse dose-response relationship occurs between Apgar score level and the risk of adverse neurologic outcome. In spite of the increased risk, however, most children with low Apgar scores survive and do not manifest neurologic or developmental disability. Through proper interpretation of the results of this cohort study, the pediatrician in the Patient Profile can inform the baby's parents that, although their child faces an increased risk of certain disabilities, there is about an 80% chance that no neurologic handicaps will develop.

STUDY QUESTIONS

Directions: For each question, select the single best answer.

Questions 1–5: A cohort study is conducted to evaluate the relationship between dietary calcium supplementation and the occurrence of hip fractures in post-menopausal women. A total of 100 women who are taking calcium supplements and 100 women who are not taking the supplements are followed over 3 years. During the follow-up period, there are 5 women with hip fractures in the calcium group and 10 women with hip fractures in the group not taking calcium.

1. What is the risk of hip fractures in the calcium group?
   A. 0.05
   B. 0.10
   C. 0.15
   D. 0.20
   E. 0.25

2. What is the risk of hip fractures in the group not taking calcium supplements?
   A. 0.05
   B. 0.10
   C. 0.15
   D. 0.20
   E. 0.25

3. What is the risk ratio for the occurrence of hip fractures?
   A. 0.05
   B. 0.10
   C. 0.30
   D. 0.50
   E. 0.60

4. The correct interpretation of these study results is that the point estimate for the risk ratio indicates that calcium supplementation with respect to hip fractures is
   A. Protective
   B. Deleterious
   C. Neutral
   D. Cannot be determined

5. The 95% confidence interval is 0.18–1.41. The correct interpretation of these results is that
   A. A statistically significant association exists between calcium supplementation and a lowering of the risk for hip fractures.

Table 8–10. Checklist for the evaluation of published cohort studies.

Hypothesis
A. Is the study hypothesis clearly stated?
B. Does it address a question of clinical interest and importance?

Design
A. Is the cohort design appropriate for the question to be answered?
B. Is it feasible to perform a cohort study?

Study Population
A. Will the study yield a fair comparison between the exposed and unexposed subjects?
B. Is the sample size adequate to answer the question of interest?
C. Do the exposed and unexposed subjects come from the same or different populations?
D. Are the exposed and unexposed subjects examined concurrently?
E. Does the investigator present a rationale for the choice of study population?
F. Is the study population similar to the type seen in clinical practice?

Exposure
A. Has the exposure been defined?
B. What is the source of exposure information?
C. Has the exposure been measured appropriately?
D. Are there objective measures or markers to substantiate subjective measures?
E. Is the exposure an acute or chronic one?
F. For chronic exposures, is there remeasurement during the course of the study?
G. Is it possible to examine a dose-response relationship?

Disease
A. Is the disease clearly defined?
B. What is the source of information about the disease?
C. Is there pathologic or other confirmation of disease?
D. Has the presence of disease been assessed in a similar fashion for the exposed and unexposed groups?
E. Were those who assessed disease status blind to subject exposure status?

Follow-up
A. Was the period of follow-up adequate for the development of disease?
B. Were appropriate measures taken to maintain subjects in the study?
C. Is there discussion of losses to follow-up?

Analysis
A. Was an appropriate analysis performed?
B. Are the results statistically significant?
C. Are the results clinically meaningful?

B. A statistically significant association exists between calcium supplementation and a raising of the risk for hip fractures.

C. The risk of hip fractures with calcium supplementation is not significantly different from the risk without supplementation.

D. One can conclude with 95% confidence that calcium supplementation protects against hip fractures.

E. One can conclude with 95% confidence that calcium supplementation increases the risk of hip fractures.

Questions 6–10: In a cohort study, 500 individuals with hypertension and 500 persons without hypertension are followed over a 10-year period for cerebrovascular accidents. During the study, 80 of the hypertensive subjects suffer a newly-diagnosed stroke, while 30 of the normotensive subjects have such an event. Assuming no losses to follow-up and no deaths from other causes, answer the following questions.

6. The incidence rate (per 10,000 person-years) for a stroke among persons with hypertension is closest to
   A. 60
   B. 100
   C. 120
   D. 160
   E. 200

7. The incidence rate (per 10,000 person-years) for a stroke among persons without hypertension is closest to
   A. 60
   B. 100
   C. 120
   D. 160
   E. 200

8. The (incidence) rate ratio for strokes is
   A. 0.37
   B. 1.33
   C. 2.67
   D. 3.15
   E. 3.75

9. The 10-year risk difference is
   A. 0.05
   B. 0.10
   C. 0.15
   D. 0.20
   E. 0.50

10. The attributable risk percent is
    A. 25.5%
    B. 35.0%
    C. 47.5%
    D. 55.5%
    E. 62.5%

FURTHER READING

Feinleib M, Breslow NE, Detels R: Cohort studies. In: *Oxford Textbook of Public Health,* 2nd ed, Vol 2. Holland WW, Detels R, Knox G (editors). Oxford Univ Press, 1991.

REFERENCES

Study Design
Feinleib M: The Framingham Study: Sample selection, follow-up, and methods of analysis. In: *National Cancer Institute Monograph,* No. 67. Greenwald P (editor). US Department of Health and Human Services, 1985.

Nelson KB, Ellenberg JH: Apgar scores as predictors of chronic neurologic disability. Pediatrics 1981;**68:**36.

Timing of Measurements
Greenberg RS: Prospective studies. In: *Encyclopedia of Statistical Sciences,* Vol 7. Kotz S, Johnson NL (editors). Wiley, 1986.

Greenberg RS: Retrospective studies (including case-control). In: *Encyclopedia of Statistical Sciences,* Vol 8. Kotz S, Johnson NL (editors). Wiley, 1988.

Analysis
Dyer AR, Stamler J, Shekelle RB: Serum cholesterol and mortality from coronary heart disease in young, middle-aged, and older men and women in three Chicago epidemiologic studies. Ann Epidemiol 1992; **2:**51.

Kleinbaum DG, Kupper LL, Morgenstern H: *Epidemiologic Research.* Lifetime Learning, 1982.

Case-Control Studies

PATIENT PROFILE

A 55-year-old woman was in excellent health until 2 weeks before admission, when she developed malaise, low-grade fever, cough, and generalized muscle pain. Despite taking aspirin, the woman experienced worsening symptoms over the next several days, in particular, increasing muscle pain which made it very difficult for her to rise from a chair. She then consulted her personal physician, who performed a thorough evaluation. The patient's history was unremarkable except for insomnia over the previous year, which she treated with self-prescribed L-tryptophan. On physical examination, she had mild, diffuse muscle tenderness and a mild, erythematous maculopapular rash over much of her body. Laboratory examination was remarkable for elevations of her blood eosinophil count (2,000 cells per mm³, normal < 250 cells per mm³) and mildly elevated aldolase levels. She was diagnosed as having eosinophilia myalgia syndrome (EMS).

CLINICAL BACKGROUND

In November 1989, researchers from the Centers for Disease Control and Prevention (CDC) and local health departments published the first description of EMS. This newly recognized syndrome is characterized by incapacitating myalgias (muscle pains), elevated eosinophil counts and, in some patients, athralgias (joint pains), skin thickening, hair loss, and interstitial lung disease.

Recognition of EMS was prompted in October 1989, when astute physicians recognized that three people with unexplained myalgias and eosinophilia had consumed L-tryptophan, an essential amino acid available without prescription in drug and health food stores. Prompt response by health departments led quickly to case-control studies that suggested ingestion of L-tryptophan as the cause of EMS. L-tryptophan containing products were taken off the market in November 1989.

EMS occurs predominantly in women and is relatively rare. Nationwide disease surveillance conducted by the CDC led to identification of about 40 deaths and 1500 cases of EMS; nearly all cases occurred between mid-1988 and the end of 1989, although the actual number of cases was probably several times higher than the reported number. In 1990, after the recall of L-tryptophan, the number of reported cases fell to near zero.

Further case-control studies showed that nearly every studied person with EMS (case) had consumed L-tryptophan produced by one particular manufacturer, whereas only about half of the sampled L-tryptophan users without EMS (controls) had ingested L-tryptophan produced by that manufacturer. Further inquiry disclosed that the implicated producer had changed manufacturing conditions in several ways prior to and during the epidemic period. Risk among those consuming L-tryptophan from the implicated manufacturer was estimated to be 20 to 40 times higher than the risk among consumers of L-tryptophan from other sources. The epidemic was attributed to contamination of the L-tryptophan produced during manufacture by the implicated producer. Although many contaminants have been identified chemically in L-tryptophan produced by that manufacturer, the search to identify the specific contaminant or contaminants that cause EMS has been hampered by the lack of an animal model which can reproduce the full spectrum of EMS seen in humans.

The history of EMS illustrates the importance of astute clinical observations and the value of a rapid public health response, which led to the timely recall of L-tryptophan and the prevention of an even larger outbreak of disease. The initial study, as well as most of the subsequent investigations, that linked L-tryptophan use with the occurrence of EMS were based upon a case-control design. In this chapter, case-control studies are described in detail.

INTRODUCTION

As with cohort studies, case-control investigations typically are designed to assess the association between disease occurrence and an exposure suspected of causing (or preventing) that disease. In many situations, however, a case-control study is more efficient than a cohort study because a smaller sample size is required. The key feature of a case-control study that distinguishes it from a cohort study is selection of subjects based upon their disease status. The investigator selects cases from among those persons who have the disease of interest and controls from among those who do not. In a well-designed case-control study, cases are selected from a clearly defined population, sometimes called the **source population.** The investigator then chooses controls from the same population that yielded the cases. The prior exposure histories of cases and controls are examined in order to assess relationships between exposure and disease. The basic design of a case-control study is shown in Figure 9–1.

The approach to the design of a case-control study can be illustrated by one study of the association between L-tryptophan use and the risk of EMS conducted in Minnesota (Belongia et al, 1990). In this study, investigators contacted physicans in an attempt to identify all cases of EMS in the metropolitan area of Minneapolis–St. Paul. To select controls, they called randomly selected telephone numbers in the same area. Researchers interviewed subjects and asked about potential risk factors and about their use of L-tryptophan. They asked cases about L-tryptophan use immediately prior to onset of illness, and asked controls about recent use. For each suject who reported use of L-tryptophan, the investigators also obtained the brand of L-tryptophan and lot number, so that the manufacturer could be traced. L-tryptophan was taken significantly more frequently by cases than by controls—61 of 63 case subjects (97%), but only 101 of

5188 control subjects (2%). Since other studies already had demonstrated this kind of strong association between EMS and use of L-tryptophan in general, the main contribution of this study was the finding that risk was strongly associated with use of L-tryptophan from a particular manufacturer. Among subjects who used L-tryptophan and for whom the manufacturer could be determined, 29 of 30 cases (97%) but only 5 of 9 controls (56%) had used L-tryptophan from the implicated manufacturer. The design of this study is illustrated schematically in Figure 9–2.

This investigation illustrates several important features of case-control studies. First, the design provides an efficient means to study rare diseases like EMS. Case-control studies tend to be more feasible than other types of epidemiologic investigations, eg, cohort studies because fewer subjects are required. The smaller sample size requirement is accompanied by a reduction in cost. Second, case-control studies allow the researcher to investigate several risk factors. In this example, the investigators evaluated L-tryptophan and other factors as possible causes of EMS. Third, as with other nonexperimental or observational studies, a single case-control investigation does not "prove" causality, but it can provide suggestive evidence of a causal relationship that warrants public health intervention to reduce exposure to the risk factor. In this context, the removal of L-tryptophan-containing products from the market resulted in the virtual elimination of reported cases of EMS.

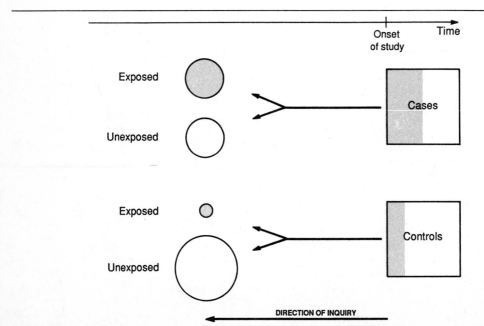

Figure 9–1. Schematic diagram of the design of a case-control study. Shaded areas represent subjects who were exposed to the risk factor of interest.

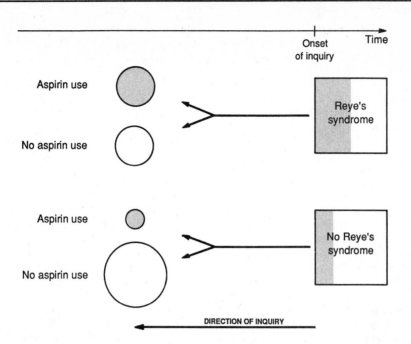

Figure 9–2. Schematic diagram of a case-control study of a specific brand of L-tryptophan use and the subsequent risk of developing eosinophilia-myalgia syndrome (EMS).

DESIGN OF CASE-CONTROL STUDIES

In this section, several aspects of case-control design are discussed, including sources of cases, sources of controls, and collection of information.

Cases

One of the first steps in a case-control study is to identify and select cases—a step that also determines the source population. Case identification should be complete, and the source population—ie, the population from which cases arise—should be well defined. For example, cases might be sampled at random from all patients who are diagnosed with EMS during the study period and who reside within a certain geographic region, such as a state of the United States, or from all cases that occur among subscribers to a health maintenance organization. The source population consists of state residents, in the first instance, and subscribers to the health maintenance organization, in the second instance. In the previously cited study of EMS, the source population consisted of residents of the metropolitan area of Minneapolis–St. Paul, Minnesota. These cases may be identified by a surveillance system or by reviewing hospital records, other medical records, or death certificates available through institutional or population-based disease registries.

In some situations, complete identification of cases in a well-defined source population may be too time-consuming or otherwise infeasible. If so, a common

alternative involves use of a "convenience sample." Cases might be sampled from patients admitted to particular hospitals or from those seen in certain clinics. Although such cases often can be identified easily, the underlying source population may not be well defined, thus making it difficult to generalize results.

The investigator typically studies newly diagnosed or **incident cases,** although sometimes it is necessary to include previously existing or **prevalent cases.** The main reason to exclude prevalent cases is that the exposure may affect the prognosis or the duration of the illness. When this effect occurs, the exposure status of existing prevalent cases tends to differ from that of all cases. For example, suppose that prior L-tryptophan use either prevents death or prolongs the duration of EMS. Prevalent cases of EMS might then have a higher reported use of L-tryptophan than would all cases with this disease. Consequently, a case-control comparison of L-tryptophan use would tend to be distorted by an inflated estimate for cases. The general principle involved is that the likelihood of a case being included in the study must not depend on whether that case was exposed to the risk factor of interest.

Another important step in designing a case-control study is to specify the case definition. The criteria should minimize the likelihood that true cases are missed (ie, the criteria must be **sensitive**). At the same time, falsely classifying a nonaffected person as a case should be avoided (ie, the criteria must be **specific**). In general, there is a trade-off between the desire to include all cases (especially when the disease is extremely rare, as is EMS) and the desire to prevent dilution of the case group with nonaffected persons. Moreover, restrictive criteria may require information that is unavailable for some subjects, so that such subjects could not be classified fully. In practice, inclusion criteria are chosen to minimize misclassification yet retain feasibility. For example, in the previously cited study of EMS in Minneapolis–St. Paul, cases met specific criteria including the following: elevated eosinophil counts, myalgia or muscle weakness, and residence in the study area.

Controls

The next key step in a case-control study design is to identify and select controls. Ideally, controls are chosen at random from the source population. If the source population is a state, city, or other well-defined area, controls in that area might be contacted by dialing telephone numbers at random (random-digit dialing), by visiting residences, by mailing letters soliciting participation, or by other means. An important goal is to select controls so that participation does not depend on exposure. That is to say, the sample of controls should have the same prevalence of exposure as the source population of unaffected persons. If participation does depend on exposure, then the case-control comparison may be distorted. In the previously cited study of EMS, the investigators selected controls by random digit dialing in the Minneapolis–St. Paul area (the source population). Since the population of Minneapolis–St. Paul has fairly complete telephone coverage, this approach to selecting controls is unlikely to be influenced by use of L-tryptophan (the exposure) or, among users, by the manufacturer of L-tryptophan. Accordingly, manufacturer of L-tryptophan within the control group selected by random digit dialing should be comparable to that of the source population.

Determination of Exposure

Once cases and controls are selected, information must be collected on prior exposure to the risk factor of interest, as well as to other exposures. The goal is to obtain as accurate information as possible about each individual's exposure to the main risk factors and to other exposures. The information concerning other exposures is used to determine whether association of disease with a risk factor is due to the exposure of interest or to other characteristics of exposed persons. Since factors cannot affect risk after the disease occurs, the timing of exposures is critical. With slowly developing diseases that lack early evidence of involvement, establishing the temporal sequence of exposure and disease onset can be difficult or impossible.

Interviews and questionnaires are the most common means of determining a subject's exposure history. Interviews can be conducted face-to-face or by telephone. To ensure that information from cases and controls is obtained in the same manner, interviews should be standardized, monitored, and conducted by trained interviewers. Interviews are useful for collecting data because (a) questions may cover a wide range of potential risk factors, (b) costs are relatively low, and (c) information can be obtained on exposures that occurred years prior to the onset of illness. Occasionally, there is concern that cases and controls may recall exposures differently, perhaps distorting case-control comparisons. For example, cases—perhaps in an attempt to explain their illnesses—may overreport exposures. This is of particular concern when there has been a great deal of publicity about the association between the exposure and the disease of interest. For instance, after the L-tryptophan association with EMS was first identified and publicized, knowledge of this association could have affected the reported exposures of cases in subsequent investigations.

In order to minimize problems associated with subject recall, one can attempt to verify exposures through other methods. In the context of the association between L-tryptophan use and EMS, eg, the interviewer might request that the subject produce the L-tryptophan package. By inspecting the package, the interviewer can confirm that it was opened (and therefore the product was presumably used); the manufacturer and the lot number can also be identified.

Information concerning risk factors may be obtained also from medical, occupational, or other records. These methods of obtaining information are not based upon self-reporting and consequently should avoid the reporting bias that may occur when information is obtained by interviewing. The amount of information found in records often is limited, however, so that all of the data of interest may not be available. Furthermore, this information may not be recorded in a standardized manner, leading to variability in subject classification.

The most objective means of characterizing exposure is through the use of a biologic marker, such as measurement of an agent—or an indicator of an agent—in blood or other specimens. There are several difficulties inherent in the use of biologic markers, however. First, obtaining the specimens can involve an invasive procedure that discourages subject participation. Second, many exposures do not have known biologic markers. Third, even if a marker exists, it may be transient and thus not present when the measurement is taken. For example, L-tryptophan levels in blood would reflect only relatively recent exposure and would decline rapidly after exposure is stopped. Finally, the disease state may alter metabolism, thereby distorting case-control comparisons.

The type of case-control study described in the Minneapolis-St. Paul investigation of L-tryptophan and EMS, in which newly diagnosed cases and controls are sampled from a source population, is used quite commonly. It is often called a **population-based** study because cases and controls are sampled from a defined population.

HOSPITAL-BASED CASE-CONTROL STUDIES

Other types of case-control studies differ from the population-based study primarily in the way the samples of cases and controls are selected. Variations include the use of prevalent rather than incident cases and sampling of controls from a readily available, convenient group such as hospital inpatients. The **hospital-based** case-control study is used so often that it merits mention. In this type of study, the investigator typically selects cases from persons with the disease of interest who are admitted to a particular hospital or hospitals; controls are selected from persons admitted with other conditions but with no evidence of the disease of interest. The researcher then obtains information from cases and controls, often by interviewing them in the hospital.

The hospital-based approach can be illustrated by a case-control study of Reye's syndrome, a condition characterized by acute encephalopathy associated with fatty degeneration of the liver. This illness occurs almost exclusively in children and typically follows a viral illness. To study the association between Reye's syndrome and use of various medications during an antecedent viral illness, researchers in this study selected cases from children admitted with Reye's syndrome to any of a preselected group of referral hospitals. Investigators selected controls from children admitted to these same hospitals with an antecedent illness, presumably of viral origin. Parents were interviewed to assess prior aspirin exposure. Twenty-six of the 27 cases—but only 6 of the 22 hospitalized controls—had been exposed to a salicylate-containing medication. In nearly every instance, the salicylate was aspirin.

The hospital-based case-control study can be very convenient, since cases and controls are found in the same institutions. Moreover, potential subjects, if not too ill, may be particularly willing to participate. For example, they may have more time than would normally be available. Within a hospital-based case-control study, factors that might influence hospitalization at a particular facility, eg, socioeconomic status, tend to be balanced between cases and controls. Although hospital-based studies can be convenient, they also are susceptible to distorted results. First, cases and controls in a hospital-based study may not arise from a single, well-defined population—in contrast to the population-based case-control studies described previously. This could happen, eg, if referral patterns to particular hospitals varied across different diagnoses. Moreover, controls in a hospital-based case-control study are in a hospital because they are ill, and the condition or conditions for which they are hospitalized may be associated with—and even caused by—the exposure of interest. If so, the exposure histories of controls may differ from those of the source population, and a distorted case-control comparison may result. Several selection criteria for hospital-based controls may help to reduce this type of distortion; those criteria are listed in Table 9–1.

These difficulties probably underlie a decline in popularity of hospital-based case-control studies. Despite these problems, however, hospital-based case-control studies are still performed. Typically, they are easier and quicker to conduct than population-based studies, since cases and controls are identified efficiently. Consequently, hospital-based case-control studies may be less expensive. Furthermore, the collection of exposure information from medical records and biologic markers is easier in the hospital environment. Subjects in the hospital are more accessible for interview than persons in the community. As already noted, hospital-based controls may be more cooperative with investigators since they are ill and may want to advance medical knowledge.

Despite these differences in approach and the subtle differences in interpretation that may result, the basic case-control design remains intact. Cases are selected from those with the disease of interest and controls from those without that disease. The relative strengths of population-based and hospital-based case-control studies are summarized in Table 9–2. In brief, the hospital-based approach offers logistical advantages, whereas the population-based approach tends to characterize more accurately the exposure history of the source population.

SELECTION BIAS

Bias is a systematic error in a study that distorts the results and limits the validity of conclusions, as will be discussed in Chapter 10. Bias can occur for a variety of reasons, most of which can affect any type of study.

Table 9–1. Approaches to sampling of controls in hospital-based case-control studies.

Selection Criteria for Hospital-Based Controls	
To Do	**To Avoid**
Select controls from various diagnostic groups so no particular risk factors will be overrepresented.	Do not select patients who have multiple concurrent conditions.
Select controls from patients with acute conditions so earlier exposures could not have been influenced by the condition.	Do not select patients with diagnoses known to be related to the risk factor of interest.

Table 9–2. Relative strengths of population-based and hospital-based case-control studies.

Population-Based	Hospital-Based
Source population is better defined	Subjects are more accessible
Easier to make certain that cases and controls derive from the same source population	Subjects tend to be more cooperative
Exposure histories of controls more likely to reflect those of persons without the disease of interest	Background characteristics of cases and controls may be balanced
	Easier to collect exposure information from medical records and biologic specimens

One form—selection bias—poses a particular threat to case-control studies. This form of bias, as suggested by its name, reflects systematic errors that arise from the way in which subjects are selected. If selection of cases, controls, or both is influenced by prior exposure, this bias may be present. In particular, if the exposure of the cases studied differs from that of all cases arising from the source population—or if exposure of controls differs from that of persons in the source population without the disease—selection bias may be present. The particular susceptibility of case-control studies to selection bias reflects the need to obtain two samples: a sample of cases and a sample of controls. Unless each sample is obtained without regard to exposure, results may be biased.

The development of selection bias is illustrated schematically in Figure 9–3. The shaded figures represent persons who were exposed and the unshaded figures represent those who were not. In the source population, one-third of persons with disease were exposed. Among the cases included in the study, however, two-thirds were exposed. That is to say, exposed persons with disease were more likely than unexposed persons with disease to be selected for the study. In this illustration, an opposite sampling pattern is displayed for persons without disease. In this group, ex-

posed persons were less likely to be selected for study than were unexposed persons. Obviously, comparison of exposure histories of sampled cases and controls in this study would yield a result different from that achieved by contrasting exposure histories of persons with and without disease in the source population.

There are at least three ways in which this type of bias could arise in case-control studies of EMS:

(1) Preferential diagnosis of exposed cases may lead to selection bias. After the initial publicity concerning the suspected association of EMS with L-tryptophan use, physicians may have been more inclined to suspect the diagnosis of EMS among those who were known to have used L-tryptophan. If so, subjects with EMS who did not take L-tryptophan could have been underrepresented within the case group, thus leading to selection bias.

(2) Low participation may lead to selection bias. For example, eligible subjects may refuse to participate, or physicians may advise their patients not to participate. If L-tryptophan use of those who did not participate differed from that of participants, selection bias must be suspected.

(3) Errors in sampling controls from the source population can also create selection bias. For example, if sampled controls had a condition like insomnia that would make them more likely than other people to use L-tryptophan, selection bias could occur.

Studies of EMS and use of L-tryptophan raise an interesting point concerning susceptibility of different studies to selection bias due to preferential diagnosis of exposed cases. Selection bias could have affected any case-control study of the association between EMS and *any* use of L-tryptophan that was conducted after the extensive media publicity. Nearly all the published case-control studies, however, were designed to investigate the association between risk of EMS and the manufacturing *source* of the L-tryptophan. These studies were less susceptible to selection bias. For example, consider the possibility that preferential diagnosis of exposed cases led to underrepresentation of unexposed subjects in the case series. This type of problem was unlikely in the studies of the source

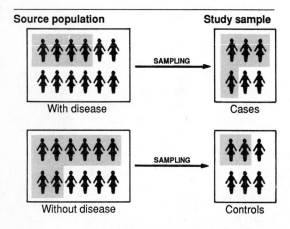

Figure 9–3. Schematic diagram of the origin of selection bias in a case-control study. The shaded figures represent persons who were exposed, and the unshaded figures indicate persons who were unexposed.

of L-tryptophan because most physicians would not have known the source, nor would they have been aware of the link between a particular manufacturer and risk of L-tryptophan. Thus, preferential diagnosis of exposed cases (those who used L-tryptophan from the implicated manufacturer) should not have occurred to any important extent, and they should not been overrepresented in the case group.

MATCHING

Confounding, is a distortion of results that occurs when the apparent effects of the exposure of interest actually are attributable entirely or in part to the effects of an extraneous variable. Confounding is likely to occur when persons exposed to the risk factor of interest differ from the nonexposed with respect to the prevalence of other risk factors. Confounding is discussed in more detail in Chapter 10.

In this chapter, several possible ways to control confounding are presented, including matched sampling. **Matching** is a popular approach to control confounding in case-control studies. Its popularity reflects the sense that matching cases and controls forces these groups to be similar with respect to important risk factors, and thereby makes case-control comparisons less subject to confounding. This perception about matching is true, provided one conducts the appropriate matched analysis.

The first step in matching is to identify a case. Then investigators select from the source population one or more potential controls who have the same values that the case has for each matching factor. The process of matching by race and gender is illustrated schematically in Figure 9–4. In order to match on a continuous variable like age, it typically is necessary to form categories, such as 5-year intervals (years 10–14, 15–19, 20–24, etc). In a study with matching on race, gender, and age in 5-year intervals, eg, a 17-year-old black female case would be matched to a black female control aged 15–19 from the source population. As in an unmatched study, these controls would come from the defined source population. More than one control can be matched to each case, but the ratio of controls to cases rarely exceeds 4:1 because additional controls beyond this ratio add relatively little to the statistical power of the study.

The use of matching is common in clinical studies, especially when the disease of interest is extremely rare, as is EMS. In this situation, there are a small number of potential cases and a large number of potential controls. Matching can increase the statistical efficiency of case-control comparisons and thus achieve a specified level of statistical power with a smaller sample size. The matching protocol often simplifies decisions about how to sample controls. In addition, matching tends to ensure that case-control differences in the risk factor of interest cannot be explained by reference to the matched variables.

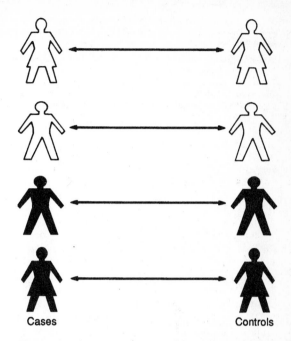

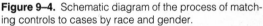

Cases   Controls

Figure 9–4. Schematic diagram of the process of matching controls to cases by race and gender.

These advantages of matching must be weighed against a number of disadvantages, however. As indicated in Table 9–3, matching can be time-consuming and therefore expensive. Any potential cases or controls that cannot be matched must be discarded, which can be viewed as a wasteful process. Any variable that is matched in a study cannot be evaluated as a risk factor in that investigation. Finally, matching on ordinal or continuous variables may result in categories that are too broad to remove completely the effects of the matched variables from the exposure-disease relationship.

Another investigation of EMS and L-tryptophan use conducted by researchers in Minnesota illustrates the use of a matched case-control study design (CDC, 1989). In that study, researchers contacted area physicians to identify people with unexplained eosinophilia and severe myalgia. They also required that a muscle biopsy, if done, show eosinophilic perimyositis or perivasculitis. For each case, they identifed a control who matched the case on age, sex, and telephone exchange. They interviewed subjects and asked about L-tryptophan use, selected other medications, and diet. For each of the 12 case-control pairs, the case had consumed L-tryptophan prior to onset of illness, but none of the matched controls had consumed L-tryptophan. Results of this study indicated a strong association between ingestion of L-tryptophan and risk of EMS.

Table 9–3. Advantages and disadvantages of matching in case-control studies.

Advantages	Disadvantages
May increase the precision of case-control comparisons and thus allow a smaller study	May be time-consuming and expensive to perform
The sampling process is easy to understand and explain	Some potential cases and controls may be excluded because matches cannot be made
If analyzed correctly, provides reassurance that matched variables cannot explain case-control differences in the risk factor of interest	The matched variables cannot be evaluated as risk factors in the study population
	For continuous or ordinal variables, matching categories may be too broad, and residual case-control differences in these variables may persist

ANALYSIS

The type of analysis employed in a case-control study depends upon whether subjects were sampled in an unmatched or in a matched approach. These two analytic strategies are described in the following sections.

Unmatched Design

The data obtained in an unmatched case-control study can be summarized as indicated in Table 9–4. For simplicity, only two levels of exposure are discussed here, though the basic methods can be expanded to include multiple levels of exposure. Each subject can be classified into one of the four basic groups defined by disease and prior exposure status:

A. Cases who were exposed.
B. Cases who were not exposed.
C. Controls who were exposed.
D. Controls who were not exposed.

The format of Table 9–4 should appear familiar, since it resembles that of Table 8–6. Although the summary tables for cohort and case-control studies are similar, it is important to remember that the underlying approaches to sampling differ, and the analysis must account for these differences. In a cohort study, sampling is based upon exposure status, and the investigator thus determines the total numbers of exposed ($A + C$) and unexposed subjects ($B + D$) included in the study. Then risk of disease development can be estimated separately for exposed and unexposed groups, and these two risks can be compared in a risk ratio (*RR*).

A case-control study, on the other hand, begins with sampling of persons with the disease of interest and individuals without the disease ($A + B$ and $C + D$, respectively). With this approach, the proportion of

Table 9–4. Summary of data collected in an unmatched case-control study.

	Exposed	Unexposed	Total
Case	A	B	A + B
Controls	C	D	C + D
Total	A + C	B + D	A + B + C + D

persons in the study who have the disease is no longer determined by the disease risk in the source population, but rather by the choice of the investigator. That is, a disease that occurs infrequently in the source population can be oversampled, so that affected individuals constitute a large proportion of the study sample. This ability to oversample affected individuals is why case-control studies are statistically efficient for the study of rare diseases.

Since in a case-control study the investigator determines the ratio of persons with the disease to persons without it, the proportion of study subjects who have disease does not provide an estimate of disease risk. As shown in the following section, however, an indirect estimate of the incidence rate ratio can still be obtained in a case-control study.

Odds Ratio

With the notation introduced in Table 9–4, the probability that a case was exposed previously is estimated by:

$$\text{Case exposure probability} = \frac{\text{Exposed cases}}{\text{All cases}}$$

$$= \frac{A}{A + B}$$

The odds of exposure for cases represent the probability that a case was exposed divided by the probability that a case was not exposed. The odds then are estimated by:

Odds of case exposure

$$= \frac{\text{Exposed cases}}{\text{All cases}} \bigg/ \frac{\text{Unexposed cases}}{\text{All cases}}$$

$$= \frac{A}{A + B} \bigg/ \frac{B}{A + B} = \frac{A}{B}$$

Similarly, the odds of exposure among controls are estimated by:

$$\text{Odds of control exposure} = \frac{C}{D}$$

The odds of exposure for cases divided by the odds of exposure for controls are expressed as the **odds ratio (OR).** Substituting from the preceding equations, the *OR* is estimated by:

$$\text{Odds ratio} = \frac{\text{Odds of case exposure}}{\text{Odds of control exposure}}$$

$$= \frac{A}{B} \bigg/ \frac{C}{D} = \frac{A \times D}{B \times C}$$

The *OR* is sometimes termed the exposure odds ratio or the cross-product of Table 9–4, because it results from dividing the product of entries on one diagonal of this table by the product of entries on the cross-diagonal.

When incident cases and controls are sampled from the same source population (with selection independent of prior exposure), the exposure *OR* provides a valid estimate of the incidence rate ratio (See Appendix D). In other words, if properly designed, a case-control study can yield a measure of association between exposure and disease that approximates the incidence rate ratio.

The calculation of the *OR* can be illustrated by data from a case-control study of EMS in which risk associated with use of particular brands of L-tryptophan was studied. Among those who took L-tryptophan, 22 of 48 cases took one particular retail lot (lot A), compared with 7 of 93 controls, as summarized in Table 9–5. The *OR* for these data is as follows:

$$\text{Odds ratio} = \frac{A \times D}{B \times C} = \frac{23 \times 86}{36 \times 7} = 7.5$$

In other words, the odds of using lot A for patients with EMS were over seven times larger than the odds for use of lot A among controls in this study. To the extent that the *OR* provides a valid estimate of the incidence rate ratio, one could conclude from this investigation that use of Brand A increased the likelihood of developing EMS more than sevenfold.

As with the risk ratio, a 95% confidence interval around the point estimate of the *OR* can be calculated. A formula to calculate an approximate 95% confidence interval is given in Appendix E. With the data presented in Table 9–5, the approximate 95% confidence interval for the *OR* is 2.9 to 19.1. That is, the data from this study are consistent with a moderately-to-strongly-positive association between the use of a particular lot of L-tryptophan and the development of EMS. This association is unlikely to have occurred by chance alone, since the null value of the *OR* (null value = 1) is well outside of the 95% confidence interval. The point estimate and confidence interval for this odds ratio are illustrated in Figure 9–5.

Matched Design

In a matched case-control study, the analysis must account for the matched sampling scheme. When one control is matched to each case, summary data can be presented in the format shown in Table 9–6. An extension of this basic format can be employed for situations in which the ratio of controls to cases differs from 1:1. Although there are four cells in Table 9–6, the entries into this format are quite different from what we find in previous tables. Each entry into Table 9–6 represents not one subject but two (a matched case-control pair). That is, each case-control pair can be classified into one of the four basic combinations of exposure status:

W—Both case and control exposed.
X—Case exposed but control unexposed.
Y—Case unexposed but control exposed.
Z—Both case and control unexposed.

Case-control pairs that are entered into cells *W* and *Z* are referred to as **concordant pairs,** because the exposure status of cases and controls in these pairs are the same. Case-control pairs that are entered into cells *X* and *Y,* in contrast, are referred to as **discordant pairs** since, in these pairs, the exposure status of cases and controls differs.

The *OR* for a pair-matched case-control study is given by a simple ratio:

$$\text{Odds ratio} = \frac{X}{Y}$$

This odds ratio can be interpreted in the same manner as the *OR* for unmatched studies.

To illustrate the calculation of the *OR* from a matched study, the results of a hypothetical matched study with 200 matched case-control pairs are shown in Table 9–7. The *OR* from this study is as follows:

$$\text{Odds ratio} = \frac{X}{Y} = \frac{57}{5} = 11.4$$

A 95% confidence interval around the point estimate of the matched *OR* can be calculated. A formula to calculate an approximate 95% confidence interval is given in Appendix E. With the data presented in Table 9–7, the approximate 95% confidence interval for the *OR* is 4.6 to 28.3. That is, the data from the hypothetical matched case-control study are consistent with a strong to a very strong positive association between the use of L-tryptophan and the development of EMS. This association is highly unlikely to have occurred by

Table 9–5. Summary of data from the study of eosinophilia myalgia syndrome (EMS) and use of Brand A.

	Use Brand A	Use Other Brand	Total
Cases	22	36	58
Controls	7	86	93
Total	29	122	151

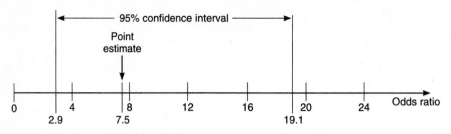

Figure 9–5. Point estimate and 95% confidence interval for odds ratio comparing lot A L-tryptophan use patients with eosinophilia-myalgia syndrome (EMS) and controls.

chance, since the null value of the *OR* (null value = 1) is far outside the 95% confidence interval.

To further illustrate analysis of matched case-control studies, consider again the matched case-control study of L-tryptophan conducted by the researchers in Minnesota (CDC, 1989). The results of that study, summarized in Table 9–8, indicate that for every case-control pair, the case but not the control had taken L-tryptophan. Therefore, the *OR* from this study is as follows:

$$\text{Odds ratio} = \frac{X}{Y} = \frac{12}{0}$$

This odds ratio is undefined or infinite, since the denominator is zero. This suggests a very strong association between L-tryptophan and risk of EMS. The 95% confidence interval for the odds ratio is 2.8 to infinity. It is highly unlikely that this association occurred by chance, since the null value of the *OR* (null value = 1) is well outside the 95% confidence interval. (In this example, the small number of case-control pairs in the **Y** category violates the large sample assumptions of the approximate confidence interval formula in Appendix E. Therefore, a more complicated exact formula was used to estimate this 95% confidence interval.)

SUMMARY

In this chapter, the basic approach to the design and analysis of case-control studies is presented, with illustrations drawn primarily from the literature on the relationship between the use of contaminated L-tryptophan and risk of EMS. A case-control study is a type of observational investigation in which subjects are enrolled on the basis of the presence or absence of a particular disease (eg, EMS) and then evaluated to determine their history of exposure to risk factors of interest (eg, L-tryptophan use).

The advantages and disadvantages of the case-control approach are summarized in Table 9–9. The advantages of this design are chiefly logistical. In particular, rare diseases (EMS is an example) and those with long latency periods can be studied efficiently. The sample size required for a case-control study tends to be smaller than would be needed for an alternative design, such as a cohort study. As a result, the expense of conducting a case-control study may be substantially less than the cost of a cohort study. Furthermore, reliance on historical information allows rapid completion of a case-control study. The ability to reach a prompt conclusion is particularly important if the disease is potentially life-threatening, as is EMS, because future cases might be prevented by authoritative action to limit exposure to a suspected risk factor.

The disadvantages of case-control studies relate primarily to their susceptibility to systematic errors. Since cases and controls are sampled separately, it is possible that these groups may not arise from the same source population. Bias can be introduced into the study results if exposure status is associated with the likelihood of including cases or controls into the study. Reliance upon subject recall of earlier exposures or the use of historical records can lead to imprecise or inaccurate classification of exposure.

The decision to conduct a case-control study typically is motivated by a desire to explore the relationship between a specific risk factor and a particular disease. Ideally, the cases and the controls should derive from a single well-defined source population, such as a state or metropolitan area (a **population-based** sam-

Table 9–6. Summary data format for a matched case-control study with one control per case.

	Control Exposed	Control Unexposed	Total
Case exposed	*W*	*X*	*W* + *X*
Case unexposed	*Y*	*Z*	*Y* + *Z*
Total	*W* + *Y*	*X* + *Z*	*W* + *X* + *Y* + *Z*

Table 9–7. Summary data from a hypothetical matched case-control study of L-tryptophan use and risk of eosinophilia myalgia syndrome (EMS).

	Control Exposed	Control Unexposed	Total
Case exposed	132	57	189
Case unexposed	5	6	11
Total	137	63	200

pling scheme). An attempt may be made to identify all newly diagnosed cases (**incident cases**) within the source population, particularly when the disease is rare or the source population is modest in size. Cases may be identified from hospital records, surveillance systems, death certificates, or other sources. Careful criteria for the presence of disease must be established to minimize false inclusions or exclusions.

Controls typically are sampled from the population that gave rise to the cases. Occasionally, for purposes of convenience, **hospital-based samples** of cases and controls are selected. The hospital-based approach tends to have the advantages of accessibility to the subjects and cooperative study participants. On the other hand, cases and controls may derive from dissimilar source populations in a hospital-based study, and exposure status might influence the likelihood of inclusion in this type of investigation.

Matching of controls to cases on the basis of known risk factors for the disease of interest is a common practice in case-control studies. The intent of matching is usually to decrease the possibility of **confounding,** or mixing of the effect of interest with the effects of other risk factors. Matching can increase the statistical precision of estimates and thereby allow a smaller sample size. On the other hand, matching can be time consuming, and subjects who are not successfully matched can produce useless information that must be discarded.

The process of subject selection in a case-control study precludes the estimation of risks (or rates), and the risk ratio therefore cannot be calculated directly from case-control data. An indirect estimate of the risk ratio, however, can be calculated in a case-control study. This measure is referred to as the **odds ratio** and is defined as the odds of exposure among cases, divided by the odds of exposure among controls. The approach to calculating the odds ratio depends upon whether subjects were sampled in an unmatched or matched fashion. In either instance, a point estimate and 95% confidence interval for the odds ratio can be

Table 9–8. Results of a matched case-control study of L-tryptophan use and eosinophilia myalgia syndrome (EMS).

	Control Exposed	Control Unexposed	Total
Case exposed	0	12	12
Case unexposed	0	0	0
Total	0	12	12

calculated as a measure of association between exposure and disease occurrence.

A number of case-control studies of EMS are discussed. In those studies, cases and controls were sampled using various approaches. The most consistent risk factor that emerged from the studies was the use of L-tryptophan from one manufacturer. The strength of the association between L-tryptophan from the implicated manufacturer and EMS, the dose-response, and the consistency of results across studies—as well as other considerations such as biologic plausibility—suggest that a cause-and-effect relationship exists between the exposure in question and the occurrence of disease. The decline in the incidence of reported cases of EMS after withdrawal from the market of L-tryptophan-containing products further supports this explanation.

STUDY QUESTIONS

Questions 1–3: For each measure described below, select the most appropriate calculation from the following lettered options. Each option can be used once, more than once, or not at all.

A. 15/85
B. (15/100)/(85/100)
C. (15/100)/(10/200)
D. (15 × 190)/(85 × 10)
E. (85 × 10)/(15 × 190)
F. 10/190
G. (10/200)/(190/200)

1. The odds of exposure among cases in an unmatched case-control study of risk factors for congenital defects of the neural tube, in which maternal folate deficiency was found in 15 of 100 mothers of cases and 10 of 200 mothers of controls.

2. The odds of exposure among controls in the unmatched case-control study described in question (1).

3. The odds ratio for exposure in the unmatched case-control study described in question (1).

Questions 4–5: For each confidence interval below, select the most appropriate lower bound from the following lettered options. Each option can be used once, more than once, or not at all.

A. 1.7%
B. 6.1%
C. 17%
D. 61%
E. 70%
F. 1.5%
G. 11%
H. 35%
I. 100%

Table 9–9. Advantages and disadvantages of case-control studies.

Advantages	Disadvantages
Efficient for the study of rare diseases	Risk of disease cannot be estimated directly
Efficient for the study of chronic diseases	Not efficient for the study of rare exposures
Tend to require a smaller sample size than other designs	More susceptible to selection bias than alternative designs
Less expensive than alternative designs	Information on exposure may be less accurate than that available in alternative designs
May be completed more rapidly than alternative designs	

4. The minimal percentage increase in the odds of high stress levels at a 95% confidence level in an unmatched case-control study of risk factors for migraine headaches, with an odds ratio of 3.2 for high stress levels (95% confidence interval: 1.7, 6.1).

5. The minimal percentage increase in the odds of high levels of daily stress for cases compared to controls if the sample size in question (4) were doubled, but the odds ratio estimate were to remain 3.2.

Questions 6–7: For each study result described below, select the most appropriate interpretation from the following lettered options. Each option can be used once, more than once, or not at all.

    A. Protective
    B. Harmful
    C. No association
    D. Uncertain without the results of an hypothesis test
    E. Not appropriately assessed by statistical significance because randomization was not performed

6. The single best estimate of the association between fresh fruit consumption and risk of oral cancer in a case-control study that has an odds ratio of 0.6 with a 95% confidence interval of 0.4 to 0.9.

7. The interpretation implied by the 95% confidence level in the study result described in question (6).

Questions 8–9: For each numbered situation below, select from the following lettered options the most appropriate advantage of the case-control design. Each option can be used once, more than once, or not at all.

    A. Confounding unlikely because of randomization
    B. Efficient for the study of rare diseases
    C. Efficient for the study of diseases that develop slowly
    D. The risk among exposed persons can be determined directly
    E. The temporal relationship between exposure and disease is better refined

8. Assessing risk factors for the development of toxic shock syndrome.

9. Assessing risk factors for the development of osteoarthritis.

Questions 10–12: For each numbered situation below, select the most likely type of bias from the following lettered options. Each option can be used once, more than once, or not at all.

    A. Ecologic fallacy
    B. Confounding
    C. Random error
    D. Misclassification
    E. A cohort effect
    F. Selection bias

10. The cases tend to overreport use of an intrauterine device (IUD) in a case-control study of IUD use and risk of ectopic pregnancies.

11. The cases are identified from emergency room visits, and the controls are sampled from fertility clinic patients in a case-control study of IUD use and risk of ectopic pregnancies.

12. Low socioeconomic status is associated with both exposure and disease occurrence in a case-control study of IUD use and ectopic pregnancy.

FURTHER READING

Austin H et al: Limitations in the application of case-control methodology. Epidemiol Rev 1994;**16**:65.

Correa A et al: Exposure measurement in case-control studies: Reported methods and recommendations. Epidemiol Rev 1994;**16**:18.

Dwyer DM et al: Use of case-control studies in outbreak investigations. Epidemiol Rev 1994;**16**:109.

Lasky T, Stolley PD: Selection of cases and controls. Epidemiol Rev 1994;**16**:6.

REFERENCES

Belongia EA et al: An investigation of the cause of the eosinophilia-myalgia syndrome associated with tryptophan use. New Engl J Med 1990;**323:**357.

CDC: Eosinophilia-myalgia syndrome and L-tryptophan-containing products—New Mexico, Minnesota, Oregon, and New York, 1989. MMWR 1989;**38:**785.

Hertzman PA et al: Association of the eosinophilia-myalgia syndrome with the ingestion of tryptophan. New Engl J Med 1990;**322:**869.

Hurwitz ES et al: Public Health Service study of Reye's syndrome and medications. JAMA 1987;**257:**1905.Kilbourne EM: Eosinophilia-myalgia syndrome: Coming to grips with a new illness. Epidemiol Reviews 1992;**14:**16.

Slutsker L et al: Eosinophilia-myalgia syndrome associated with exposure to tryptophan from a single manufacturer. J Am Med Assoc 1990;**264:**213.

Swygert LA et al: Eosinophilia-myalgia syndrome. Results of national surveillance. JAMA 1990;**264:**1698.

Variability & Bias

10

PATIENT PROFILE

A 45-year-old man began working as a production supervisor, and his employer required that he undergo a complete medical examination. His physician learned that the patient's father had died of myocardial infarction at age 65. On physical examination, the patient was moderately obese, and his blood pressure was 140/86. The remainder of the examination revealed no notable abnormalities. The patient's total serum cholesterol level (nonfasting) was 242 mg/dL.

According to the National Cholesterol Education Program (NCEP) guidelines, a total serum cholesterol concentration greater than 240 mg/dL is an indication for possible pharmacologic lowering of serum cholesterol. A value of 200–239 mg/dL is considered borderline and should trigger dietary intervention, and a value less than 200 mg/dL is considered normal.

Based on the initial cholesterol results, the physician asked the patient to return in 2 weeks for further testing. On repeat measurement, the total serum cholesterol was 198 mg/dL on a fasting lipid profile. Table 10–1 lists several different factors that could explain the observed variability in measured total serum cholesterol. The source of this variability in the measured total cholesterol level had important implications for how the physician treated this patient.

VARIABILITY IN MEDICAL RESEARCH

Difficulties in the interpretation of test results of individual patients are magnified when groups of patients are studied. The sources of variability in test results and errors in medical research are discussed in this chapter. Appreciation of these issues is important for the interpretation and appropriate application of research findings in the clinical setting.

Variability in measurements can be either random or systematic. A schematic representation of random and systematic variation is shown in Figure 10–1. The shots at the targets in both A and B are centered around the middle, but in A the shots are less scattered and have less variability, or more **precision.** In targets C and D the scatter is similar, but in target D the cluster

of shots is off center. This might occur, eg, if the sight of the gun were bent. The precision is comparable, but the result in D is systematically off target or **biased.** The results in target C are accurate, or valid. It is important to consider the accuracy and precision of any measurements made in the medical setting. In clinical medicine and medical research, variability can occur at a number of different levels (eg, at the level of the individual or the population) (Table 10–1). At each level, the variability inherent in the method of measurement is important.

Variability Within the Individual

The first level of concern is variability in the true value of a person's characteristics over time. This was a source of concern for the clinician in the Patient Profile. Some potential sources of individual variability are listed in Table 10–2. The source of this variation can be the individual being measured, the instrument used to perform the measurement, the technician taking the measurement, or the person interpreting the result. Variation can occur because of biologic changes in an individual over time. These changes may (a) occur on a minute-to-minute basis (eg, heart rate), (b) follow a regular diurnal pattern (eg, body temperature), or (c) progress with normal development (eg, height or weight).

When the variation within a subject is large, a single measurement may not adequately represent the "true" status of that individual. By repeating a test, the physician may obtain a better understanding of the true value and its variability. This may also give the clinician a clue about variability or error due to the measurement technique. In the Patient Profile, different results were obtained when the total serum cholesterol was measured a second time, ie, when the patient was fasting. It is unlikely, however, that the fasting state alone could cause such a drop in total serum cholesterol. Furthermore, it is unlikely that the patient could have made the kind of dietary or other alterations in 2 weeks that would lead to the observed change in total serum cholesterol.

Variability Related to Measurement

Laboratory measurements of total serum cholesterol are notorious for both variability and error. In order to determine which value—198 mg/dL or 242 mg/dL—

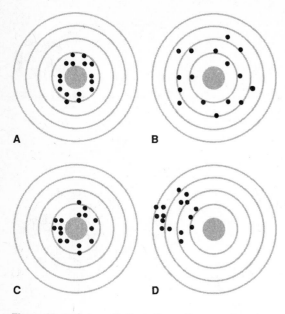

A   B

C   D

Figure 10–1. Schematic illustrations of increased random error (target B versus target A) and systematic error (target D versus target C).

is closer to the truth, the physician in the Patient Profile would need to know whether or not both measurements were obtained in the same laboratory. For example, the first result may have been obtained from a desktop analyzer in the physician's office, while the lipid profile may have been measured in a standardized laboratory. In reality, the physician may not be able to discern readily which value is closer to the truth. This is one reason that programs with guidelines that support cutoff points for clinical decision-making, such as the NCEP, often recommend that elevated values be confirmed by repeated measurements over time before treatment is instituted.

Variations Within Populations

Just as there is variation in individuals, there is also variability in populations (see Table 10–2), which can be considered the cumulative variability of individuals. Since populations are made up of individuals with different genetic constitutions who are subject to dif-

ferent environmental influences, populations often exhibit more variation than individuals. Physicians use knowledge about variability in populations to define what is "normal" and "abnormal." The physician in the Patient Profile could refer to population survey data to learn that, for 45-year-old males, a total serum cholesterol value of 200 mg/dL is close to the 50th percentile, and a value of 240 mg/dL is equivalent to the 75th percentile. Accordingly, the patient falls generally in the upper half of the population distribution of total serum cholesterol values. Assuming that the measurement is correct, this could be a result of genetic factors, environmental factors, or both.

Variability in Research Studies

It is worthwhile to ask how the clinician would know that a total serum cholesterol value in the upper end of the population distribution is disadvantageous. Are these values really unhealthy? Answers may be found in studies that have linked the level of total serum cholesterol with an increased risk of cardiovascular mortality. In cohort studies like the Framingham Heart Study, groups of subjects were followed and compared according to their different levels of total serum cholesterol and the associated frequency of death from myocardial infarction or stroke. In these investigations, a higher level of total serum cholesterol was associated with an increased risk of death from cardiovascular disease.

When investigators perform such studies, they cannot usually study the entire population. Instead they study subsets or samples of the population. This introduces another source of variability—sampling variability—that is important in medical research. Using a single sample of subjects to represent the population is analogous to using a single measurement to characterize an individual. Repeated samples from the population will give different estimates of the true population values. Sampling variability is illustrated in Figure 10–2. In the source population of 20 persons, there are 5 individuals (25%) with total serum cholesterol values above 240 mg/dL. In the three different samples of 5 subjects drawn from the source population by chance, the proportion of individuals with total serum cholesterol values above 240 mg/dL ranges from 0–40%. Each of these small samples presents a different picture of the source population. A larger sample size would result in less variability and would more likely represent the source population.

Variability can be important in other ways when two groups are compared in a study. The goal of such studies often is to determine whether a measurable difference exists between the groups. When a research paper reports no statistically significant difference between groups, the reader must ask the following question: Was there no difference between the two treatments in truth, or was the estimate of effect so imprecise that the investigator could not distinguish differences between the two groups (ie, a type II error)?

Table 10–1. Levels of variability.

Levels	Features
Individual	Individual variability
	Measurement variability
Population	Genetic variability between individuals
	Environmental variability
	Measurement variability
Sample	Manner of sampling
	Size of sample
	Measurement variability

Table 10–2. Potential sources of variability in measurements of individuals.

Sources of Variability	Features
Individual characteristics	Diurnal variation
	Changes related to factors such as age, diet, and exercise
	Environmental factors such as season or temperature
Measurement characteristics	Poor calibration of the instrument
	Inherent lack of precision of the instrument
	Misreading or misrecording information from the instrument by the technician

A graphic display of the results of two hypothetical studies of the same question is presented in Figure 10–3. In each study, the investigators attempted to determine whether a cholesterol-lowering drug had a favorable effect on the risk of myocardial infarction. The measure of effect that was estimated in each study was the risk ratio. Each study compared a group of patients randomly allocated to receive the cholesterol-lowering drug with a group chosen to receive dietary modification alone. The researchers reached different conclusions. In the study with the smaller sample, the report indicated that the drug had no beneficial effect on risk of myocardial infarction, when compared with diet therapy. In the study with the larger sample, the investigators concluded that the drug decreased the risk of myocardial infarction, when compared with dietary management.

As shown in Figure 10–3, Study A had a small sample size, which resulted in imprecise estimates (ie,

wide confidence intervals) of the risk of myocardial infarction in the two groups. Consequently, the two estimates overlapped, and the statistical test was not capable of distinguishing between the effects of the two treatments. The investigators concluded that there was no difference in risk of myocardial infarction between patients who received the cholesterol-lowering drug and those who received dietary therapy. In Study B, the investigator used a larger sample size yielding the same point estimates of risk in the two groups but with much more precision (ie, narrower confidence intervals) in the estimate of the effects of the drug. With this gain in precision, the statistical test was able to distinguish between the two groups, and the investigator was able to infer correctly that the cholesterol-lowering drug was superior to dietary therapy. Generally, the larger the sample size, the more precise the estimate of effect and the smaller the detectable differences between groups. In studies with very large sample sizes, small differences between groups may be judged to be statistically significant but have little biologic or clinical meaning. For example, a study of 20,000 subjects might have concluded that a 1% difference in risk of myocardial infarction was statistically significant. It is unlikely, however, that a difference in risk this small would justify prolonged use of the cholesterol-lowering agent.

VALIDITY

The concept of validity concerns the degree to which a measurement or study reaches a correct conclusion. A measurement or study may lead to an incorrect (invalid) conclusion because of the effects of **bias.** The variability seen with bias is systematic or nonrandom and distorts the estimated effect. In Figure 10–1, the amount of bias can be determined by the degree to which the shots are off target in D. Unfortunately, in medical research the truth (bulls-eye) may not be known, or there may no "gold standard" for comparison. Consequently, the degree of bias often is difficult to determine. Two different types of validity, internal validity and external validity, are described in this chapter.

Internal Validity

Internal validity is the extent to which the results of an investigation accurately reflect the true situation of

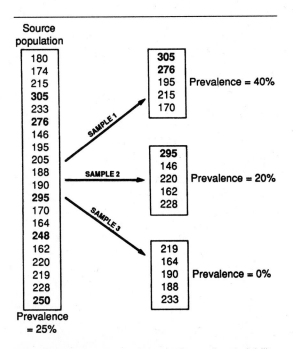

Source population

180	
174	
215	
305	
233	
276	
146	
195	
205	
188	
190	
295	
170	
164	
248	
162	
220	
219	
228	
250	

Prevalence = 25%

SAMPLE 1
| 305 |
| 276 |
| 195 | Prevalence = 40%
| 215 |
| 170 |

SAMPLE 2
| 295 |
| 146 |
| 220 | Prevalence = 20%
| 162 |
| 228 |

SAMPLE 3
| 219 |
| 164 |
| 190 | Prevalence = 0%
| 188 |
| 233 |

Figure 10–2. Schematic diagram of sampling variability. The source population of 20 persons has a 25% prevalence of hypercholesterolemia (elevated cholesterol values are presented in bold). Each of three random samples of 5 persons yields prevalence estimates ranging from 0–40%.

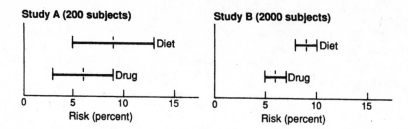

Figure 10–3. The effect of sample size on precision of risk estimates. Point estimates are shown as dashed vertical lines and 95% confidence intervals are shown as solid horizontal lines. In both studies, the 5-year risk of myocardial infarction was 9% among persons receiving dietary therapy and 6% among persons treated with a cholesterol-lowering drug. In the larger study, however, the 95% confidence intervals are narrower, and the difference in risk between treatment groups is statistically significant.

the study population. If the results are not valid in the study population, there is little reason to suspect that those results will apply to other populations. Internal validity is defined by the boundaries of the study itself. Therefore, a study is internally valid if it provides a true estimate of effect, given the limits of the population studied. Measures that can be used to improve internal validity often involve restricting the type of subjects and the environment in which the study is performed. These measures decrease the impact of factors extraneous to the question of interest.

External Validity

A result obtained in a tightly controlled environment, however, may not be applicable to more general situations. *External validity is the extent to which the results of a study are applicable to other populations.* External validity addresses the question: Do these results apply to other patients, such as patients who are older, sicker, or less economically advantaged than subjects in the study?

External validity often is of particular interest to clinicians who must decide if a research finding is applicable to their clinical practice. Determining whether the results of a study can be generalized involves a judgment regarding the following:

(1) The type of subjects included in the investigation.
(2) The type of patients seen by the clinician.
(3) Whether there are clinically meaningful differences between the study population and other populations.

An example of the kind of difficulty that can occur when study results are generalized is the criticism that too many clinical studies focus on white males. One such study is the Lipid Research Clinics-Primary Prevention Trial, which demonstrated a significant reduction in cardiovascular mortality for hypercholesterolemic white men aged 35–59 years who were placed on a cholesterol-lowering diet and medication. Do the results also apply to women, as well as to men

of different ages with or without lower, but still abnormal, cholesterol levels? This question has led to the suggestion that federally funded research should include women and minorities in the study populations.

Bias

Bias is a systematic error in a study that leads to a distortion of the results. Bias, a threat to validity, can occur in any research but is of particular concern in observational studies, because the lack of randomization increases the chance that study groups will differ with respect to important characteristics. Bias often is subdivided into different categories, based upon how bias enters the study. The most common classification divides bias into three categories:

(1) Selection bias.
(2) Information bias.
(3) Confounding.

Although these categories overlap, this classification is useful because it provides the reader with a systematic approach to evaluate bias. It should be remembered that—with the exception of confounding, which can be quantitated—the evaluation of bias is subjective and involves a judgment regarding the likelihood of (a) the presence of bias and (b) its direction and potential magnitude of effect on the results. Even though the magnitude of bias cannot be quantified, often its influence on the results of a study can be inferred. It is important to discern whether the suspected bias is likely to make an association appear stronger or weaker than it really is. Overestimation of a risk ratio for a protective exposure and a separate hazardous exposure is demonstrated schematically in Figure 10–4. Underestimation of a risk ratio for a protective exposure and a hazardous exposure is shown in Figure 10–5.

Selection Bias

A variety of procedures can be used to select subjects for a study. Usually, it is not possible to include all individuals with a particular disease or exposure in

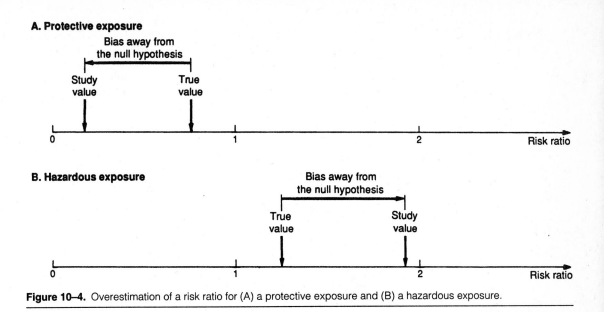

Figure 10–4. Overestimation of a risk ratio for (A) a protective exposure and (B) a hazardous exposure.

a study, so a sample of subjects must be chosen. The procedures used for the selection of subjects depend on a number of factors, including:

(1) The design of the investigation.
(2) The setting of the study.
(3) The disease and exposure of interest.

Often subjects are selected in a manner that is convenient for the investigator. Under optimal circumstances, the method for inclusion of subjects leads to a valid comparison that, in turn, yields correct informa-

tion regarding a disease process or treatment. The selection process itself, however, may increase or decrease the chance that a relationship between the exposure and disease of interest will be detected. A schematic diagram of the steps involved in recruiting and maintaining a study population is shown in Figure 10–6. From this diagram, it is easy to see that selection factors could lead to biased results at several different steps in the process.

Some aspects of the selection of subjects lead primarily to problems with the generalization (extrapolation) of the results (ie, external validity). Subjects must

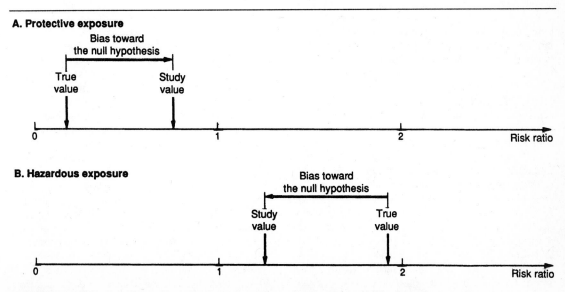

Figure 10–5. Underestimation of a risk ratio for (A) a protective exposure and (B) a hazardous exposure.

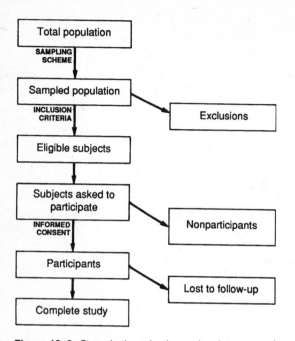

Figure 10–6. Steps in the selection and maintenance of subjects in a study.

agree to participate in a study, and this causes one of the most common problems. Volunteers for a study may differ from individuals who do not volunteer in various characteristics such as age, race, economic status, education level, and gender. Moreover, volunteers may be healthier than those who decline to participate. A study of a population limited to individuals who are employed may also make it difficult to generalize the results, since people who work are generally healthier than those who do not. A comparison of health outcomes between workers and the general population may show that the workers have a more favorable outcome simply because they are healthy enough to be employed (the "healthy worker" effect).

Referral of patients to clinical facilities also can lead to distorted study conclusions. Selective referral patterns can be seen in the study of children with febrile seizures. Febrile seizures are brief, generalized seizures that occur in conjunction with temperature elevation in children aged 6 months to 6 years. There is some disagreement about whether these febrile convulsions are predictive of future seizures and other unfavorable neurologic sequelae. Ellenberg and Nelson (1980) compared the results of a number of studies on the long-term outcome of patients with febrile seizures. Studies of geographically defined populations in which affected children were followed, regardless of whether medical care was sought, consistently revealed a relatively low rate of unfavorable sequelae. Clinic-based studies tended to report a high frequency of adverse outcomes. Accordingly, it was concluded that clinic-based studies selectively in-

cluded children at the more severe end of the clinical spectrum. The inferences that one might draw regarding the prognosis of a child with febrile seizures might be very different based upon whether a clinic-based or population-based sample was studied.

Other aspects of the selection process can diminish internal validity. *In a clinical trial or cohort study, the major potential selection bias is loss to follow-up.* Once subjects are enrolled in the study, they may decide to discontinue participation. Certain types of subjects are more likely than others to drop out of a study. Furthermore, during the course of the study some subjects may die from causes other than the outcome of interest. At first glance, these losses may not appear to be related to selection because the subject already was enrolled in the study. If the lost subjects differ, however, in their risk of the outcome of interest, biased estimates of risk may be obtained.

If the unrecognized early manifestations of the disease of interest cause exposed persons to leave the study more or less frequently than unexposed persons, a distorted conclusion might be reached. For example, in a randomized controlled trial of the effects of a cholesterol-lowering drug vs diet on prevention of myocardial infarctions, bias might be introduced if drug-treated patients with coronary insufficiency were more likely to develop side effects from treatment and withdrew from participation, while patients with coronary insufficiency receiving dietary therapy remained in the study.

Selection bias is of particular importance in case-control studies (see Chapter 9) where the investigator must select two study groups, cases and controls, in a setting in which the exposure has already occurred. For example, it must be decided whether to use existing (prevalent) cases who are available at the time of study, regardless of the duration of their disease, or to limit eligibility to newly diagnosed (incident) cases. If the risk factor of interest also is a prognostic factor, the use of prevalent cases can lead to a biased conclusion. Consider, eg, a case-control study of total serum cholesterol as a risk factor for myocardial infarction. Suppose that myocardial infarction patients with very high total serum cholesterol levels are more likely than those with lower cholesterol levels to die suddenly. Under these circumstances, a comparison of surviving myocardial infarction patients against controls will underestimate the true association between total serum cholesterol elevation and risk of myocardial infarction.

Another potential type of selection bias can occur when a case-control study involves subjects who are hospitalized. Patients with two medical conditions are more likely to be hospitalized than those with a single disease. Thus, a hospital-based case-control study might find a link between two diseases or between an exposure and a disease, when there is no association between them in the general population. This type of bias, often called Berkson's bias, was demonstrated in a study that showed that respiratory and bone diseases were associated in a sample of hospitalized patients but not in the general population. Thus, in a hospital-based study, an exposure such as cigarette smoking, which is correlated with respiratory disease, may also appear to occur together with bone disease because those diseases are related in hospitalized patients.

Information Bias

Information (or misclassification) bias can occur when there is random or systematic inaccuracy in measurement. This can be visualized best in epidemiological studies that involve dichotomous exposure and disease variables, such as elevated total serum cholesterol and myocardial infarction. Subjects are classified according to whether they have had high cholesterol and whether they have had a myocardial infarction. The investigator either can be correct or incorrect, resulting in true-positive and true-negative findings, as well as false-positive and false-negative classifications of subjects with respect to either exposure or disease.

If the errors in classification of exposure or disease status are independent of the level of the other variable, then the misclassification is termed nondifferential. Nondifferential misclassification may occur in a case-control study, if the subject's memory of exposure status is unrelated to whether the subject has the disease of interest. An example of nondifferential misclassification is sometimes referred to as unacceptability bias. Subjects may answer a question about the exposure with a socially acceptable but sometimes inaccurate response, regardless of whether they have the disease of interest. Consider a case-control study of myocardial infarction in which the exposure of interest is prior intake of foods high in saturated fats. Regardless of disease status, respondents may underreport intake of foods with high fat content because they think low-fat diets are more acceptable to the investigator. In most instances, when nondifferential misclassification occurs, it blurs differences between the study groups, making it more difficult for the investigator to detect an association between the exposure and the disease. This is often referred to as a bias toward the null hypothesis or toward no association.

Differential misclassification occurs when the misclassification of one variable depends upon the status of the other. In a case-control study, this type of misclassification could occur if the information on exposure status depends on whether the subject has the disease. If a case with a myocardial infarction is more likely to overestimate the level of dietary fat intake than a control subject, then a biased result may occur. In this instance, the bias would lead to an overestimate of the relationship between dietary fat intake and myocardial infarction.

The difference between nondifferential and differential misclassification can be demonstrated by examining the data in Figure 10–7. Consider a case-control study of the relationship between high-fat diets and myocardial infarction in which the true odds ratio (OR) is 2.3. With nondifferential misclassification, the subjects did not recall the amount of fatty foods eaten,

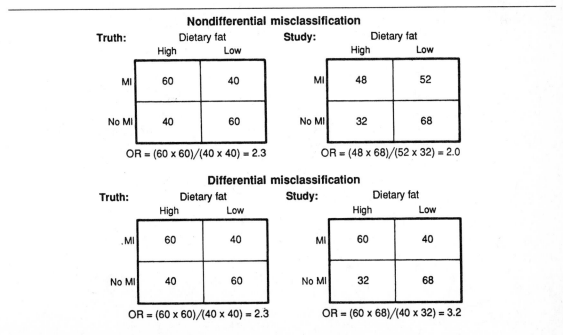

Figure 10–7. Illustration of nondifferential and differential misclassification of exposure to high-fat diets in a case-control study of myocardial infarction (MI). (OR = odds ratio.)

but the errors in recall did not depend upon whether they had a myocardial infarction. In this situation, 20% of both cases and controls who ate high-fat diets underreported fat intake. The resulting OR of 2.0 was an underestimate of the true OR. On the other hand, if all the myocardial infarction patients correctly recalled their dietary fat exposure status, but only 80% of the exposed controls correctly reported their exposure, then differential misclassification would occur. This type of misclassification can result in either an underestimate or overestimate of the true OR. In this example, the investigator overestimated the OR.

Two common types of differential information bias are often referred to as **recall bias** and **interviewer bias.** Recall bias results from differential ability of subjects to remember previous activities and exposures. Patients who have a serious disease may search their memory for an exposure in an attempt to explain or to understand why they acquired the illness. Control subjects, who do not have the disease, may be less likely to remember an exposure because it has less meaning and is less important for them.

When interviewers are employed to determine exposures in case-control studies, results may be influenced by how the interviewers collect information. If they are aware of the research hypothesis, the interviewers intentionally or unintentionally may influence the responses of the subjects. They may probe more deeply for responses from cases than from controls. If a dietary exposure is examined, the interviewers may ask certain subjects specific questions about particular food items. Interviewers may also give the subjects subtle clues by tone of voice or body language that suggest a preference for certain responses. Generally, it is desirable to blind the interviewers to the research hypothesis under investigation. In a case-control study, however, it may be difficult to blind the interviewers to the disease status of cases and controls. Nevertheless, if the interviewers are not aware of the exposure of primary interest, biased data collection still can be minimized.

As a way to reduce misclassification and to improve accuracy of study measurements, investigators increasingly are using **biologic markers.** As shown in Table 10–3, these markers can measure many facets of

disease and exposure—or the relationship between the two. For example, biologic markers can measure:

(1) Susceptibility (biologic markers can be used to identify subjects with particularly high risk due to a particular biologic predisposition).
(2) Internal dose (biologic markers can be used to measure the amount of a chemical or other exposure in the body).
(3) Biologically effective dose (biologic markers can be used to measure the amount of a substance that reaches the target sites).
(4) Biologic effect (biologic markers can be used to quantify a deleterious effect of a particular exposure).

Biologic markers find use in most substantive areas of investigation, including nutritional, cardiovascular, reproductive, cancer, and infectious disease epidemiology.

Use of biologic markers is important in observational studies for several reasons. These markers are important methodologically because they can serve to reduce misclassification by allowing more accurate assessment of exposure or disease status. Furthermore, they may allow the investigator to define more homogeneous disease categories or to identify susceptible subjects, so that the study can focus on specific subgroups. Finally, biologic markers can help to provide insights into the underlying disease process and pathogenesis.

The use of serum dioxin levels to measure exposure of men who worked with the herbicide, Agent Orange, during the Vietnam War illustrates the use of a biologic marker to measure internal dose. After the Vietnam War, concern arose about wartime exposures of servicemen to Agent Orange, in part because of its contamination with the highly toxic trace contaminant known as 2,3,7,8 tetrachloro-dibenz-p-dioxin (TCDD). Because of this concern, Air Force researchers began epidemiologic studies to assess the health effects among Air Force veterans associated with exposure to Agent Orange and TCDD. Researchers initially used job descriptions to classify exposure to TCDD. Later, after laboratory techniques became available to mea-

Table 10–3. Uses of biologic markers in epidemiology.

Application of Marker	Example
To measure susceptibility	Those with high **aryl hydrocarbon hydoxylase** activity have higher risk of bladder cancer
To measure internal dose	Those with high **serum carotene levels** may have lower risk of lung cancer
To measure biologically effective dose	Those with greater amounts of effective dose of **polycyclic aromatic hydrocarbon-DNA adducts** have experienced greater exposure and interaction of their DNA to these carcinogenic hydrocarbons[1]
To measure biologic effect	Higher levels of the *ras* **oncogene product** may be a preclinical marker of early carcinogenic response[1]

[1]Perera F et al: Biologic markers in risk assessment for environmental carcinogens. Environ Health Persp 1991;**90**:247.

sure TCDD in minute concentrations within the blood, the researchers discovered that classification of exposure based on job descriptions was associated with substantial misclassification. In subsequent studies, the more accurate serum TCDD measurements were used to assess exposures.

Despite the importance of biologic markers and the possibility that their use may reduce information bias, they do not eliminate the possibility of systematic errors. Although it may be diminished by employing a biologic marker, misclassification remains a possibility. For example, marker instability and inter- or intra-individual variability can contribute to measurement errors. Moreover, if required biologic specimens are collected after disease occurrence, as often happens in case-control studies, the presence of disease in cases may affect the biologic marker. This possibility can make the biologic marker particularly susceptible to differential misclassification and measurement error. Bias can even be created if the investigator adjusts inappropriately for a factor that is caused by the exposure of interest and is associated with the outcome.

Case-control studies of β-carotene and cancer illustrate the potential for residual information bias. β-carotene is a fat-soluble antioxidant found in many fruits and vegetables. It acts as a provitamin (vitamin A), protects against cancer in animals, and is suspected of reducing cancer risk in humans. In a case-control study of serum levels of this antioxidant, differential misclassification could create or accentuate a protective effect, if cases with advanced cancer had altered nutritional status and a resulting lowering of β-carotene levels. Although these biases are somewhat speculative, the potential for bias in case-control studies is evident.

Thus, use of biologic markers offers many advantages, particularly improved assessment of exposure and more homogeneous definition of disease. Nevertheless, because use of these markers does not eliminate the possibility of information bias, caution in interpretation still is warranted.

Confounding

Confounding refers to the mixing of the effect of an extraneous variable with the effects of the exposure and disease of interest. Confounding can be demonstrated by the following hypothetical example. Suppose investigators undertake a case-control study of the association between high total serum cholesterol level and myocardial infarction. From the results of other studies, the researchers know that the risk of myocardial infarction is associated with obesity, and that total cholesterol levels also correlate with obesity (see Figure 10–8). Suppose that in our hypothetical case-control study, 36 of 60 patients with myocardial infarction (60%) are found to have high total cholesterol levels, and only 24 of 60 controls (40%) are discovered to have elevated cholesterol levels. This would suggest that elevated total cholesterol levels are associated with an increased risk of myocardial infarction.

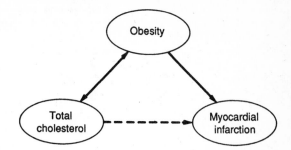

Figure 10–8. Schematic diagram of the relationship between total serum cholesterol level and risk of myocardial infarction, with confounding by obesity.

When the observed association is examined separately in obese and nonobese persons, however, a different conclusion is reached. Among obese persons, 34 of 40 patients with myocardial infarction (85%) and 18 of 20 controls (90%) are found to have elevated total cholesterol levels. Among nonobese persons, 2 of 20 patients with myocardial infarction (10%) and 6 of 40 controls (15%) have high total cholesterol levels. Thus in the case of both obese and nonobese individuals, elevated total cholesterol levels are more common in controls than in patients with myocardial infarction. Keep in mind that in the hypothetical study, obesity was associated with myocardial infarction, since 52 of 60 obese subjects (87%) had elevated total cholesterol levels, and only 8 of 60 nonobese persons (13%) had high cholesterol levels. Clearly, in this hypothetical example, the results are confounded by the extraneous variable, obesity. The results are illustrated in Figure 10–9.

For a variable—in this case, obesity—to be considered a potential confounder, it must satisfy two conditions:

(1) Association with the disease of interest in the absence of exposure.
(2) Association with the exposure but not as a result of being exposed.

Since it can be evaluated in the analysis of results, confounding differs from selection bias and information bias. The presence of confounding is demonstrated by a change in the apparent strength of association between the exposure and the disease of interest, when the effects of extraneous variables are taken into account. Confounding, which is not an all-or-none property of an extraneous variable, may occur to different degrees in different studies.

Generally, the list of potential confounders in a study is limited to established risk factors for the disease of interest. There are two accepted methods for dealing with potential confounders. The first is to consider them in the design of the study by matching on the potential confounder or by restricting the sample to

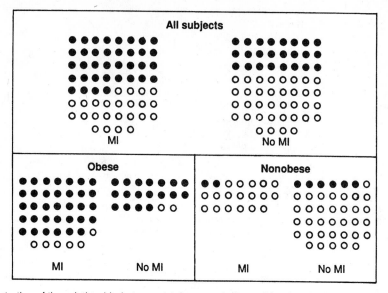

Figure 10–9. Illustration of the relationship between total serum cholesterol level and risk of myocardial infarction, with confounding by obesity. Shaded circles represent persons with elevated total serum cholesterol levels and unshaded circles represent persons with normal cholesterol levels.

limited levels of the potential confounder. The other method is to evaluate confounding in the analysis by stratification, as demonstrated schematically in Figure 10–9, or by using multivariate analysis techniques such as multiple logistic regression.

The goal of any epidemiologic study is to provide a valid conclusion. In order to accomplish this objective, complete attention must be given to all aspects of the study, from inception to design and data collection and, finally, to analysis and reporting of results. It is important to remember that bias can be introduced at any of these stages, leading to erroneous results. Thus, it is useful to look carefully for potential sources of bias and to consider their possible impact. Clinicians must judge whether results can be generalized to their particular practice. Understanding the potential problems with measurement and bias in medical research improves the physicians' ability to decide on appropriate preventive and therapeutic strategies.

SUMMARY

In this chapter, the topics of variability and systematic errors in epidemiologic measurements are discussed, with illustrative examples that focus primarily on the relationship between total serum cholesterol and the risk of myocardial infarction. A distinction is drawn between random variation, which is inversely related to precision in measurement, and nonrandom or systematic error, which is related to a distortion in measurement.

Variability can arise from (a) the subjects under study, (b) differences between individuals, (c) the approach used to sample subjects, or (d) the measurement process itself. Variability related to sampling is likely to diminish as the sample size increases. With extremely large sample sizes, a very small difference in outcome between study groups can be statistically significant. Whether the magnitude of this difference is sufficient to warrant a change in clinical practice is a separate, but equally important, question.

Validity concerns the extent to which the findings of a study reflect truth. **Internal validity** relates to the accuracy of study findings for the persons who are investigated. **External validity** concerns the extent to which study findings accurately apply to persons who are not studied.

Bias is defined as lack of validity. Conventionally, bias is classified into three major types: **selection bias, information (misclassification) bias,** and **confounding.** Selection bias refers to the introduction of systematic errors into study results through the manner in which study subjects are selected. Information bias results in systematic errors in study findings that originate in the approach to collecting information. Two kinds of information bias can exist. **Nondifferential misclassification** occurs when errors in the information about one variable are unrelated to the status of another variable. **Differential misclassification,** on the other hand, occurs when errors in the information about one variable are affected by the status of another variable.

Confounding is concerned with the mixing of the primary effect of interest with the effects of one or more extraneous factors. In experimental studies, the problem of confounding is reduced by randomization, which tends to balance the study groups with respect to known and unknown determinants of the outcome. In observational research, however, study groups may differ appreciably in factors that are (a) related to the risk of disease among unexposed persons and (b) are also associated with the exposure of interest. The influence of these potential confounders can be addressed in the study design (eg, through matching or restrictive inclusion criteria) or in the analysis (eg, through stratification or regression techniques). Only known confounders can be addressed in observational research.

No study is immune from the possibility of bias. The investigator must therefore consider potential sources of bias when sampling subjects, collecting information, analyzing results, and interpreting findings. With planning and forethought, it is possible to anticipate and avoid certain types of error and thus conduct a study that leads to a convincing and valid conclusion.

STUDY QUESTIONS

Questions 1–4: For each numbered situation below, select from the following lettered options the type of error that would most likely result. Each option can be used once, more than once, or not at all.

A. Selection bias
B. Nondifferential misclassification
C. Differential misclassification
D. Confounding
E. Ecologic fallacy
F. Random error

1. In a cohort study of hormone replacement therapy (HRT) and risk of atherosclerotic coronary artery disease (CAD), high income level is associated with both HRT use and risk of CAD.

2. In a case-control study of the relation between stressful daily events and asthmatic attacks, cases are more likely than controls to over-report the amount of stress.

3. In a cohort study of use of video display terminals (VDTs) and risk of carpal tunnel syndrome, the users of VDTs are more difficult to trace than non-users, resulting in a greater loss to follow-up of VDT users.

4. In a case-control study of beta carotene and risk of esophageal cancer, serum specimens frozen and

stored 20 years earlier are compared between cases and controls. Later it is found that the specimens deteriorated while in storage.

Questions 5–8: For each numbered situation below, select from the following lettered options the most likely effect on the study findings. Each option can be used once, more than once, or not at all.

A. Overestimation
B. Underestimation
C. No effect
D. Cannot be determined

5. In a case-control study of gestational infection as a risk factor for childhood leukemia, mothers of cases tend to give more false-positive reports of gestational infections.

6. Patients with a history of stroke within the past 10 years are enrolled in a case-control study of smoking as a risk factor for developing a stroke. Among stroke patients, the case-fatality is higher for smokers than non-smokers.

7. In a cohort study of baseline serum albumin and subsequent risk of death among patients with breast cancer, the measurement of albumin is performed without knowledge of the survival experience of individual patients.

8. In a cohort study of obesity and the risk of non-insulin dependent diabetes mellitus, the loss to follow-up is greater for obese versus non-obese persons.

Questions 9–10: For each numbered situation below, select from the following lettered options the most appropriate study design. Each option can be used once, more than once, or not at all.

A. Case-control study
B. Cohort study
C. Randomized clinical trial
D. Correlation study

9. Confounding is least likely to occur.

10. Exposure and disease can be associated across populations, without being linked within individual subjects.

FURTHER READING

Rosenbaum PR: Discussing hidden bias in observational studies. Ann Intern Med 1991;**115**:90.

REFERENCES

Byers T, Perry G: Dietary carotenes, vitamin C and vitamin E as protective antioxidants in human cancers. Annu Rev Nutr 1992;**12:**139.

Coates RJ et al: Cancer risk in relation to serum copper levels. Cancer Research 1989;**49:**4353.

Devesa SS, Silverman DT: Cancer incidence and mortality trends in the United States, 1935–1974. J Natl Cancer Inst 1978;**60:**545.

Ellenberg JH, Nelson KB: Sample selection and the natural history of disease: Studies of febrile seizures. JAMA 1980;**243:**1337.

Harris CC: Chemical and physical carcinogenesis: Advances and perspectives for the 1990s. Cancer Research 1991; **51(Suppl):**5023s.

Horwitz RI, Feinstein AR: Methodologic standards and contradictory results in case-control research. Am J Med 1979;**66:**556.

Hulka BS, Wilcosky TC, Griffith JD: *Biologic Markers in Epidemiology.* Oxford University Press, 1990.

Lipid Research Clinic Program: The Lipid Research Clinic's Coronary Primary Prevention Trial results. 1. Reduction in incidence of coronary heart disease. JAMA 1984;**251:**351.

National Heart, Lung and Blood Institute: *Recommendations for improving cholesterol measurements: A report from the laboratory standardization panel of the National Cholesterol Education Program.* US Department of Health and Human Services. NIH Publication No. 90-2964, 1990.

Perera FP: Molecular cancer epidemiology: A new tool in cancer prevention. J Nat Cancer Inst 1987;**78:**887.

Perera F et al: Biologic markers in risk assessment for environmental carcinogens. Environ Health Persp 1991;**90:** 247.

Report of the National Cholesterol Education Program Expert Panel on detection, evaluation and treatment of high blood cholesterol in adults. Arch Intern Med 1988;**148:**36.

Roberts RS, Spitzer WO, Delmore T et al: Empirical demonstration of Berkson's bias. J Chron Dis 1978;**31:**119.

Weinberg CR: Toward a clearer definition of confounding. Am J Epidemiol 1993;**137:**1.

Willett W: *Nutritional Epidemiology.* Oxford University Press, 1990.

Epidemiologic Studies of Genetics

11

PATIENT PROFILE

A 70-year-old retired car salesman is brought by his spouse of 50 years to their family physician for evaluation of "forgetfulness." Over the previous several years, the patient has had increasing difficulty with remembering recent events and with becoming lost when driving, even near his home. More recently, he has often forgotten names and has asked the same questions several times in succession. He is not taking any medications, nor is there any history of alcoholism, use of recreational drugs, exposure to toxins, high blood pressure, or stroke. The patient's family history is unremarkable, except for a similar course of progressive memory loss and cognitive disability in his mother and in the oldest of his three siblings.

The patient appears well-nourished, without evidence of systemic illness. On mental status examination, the patient does not know the year, cannot remember any of three objects 5 minutes after learning them, and cannot count backward from 100 by 7. Neurologic examination is otherwise normal. After magnetic resonance imaging and further tests to rule out specific, treatable causes of dementia, a diagnosis of Alzheimer's disease is made.

CLINICAL BACKGROUND

Dementia is characterized by impaired short- and long-term memory, along with disturbances of other cognitive functions. For a diagnosis of dementia to occur, the patient's loss of cognitive abilities must be global and of sufficient magnitude to interfere with the individual's performance of social or occupational activities. More than 60 different clinical disorders are associated with dementia, and Alzheimer's disease is the most common cause of dementia in many populations. This disease was first reported in 1907 by Alois Alzheimer, who described morphological changes in the brain of a patient who died with progressive dementia. The clinical diagnosis of Alzheimer's disease is made by excluding other possible causes of dementia, among which vascular disorders predominate.

The "gold standard" for arriving at a diagnosis of Alzheimer's disease is a histologic examination of brain tissue. Clinical diagnosis typically is rendered on the basis of the composite findings of (a) a careful history, (b) physical, neurologic, and psychiatric examinations, and (c) laboratory and radiologic assessments. When optimally applied, the standardized clinical diagnostic criteria for Alzheimer's disease can yield a positive predictive value of 85% or higher, when compared against eventual findings at autopsy.

Although signs and symptoms of Alzheimer's disease vary among patients, the onset of this disorder is typically insidious, and cognitive function deteriorates continuously over time. This form of dementia is rarely seen in patients under age 60, but thereafter the incidence rises markedly with age. Patients usually present with difficulties in new learning. With advancing disease over several years, patients also develop difficulty with attention, orientation, reasoning, and emotions.

Diagnostic imaging of the brain reveals generalized atrophy of the cerebral cortex with enlargement of the ventricles. Upon post-mortem examination, brains of patients with this disease are atrophied, especially in the neocortex. With microscopic examination of the gray matter, one can detect a loss of nerve cells and synapses, with abnormally staining neurons, neurofibrillary tangles, and neuritic plaques with a protein fragment, beta-amyloid, at their core. Beta-amyloid is an abnormal breakdown product of amyloid precursor protein, which is routinely produced by many cells, including neurons. A variety of neurochemical deficits occur in conjunction with Alzheimer's disease, the most prominent being a loss of cholinergic neurons as reflected by a decrease in choline acetyltransferase activity.

The etiology of Alzheimer's disease and its associated morphologic and biochemical abnormalities is unknown. Research to date has emphasized genetic predisposition, as well as environmental risk factors like head trauma and aluminum exposure, but findings have been inconsistent. Recent studies in genetics and genetic epidemiology point to several genes that appear to play a role in the etiology of Alzheimer's disease, including the gene that codes for apolipoprotein E.

The prognosis for patients with Alzheimer's disease is poor. Median survival from the time of diagnosis typically falls within the range of 5–8 years. Presently, no specific treatments prevent, arrest, or reverse the

145

clinical progression of the illness. For patients with Alzheimer's disease, some symptomatic relief can be achieved by addressing the neurochemical deficits. For example, the cholinesterase inhibitor, tacrine (tetra-hydroaminoacridine) has been shown to slow the loss of cognitive function in at least subsets of patients with Alzheimer's disease.

INTRODUCTION

Researchers often use epidemiologic techniques to study genetic risk factors and interactions between genetic susceptibility and environmental factors, an application known as **genetic epidemiology.** The field of genetic epidemiology concerns the study of hereditary and environmental determinants of disease in human populations. This application of epidemiology is growing rapidly, in parallel with gains in knowledge about the human genome. As illustrated by the Patient Profile, we can apply knowledge of genetic susceptibilities to identify high risk individuals and groups. For diseases in which screening tests and effective preventive or therapeutic regimens are available, knowledge of inherited risks can be used to enhance early detection and to encourage prevention programs.

Genetic epidemiology involves principles from the field of genetics as well as epidemiology. In particular, the design, conduct, and interpretation of genetic epidemiologic studies involves the same principles that apply to other kinds of epidemiologic research. For example, most genetic epidemiologic research involves a cohort or case-control design; but such a study differs from other epidemiologic research primarily in that one of the "exposures" is a genetic factor.

In genetic applications, as in other areas of inquiry, early investigation of disease etiology often involves study of the descriptive epidemiology of the disease. Results of descriptive studies provide information about disease frequency and public health importance. Such findings may suggest an etiologic role of specific genetic, environmental, or other risk factors, and further investigation may evaluate a putative role for inherited susceptibility. Since a hereditary predisposition would give rise to clusters of disease within families, the epidemiologist may conduct studies to ascertain the degree of familial aggregation. If results of such studies document familial aggregation and suggest that genetic factors contribute to disease occurrence, subsequent investigation might involve assessing the association of disease risk with specific markers, eg, a particular gene or gene product. Thus, genetic epidemiologic study of disease etiology frequently proceeds from

(1) general descriptive studies, as part of an initial search for clues about etiology,

(2) to studies of familial aggregation, as part of a search for evidence of clustering within families,

(3) to epidemiologic studies designed to assess risk associated with specific genetic factors. An additional step in investigation, one that is more an application of population genetics than of epidemiology, may involve more complex genetic analytic methods that look for evidence of genetic etiology within pedigrees.

The basic types of investigation used in genetic epidemiology are shown in Table 11–1, along with a description of the goals of such studies and some illustrative applications. These various approaches are characterized in greater detail in the following sections of this chapter. The text is organized in a sequence that parallels the order in which these investigations might be conducted to characterize the etiology of a disease. First descriptive studies are performed, followed by research on familial aggregation, then exploration of specific genetic traits. For completeness of presentation, complex genetic analyses are mentioned briefly at the conclusion of the chapter, although these methods are often considered part of the domain of population genetics. Throughout the chapter, illustrative examples are drawn from the literature on Alzheimer's disease.

DESCRIPTIVE EPIDEMIOLOGIC STUDIES

The health researcher can use descriptive studies to shed light on the public health importance of an illness and on possible roles of genetic and environmental factors in disease occurrence. In particular, basic char-

Table 11–1. Types of studies used to elucidate genetic influences on the risk of disease occurrence in human populations.

Type of Study	Goal	Example
Descriptive studies	Study non-specific factors, eg, age, gender, ethnicity	Higher occurrence of classic hemophilia in males
Studies of familial aggregation	Study recurrence risks, familial aggregation, influence of inbreeding	Higher risk of breast cancer among daughters of women with breast cancer
Studies of specific genetic factors	Study risk associated with specific genetic factors, eg, enzymes or DNA sequences	Higher risk of insulin dependent diabetes among those with certain human leukocyte antigens (HLAs)
Complex genetic analyses	Study pattern of risks within pedigrees	Higher risk of Alzheimer's disease in relative who shares alleles with a case

acteristics of person, time, and place—as discussed in Chapter 3—can provide clues to possible genetic and environmental risk factors.

Personal characteristics associated with variations in incidence can provide important information. Higher occurrence among certain ethnic or racial groups can suggest lifestyle, environmental, or possibly, genetic risk factors. Higher occurrence of a disease among males can suggest hormonal risk factors, lifestyle factors, or an X-linked genetic disease. For example, the rare occurrence among females of classic hemophilia, a deficiency of functional clotting factor VIII—coupled with the 50% risk among male offspring born to certain female carriers of this disease—points to an X-linked recessive inheritance.

Geographic and temporal variation in disease occurrence can also provide important information. In particular, environmental factors that vary in parallel with disease rates may play a causal role. For example, within the United States the North to South gradient of increasing mortality from malignant melanoma, a potentially lethal form of skin cancer, parallels the North to South gradient of rising exposure to ultraviolet radiation (UVR). This pattern supports the role of UVR as a cause of malignant melanoma. Genetic factors, if they vary in parallel with disease occurrence, also may be important.

Studies of migrants can provide information about the relative roles of genetic and environmental factors (see Chapter 3). For example, the incidence of prostate cancer is much lower in Japan than in the United States. First generation migrants from Japan to the U.S. also have relatively low incidence rates, but the rates increase successively in subsequent generations. Epidemiologists interpret this pattern as supporting a causal role for environmental exposures that change as successive generations acculturate to the lifestyle patterns of the adopted country. If prostate cancer occurrence were primarily influenced by genetics, then one would not expect to find a dramatic change in disease risk within a few generations.

Of course, discovery of an important role of nongenetic factors does not preclude the contribution of genetic factors and, conversely, discovery of an important role for genetic factors does not preclude a contribution from nongenetic factors. A very brief overview of the epidemiology and pathophysiology of phenylketonuria illustrates the importance of both genetic and environmental factors in this disease. Phenylketonuria is an autosomal recessive disorder in which those who inherit two recessive genes have altered metabolism of phenylalanine and, consequently, develop mental retardation. However, special diets low in phenylalanine can prevent mental retardation, if instituted early. This strongly suggests that genetic susceptibility and diet act jointly to cause mental retardation in this disorder.

Example 1. To investigate the descriptive epidemiology of Alzheimer's disease, researchers in East Boston conducted a survey of people aged 65 and over. After testing the memory and evaluating the neurologic condition of survey participants, the researchers estimated that about 10% of participants aged 65 or over probably had Alzheimer's disease. The prevalence increased with age to a high of nearly 50% among those over age 85. Moreover, more than 80% of the cases of moderate-to-severe cognitive impairment in this population were due to Alzheimer's disease. These results point out the overall high prevalence of Alzheimer's disease, its increasing prevalence with age, and its growing public health importance as the population ages. Other aspects of the descriptive epidemiology of Alzheimer's disesase, such as the low incidence in Native Americans, suggests that genetic differences by ethnicity may affect risk of Alzheimer's disease.

EPIDEMIOLOGIC STUDIES OF FAMILIAL AGGREGATION

Epidemiologists expect to see disease aggregate in families if susceptibility is, in part, genetically determined. However, disease also can aggregate in families because nongenetic risk factors cluster among relatives. A key measure of clustering or aggregation in families is the **recurrence risk,** ie, the risk of disease experienced by relatives of a subject with disease. Clustering or familial aggregation is suggested if the recurrence risk among relatives of a person with a disease exceeds that among relatives of a comparison subject without that disease. Put another way, clustering is suggested if a value >1 is found for the risk ratio that compares recurrence risk among those with an affected relative to the recurrence risk among those without an affected family member.

To study and quantify familial aggregation, epidemiologists often use cohort studies (Chapter 8) or case-control studies (Chapter 9). To study familial aggregation with a cohort design, the epidemiologist first identifies an index group of subjects with disease and a second index group of subjects without disease (Figure 11–1). The epidemiologist then assembles an "exposed" cohort consisting of the initially unaffected relatives of the index persons with disease and an "unexposed" cohort consisting of the initially unaffected relatives of the persons without disease. To simplify interpretation, the cohorts often consist of first degree relatives of those in the index groups. One then follows these two groups to determine subsequent disease occurrence and to calculate incidence rates and rate ratios in the usual way. The (incidence) rate ratio estimates the extent to which people with an affected family member have a rate of disease that differs from those without an affected family member. Accordingly, a rate ratio greater than unity suggests familial aggregation, whereas the absence of familial aggregation is indicated by a rate ratio of unity or less.

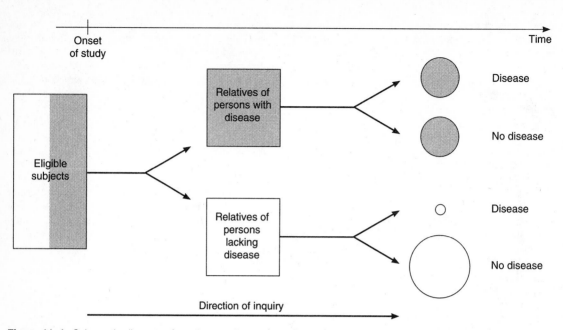

Figure 11–1. Schematic diagram of a cohort study to assess familial aggregation. Shaded areas represent "exposed" persons, ie, those who are initially unaffected family members of index persons with the disease. Unshaded areas represent "unexposed" persons, ie, those who are initially unaffected family members of persons without disease.

This approach is illustrated by a study of Alzheimer's disease conducted by Huff and colleagues: the exposed cohort consisted of siblings and parents of index cases who had Alzheimer's disease and the unexposed cohort consisted of corresponding relatives of subjects without Alzheimer's disease (see Figure 11–2). In this study, siblings and parents of patients with Alzheimer's disease had nearly a 50% lifetime risk of the illness, compared to a risk of about 10% among the corresponding relatives of comparison subjects. In other words, the lifetime risk of Alzheimer's disease was increased about fivefold (a risk ratio ie, of about 5), for family members of patients with Alzheimer's disease. The authors noted that their results were consistent with an autosomal dominant pattern of transmission, but that other factors, such as a shared environment, also could explain the familial aggregation they found. Example 2 further illustrates use of the cohort design to study familial aggregation.

Example 2. As noted in Example 1, the incidence of Alzheimer's disease varies across ethnic and racial groups. To study familial risk factors for Alzheimer's disease, Payami and coworkers studied risk of this disease among three groups: parents and siblings of patients with Alzheimer's disease, parents and siblings of healthy elderly controls, and parents and siblings of randomly identified controls. The healthy elderly controls underwent neurologic examination and magnetic-resonance imaging to ensure that they did not have dementia. The subjects and family members were interviewed to obtain histories of Alzheimer's disease and other dementia in relatives. The investigators

found the risk of dementia by age 90 to be .44 for relatives of Alzheimer's disease patients, .20 for relatives of randomly sampled controls, and .06 for relatives of healthy elderly controls. These observations demonstrate familial aggregation, and they are consistent with the presence in some families of genes that confer increased risk of Alzheimer's disease. The authors interpreted the lower risk of aggregation in relatives of healthy controls as possibly suggesting the presence of "protective" genes whose presence reduces risk.

Epidemiologists also use the case-control study design to study familial aggregation. The design of this type of case-control study is analogous to that discussed in Chapter 9, except that exposure is determined by family history—ie, the epidemiologist defines subjects who have one or more affected relatives to be "exposed" and subjects who do not have an affected relative to be "unexposed" (Figure 11–3). One calculates the odds ratio from this case-control study in the usual way. In this context, the odds ratio is the odds of having an affected family member among persons with the disease, divided by the odds of having an affected family member among persons without the disease. Under appropriate circumstances, as outlined in Chapter 9, the odds ratio approximates the risk ratio—the risk of disease among those with an affected family member, divided by the corresponding risk among those without an affected family member. Of course, odds ratios greater than one support familial aggregation. Interpretation can be difficult unless one specifies which relatives—and how many of them—to use in determining family history. For purposes of

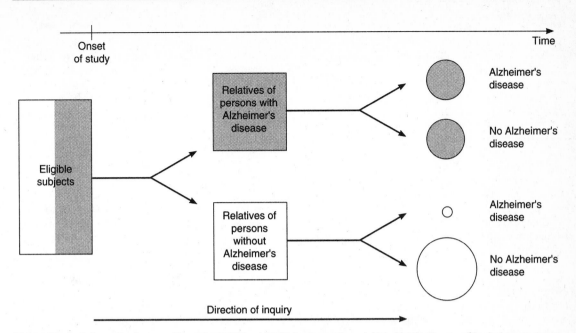

Figure 11–2. Schematic diagram of a cohort study of familial aggregation of Alzheimer's disease. Shaded areas represent "exposed" persons, ie, those who are initially unaffected family members of patients with Alzheimer's disease. Unshaded areas represent "unexposed" persons, ie, those who are initially unaffected family members of persons without Alzheimer's disease.

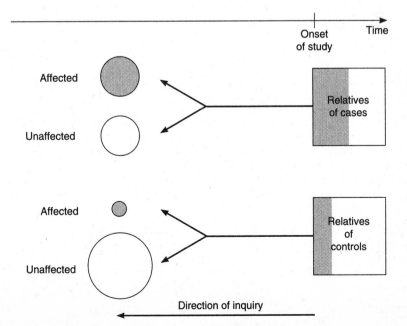

Figure 11–3. Schematic diagram of a case-control study of familial aggregation. Shaded areas represent "exposed" persons, ie, those who are affected relatives of study subjects. Unshaded areas represent "unexposed" persons, ie, those who are unaffected relatives of study subjects.

simplicity, limiting the relatives of interest to the parents of each subject avoids the problem of any systematic differences in the average family sizes of cases and controls.

Case-control and cohort studies can provide useful information by documenting the presence and quantifying the degree of familial aggregation. These studies also may identify factors that create the aggregation by evaluating and assessing the roles of specific nongenetic risk factors. For example, in estimating recurrence risk for breast cancer among those with an affected relative, many other nongenetic exposures, such as diet and reproductive history, may be assessed as well.

Documentation and quantification of familial aggregation using the case-control or cohort study provides important information and may suggest a genetic etiology. Further studies of familial aggregation may assess the pattern of disease occurrence within the family in order to separate the relative roles of genetic and nongenetic factors. We consider two such studies—twin studies and inbreeding studies.

Twin studies can provide useful information about the role of possible genetic and environmental risk factors by comparing the pattern of risk among dizygotic (fraternal) twins with that among monozygotic (identical) twins. Monozygotic twins have identical genetic constitutions, whereas dizygotic twins have no more genetic similarity than do siblings. Accordingly, a pattern in which monozygotic twins have greater concordance for disease than do dizygotic twins suggests genetically determined susceptibility. For example, twin

studies of this type have provided evidence for genetic inheritance of Alzheimer's disease. In one such study, researchers identified 20 patients with Alzheimer's disease who had a twin. Among the 12 patients who had a monozygotic twin, 4 of their co-twins had Alzheimer's disease, whereas among the 8 patients with a dizygotic twin, none of their co-twins had Alzheimer's disease (Figure 11–4). The greater concordance among monozygotic vs dizygotic twins suggests an underlying genetic predisposition to Alzheimer's disease.

In another type of twin study design, researchers study genetic and environmental factors by comparing disease concordance among twins reared together with that among twins reared apart. In this type of study, a pattern of disease risk in which twins reared together have greater concordance for disease than twins reared apart suggests the importance of nongenetic factors, including social and environmental influences.

Studies of the association of inbreeding with disease risk, so called **inbreeding studies,** also provide clues about the causes of familial aggregation. Since consanguineous marriages and the resulting inbreeding increase the risk of autosomal recessive disorders, the epidemiologist can use these studies to assess whether familial aggregation reflects an autosomal recessive pattern of inheritance. Briefly, in these studies the exposure of interest is the degree of inbreeding that measures the likelihood that a subject has inherited two copies of the same allele from a single ancestor. If subjects with a higher degree of inbreeding also have

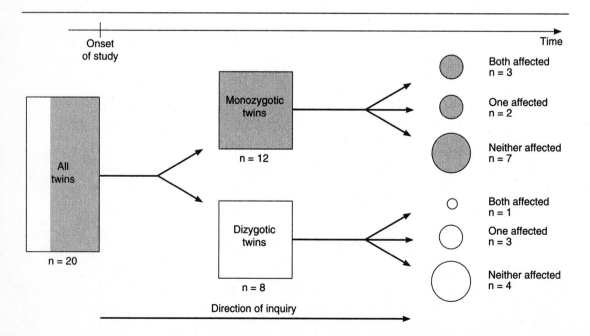

Figure 11–4. Schematic diagram of a study of concordance for Alzheimer's disease among monozygotic and dizygotic twins.

higher disease risk, autosomal recessive disease inheritance may be suggested.

EPIDEMIOLOGIC STUDIES OF SPECIFIC GENETIC FACTORS

The descriptive studies and the studies of familial aggregation considered so far can provide useful, but indirect, information about possible genetic and environmental causes of disease. If these studies suggest that the disease has, at least in part, a hereditary basis, further research can focus on the risks associated with specific genetic factors like enzymes, receptors, or structural proteins. The following sections present a direct and an indirect approach to studying the association of disease with specific genetic factors.

To understand both the direct and indirect approach, as well as the more complex genetic linkage analyses, we must first understand genetic **linkage.** Linkage between one gene and another arises because alleles that are closely situated on the same chromosome tend to be passed together as a group to offspring. Thus, if a subject inherits a particular allele, he or she will tend to also inherit other alleles present nearby on the same chromosome, a situation termed **cosegregation.**

At the population level, recombination or crossing over between genes tends to eliminate or reduce imbalances due to genetic linkage. This recombination tends to create an equilibrium in which the frequency with which two alleles (at different genes) occur together is simply the product of the frequencies with which each allele occurs in the population. Nevertheless, for some gene pairs an excess or deficiency of certain combinations of alleles occurs, a situation termed **linkage disequilibrium.** Such linkage disequilibrium can be present if a mutation (ie, a new allele) has arisen recently in a population, or if certain combinations of alleles at the two loci confer a survival advantage over other combinations.

The Direct Approach

With the direct approach, the researcher directly studies the possible increase in risk associated with a specific factor, such as an alteration in the DNA sequence or variations in enzyme activity. Using a cohort study, the researcher compares the risk among those with a specific variation in the DNA sequence or enzyme activity to that among a similar group without that variant (Figure 11–5). Following the principles outlined in Chapter 8 for cohort studies and defining the "exposure" to be those with a particular genetic trait, the researcher follows two groups of subjects— one with the genetic variant and the other without the variant—and then determines subsequent disease occurrence. The investigator then calculates risks for each group, as well as the risk ratio that measures the increase (or decrease) in risk associated with the genetic variant. As in other cohort studies, subjects should be free of disease at the start of follow-up and should be comparable except for the genetic variant of interest.

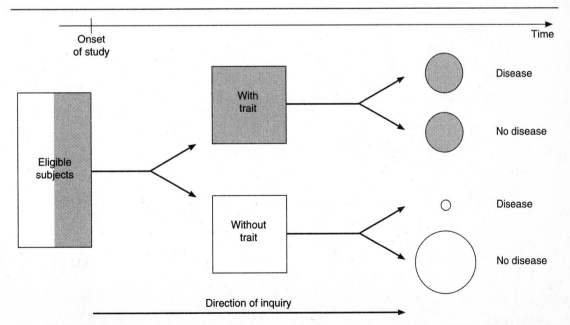

Figure 11–5. Schematic diagram of a cohort study of a specific genetic factor and risk of a particular disease. Shaded areas represent "exposed" persons, ie, those with the specific genetic factor of interest. Unshaded areas represent "unexposed" persons, ie, those who lack the specific genetic factor of interest.

Alternately, the researcher can use a case-control design to study the association between disease and a specific genetic factor. In this type of case-control study, the "exposure" is the genetic factor of interest (Figure 11–6). As in other types of case-control studies (Chapter 9), cases consist of people with the disease of interest, and investigators select controls from the source population, ie, the population which gave rise to the cases. After assembling the case and control groups, the researcher compares the frequency of the genetic factor of interest among the cases to the corresponding frequency among the controls. The odds ratio—the odds of the genetic trait among cases, divided by the odds of the trait among controls—provides an approximation to the risk ratio, as described in Chapter 9. If cases have an elevated frequency of the genetic trait, the researcher must consider the possibility that this excess could be secondary to the disease itself or its treatment, rather than a cause of the disease. This possibility could occur, eg, in a study of the association between a particular mutation and leukemia risk if the mutation was measured in blood obtained from cases after chemotherapy, since certain chemotherapeutic agents are known to be mutagens.

As with other types of epidemiologic studies, the researcher must exercise care in interpreting results of genetic epidemiologic investigations. He or she must consider the possibility of selection bias, confounding, and misclassification in the interpretation of genetic epidemiologic findings, since those biases can affect genetic epidemiologic results just as they can affect other types of research. The possibility of selection bias must be considered, particularly in case-control studies, if controls are not selected from the source population that gave rise to the cases. The possibility of confounding must be considered, particularly by factors such as race and ethnicity, since these factors relate to risks for many types of disease and also can be linked with genetic markers.

Another important consideration arises in interpreting studies of the association between disease risk and a specific DNA alteration, as measured by a marker allele. This kind of study is typified by studies of the association between insulin dependent (Type I) diabetes mellitus and certain human leukocyte antigens (HLA). These studies have documented an increased risk of diabetes mellitus in association with the presence of the HLA DR3 allele. It is possible, however, that it is not the HLA DR3 allele per se, but rather some companion alteration at a nearby genetic locus, that is responsible for increasing the risk of diabetes mellitus. This phenomenon can arise if non-causal marker alleles at one genetic locus are in **linkage disequilibrium** with alleles at the causal genetic locus. If linkage disequilibrium is present, an association between disease risk and the marker may reflect linkage disequilibrium between the marker and the gene that confers disease susceptibility—and not a causal association between the marker itself and disease risk. Nevertheless, direct evidence of increased risk in association

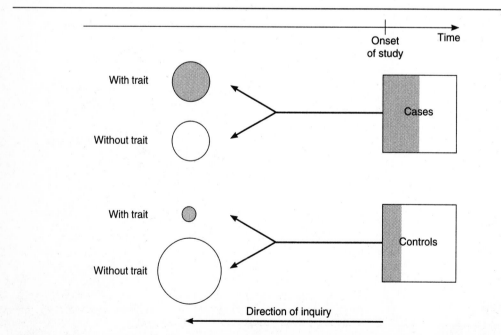

Figure 11–6. Schematic diagram of a case-control study of a specific genetic factor and risk of a particular disease. Shaded areas represent "exposed" persons, ie, those with the specific genetic factor of interest. Unshaded areas represent "unexposed" persons, ie, those lacking the specific genetic factor of interest.

with a marker allele, if valid, suggests that the marker allele or another allele linked to it relates to disease susceptibility.

Finally, it should be noted that consideration of possible gene-environment interactions is important. For example, failure to account for important environmental factors in the design or the analysis of the study can lead to an underestimate of the influence of a genetic factor. The genetic characteristic of interest may contribute to disease risk only in the presence of some environmental trigger. Accordingly, failure to account for a critical environmental trigger may obscure the role of an underlying genetic susceptibility.

The Indirect Approach

With the indirect approach, the researcher also looks for evidence of an association with a genetic factor. The indirect approach differs from the direct approach because for the genetic factor one uses a marker that may not be the same as the causal genetic factor itself. This approach depends on genetic **linkage** between the genetic marker and the disease susceptibility gene. Documentation of an association between the marker and disease risk provides evidence that a gene near the marker allele affects disease risk. Linkage analysis (a) provides information about the magnitude of risk association with a genetic marker, (b) identifies the chromosome that bears the susceptibility gene locus, and (c) provides information about the site on the chromosome of a disease susceptibility gene.

A straightforward epidemiologic approach to the study of linkage involves estimating recurrence risks in siblings of index subjects with a specific disease. For a particular marker locus, a sibling can share by descent either 0, 1, or 2 marker alleles with the case. If the marker locus is linked to a disease susceptibility locus, then a sibling who shares 2 alleles with the index case should have the highest chance of having the same disease susceptibility allele as the case—and hence the highest risk of disease. A sibling who shares 1 allele with the case should have an intermediate chance of having the same disease as the case, and a sibling who shares no alleles with the case should have the lowest chance of having the same disease susceptibility allele and hence the lowest risk of disease. If disease risk in siblings parallels the number of alleles shared with the case, the data suggest the presence of a disease susceptibility gene near the marker gene on the same chromosome. This type of study, sometimes called **sib-pair analysis,** is a simple example of genetic linkage analysis.

In more complex applications of genetic linkage analyses, the geneticist measures a genetic marker among a group of family members that is not restricted to siblings. If subjects who share the genetic marker, such as a particular allele, also tend to be concordant for disease occurrence, then the disease susceptibility gene may be located on the same chromosome near the marker allele. As with sib-pair analyses, these more

complex linkage analyses rest upon the rationale that, if the measured genetic marker is located near the disease susceptibility allele, the marker allele and the susceptibility allele will tend to be passed together, ie, to cosegregate. Cosegregation of the marker allele and the disease susceptibility allele will then create concordance between disease occurrence and presence of the genetic marker. Example 4 illustrates linkage study.

Example 3. To study the role of apolipoprotein E (Apo E), a specific genetic factor suspected of playing a role in the causation of Alzheimer's disease, Tsai and coworkers conducted a case-control study. They obtained blood from 77 cases with Alzheimer's disease and 77 matched controls, then determined the presence of three isoforms of Apo E—denoted e2, e3, and e4. About 35% of the cases had the e4 allele, compared with 13% of controls. The results support the role of Apo E as a risk factor for Alzheimer's disease. Although the mechanism remains uncertain, results of other studies suggest that Apo E may bind to β-amyloid and change it to a neurotoxic form.

Example 4. To help in the search for possible genetic factors associated with Alzheimer's disease, Schellenberg and colleagues conducted linkage analyses in a series of 14 families, each of which had at least 3 members with Alzheimer's disease in at least 2 generations. Using several markers for loci on chromosome 14, the investigators found that, within some families with early onset Alzheimer's disease, members who shared the same markers tended to be concordant for Alzheimer's disease. The evidence suggested that a gene on chromosome 14 codes for susceptibility to early onset Alzheimer's disease. If so, this would be a separate locus from the one coding for apolipoprotein E, since the Apo E gene is located on chromosome 19.

COMPLEX GENETIC ANALYSES

To study the possibility of genetic inheritance, the researcher also can apply methods from population genetics. In this section, a commonly used, powerful approach called **segregation analysis** is presented.

Briefly, segregation analysis is a complex statistical technique that geneticists use to study the pattern of disease occurrence within pedigrees. The goal of segregation analyses is (a) to provide evidence that a particular disease has, at least in part, a genetic origin and (b) to suggest the mode of inheritance. On the other hand, segregation analysis does not evaluate the role of specific genetic factors or markers. With segregation analyses, the geneticist attempts to identify which, if any, type of genetic inheritance, (eg, autosomal dominant, autosomal recessive, or multifactorial) is most consistent with the pattern of disease occurrence seen within families. Segregation analysis rests upon the rationale that disease within a family will tend to occur in different patterns for different modes of inheritance. For example, an autosomal dominant pattern of inheritance is suggested when the following types of pedigrees predominate:

- one-half of the offspring affected from marriages where only one parent has the disease,
- three-fourths of the offspring affected from marriages where both parents have the disease, and
- none of the offspring affected from marriages where neither parent has the disease.

In contrast, autosomal recessive or multifactorial patterns of inheritance will result in other characteristic patterns of disease occurrence within pedigrees.

In population studies, diseases do not tend to occur in such idealized patterns following the classical risks associated with the modes of inheritance. Segregation analysis provides a probabilistic method to assess the statistical consistency of the observed pattern of disease with the hypothesized mode of genetic inheritance.

SUMMARY

In this chapter, an overview of genetic epidemiology was presented. The field of genetic epidemiology uses the same basic principles of study design and analysis as other areas of epidemiology. Researchers in genetic epidemiology conduct three basic types of studies: descriptive studies, studies of familial aggregation, and studies of specific genetic markers. Each type of study typically involves a case-control or cohort design and differs from other types of epidemiologic studies primarily because the "exposure" of primary interest is a genetic factor.

In the initial phase of studying disease etiology, the researcher may use descriptive studies to look for characteristics that suggest genetic and nongenetic etiologies of disease—eg, person, place, and time. In a second phase, one may study familial aggregation to look for evidence of increased recurrence risks in relatives of cases and to look for further etiologic clues. Finally, one may study specific genetic characteristics, such as gene markers or products, as well as gene-environment interactions. The researcher also may apply some of the more complex analytic methods derived from population genetics, such as segregation or linkage analyses, to study patterns of genetic inheritance.

STUDY QUESTIONS

Questions 1–5: For each approach to the study of genetic factors in relation to the occurrence of a newly recognized disease, select the appropriate study design from the following lettered options. Each option can be used once, more than once, or not at all.

  A. Case-control study
  B. Inbreeding study
  C. Cohort study
  D. Migrant study
  E. Twin study
  F. Descriptive study
  G. Segregation study

1. A large population is surveyed to determine the prevalence of this newly recognized disease by age, gender, and ethnicity.

2. Concordance of the disease in twins reared together is compared with the risk among those reared apart.

3. The risk in first degree relatives of people with the disease is compared with that among first degree relatives of people without the disease.

4. The proportion of people with the disease whose father has the disease is compared with the corresponding proportion for people without the disease.

5. The pattern of disease among several large pedigrees is analyzed statistically.

Questions 6–10: The following statements refer to a case-control study designed to determine whether various serum proteins are risk factors for a certain neurologic disease. For each numbered statement, select the most appropriate bias from the following lettered options. Each option can be used once, more than once, or not at all.

  A. Reversal of causal sequence
  B. Confounding
  C. Ecologic fallacy
  D. Misclassification
  E. Linkage disequilibrium
  F. Selection bias

6. The cases are identified from an outpatient neurology clinic, and the controls are sampled from a chronic care facility.

7. After results are reported, the laboratory determines that the reagents for measuring one of the proteins had expired.

8. A drug used to treat the disease can alter levels of one of the measured proteins.

9. A particular isozyme of one of the measured proteins occurs more commonly in association with particular isozymes of a different (unmeasured) protein. Both proteins are encoded by genes on chromosome 2.

10. Cigarette smoking is associated with one of the serum proteins and also with the occurrence of the disease.

FURTHER READING

Breitner J: Clinical genetics and genetic counseling. Ann Int Med 1991;**115:**601.

Khoury MJ, Beaty TH, Cohen BH. *Fundamentals of Genetic Epidemiology.* Oxford University Press, 1993.

REFERENCES

Clinical Background
Breteler MMB et al: Epidemiology of Alzheimer's disease. Epidemiol Rev 1992;**14:**59.

Larson EB et al: Cognitive impairment: Dementia and Alzheimer's disease. Annu Rev Publ Health 1992;**13:**431.

Descriptive Epidemiologic Studies
Evans DA et al: Prevalence of Alzheimer's disease in a community population of older persons: Higher than previously reported. JAMA 1989;**262:**2551.

Epidemiologic Studies of Familial Aggregation
Huff FJ et al: Risk of dementia in relatives of patients with Alzheimer's disease. Neurol 1988;**38:**786.

Payami H et al: Evidence for familial factors that protect against dementia and outweigh the effect of increasing age. Am J Hum Genet 1994;**54:**650.

Epidemiologic Studies of Specific Genetic Factors
Khoury MJ, Beaty TH: Applications of the case-control method in genetic epidemiology. Epidemiol Rev 1994;**16:**134.

Khoury MJ et al: Commentary: The affected sib-pair method in the context of an epidemiologic study design. Genet Epidemiol 1991;**8:**277.

Khoury MJ et al: Epidemiologic approaches to the use of DNA markers in the search for disease susceptibilty genes. Epidemiol Rev 1990;**12:**41.

Khoury MJ et al: Penetrance in the presence of genetic susceptibility to environmental factors. Am J Med Genet 1988;**29:**403.

Tsai MS et al: Apolipoprotein E: Risk factor for Alzheimer's Disease. Am J Hum Genet 1994;**54:**643.

Complex Genetic Analyses
Schellenberg GD et al: Genetic evidence for a familial Alzheimer's Disease locus on chromosome 14. Science 1992;**258:**668.

Clinical Decision-Making

12

PATIENT PROFILE

A 50-year-old man presented to his physician with a high fever and severe abdominal pain. This patient worked occasionally as a house painter, and although he reported heavy use of alcohol, he had been in generally good health. There was no history of exposure to toxic substances or intravenous drug use. Upon physical examination, the patient was jaundiced, and he had severe tenderness to palpation in the right upper quadrant of his abdomen. Laboratory examination revealed leukocytosis accompanied by elevations in the serum levels of bilirubin, alkaline phosphatase, and aspartate aminotransferase (SGOT). It was considered that the patient had either alcoholic hepatitis or cholangitis (inflammation of a bile duct). It is necessary to differentiate cholangitis, which requires surgery, from alcoholic hepatitis, in which surgery is contraindicated. In fact, the postoperative mortality for alcoholic hepatitis is very high. The issue for the medical decision-maker is to choose the alternative that will carry the greatest benefit for the patient with the lowest achievable risk.

CLINICAL BACKGROUND

Cholangitis, an infection of the biliary ductal system, classically presents with a triad of fever, jaundice, and pain in the right upper quadrant of the abdomen. The clinical illness arises in the presence of bacterial colonization of the bile in conjunction with biliary obstruction. Historically, the most common underlying cause of obstruction was blockage of the biliary tract by stones, although malignant strictures have become increasingly important contributors in recent years. The increased intraductal pressure resulting from obstruction produces bacterial reflux into the hepatic veins and perihepatic lymphatics, with subsequent bacterial spread into the circulating blood stream. The bacteria associated with cholangitis include *Escherichia coli*, *Klebsiella* species, and the enterococci, with a shift more recently to include *Enterobacter* and *Pseudomonas* species.

The clinical manifestations of cholangitis range from asymptomatic illness to severe toxic symptoms, including septic shock. Fever usually is present, typically accompanied by chills and jaundice, and often associated with abdominal pain as well. Laboratory examination usually reveals leukocytosis, with moderate elevation of bilirubin and liver enzymes, including alkaline phosphatase and the transaminases.

The clinical management of patients with cholangitis is adapted to the severity of the illness, with severely ill patients requiring intensive care and monitoring. General supportive care typically includes stopping oral intake, starting intravenous fluids, and initiating antibiotics. A small proportion of patients with more severe symptoms—and those who do not respond to initial therapy—may require emergency biliary decompression. For most patients with cholangitis, definitive surgical intervention is required to address the underlying biliary tract obstruction.

Alcoholic hepatitis is an inflammatory process that occurs in persons with long-term heavy alcohol consumption. As with cholangitis, the clinical severity of alcoholic hepatitis ranges widely from asymptomatic illness at one extreme, to severe incapacitating disease at the other extreme. Patients often experience loss of appetite, nausea and vomiting, weight loss, and malaise. Fever is present in about half of patients. The physical examination typically reveals jaundice and tender enlargement of the liver. With advanced disease, patients may present with abnormal fluid collections in the soft tissues (edema) or abdominal cavity (ascites), bleeding, or impaired central nervous system functioning.

The laboratory evaluation of patients with alcoholic hepatitis often reveals leukocytosis. Bilirubin levels can be elevated to varying extents, typically accompanied by abnormal levels of alkaline phosphatase and aspartate transaminase. To the extent that hepatic function is disordered, one may also observe prolonged prothrombin time, depressed levels of serum albumin, or elevation of blood ammonia. Microscopic examination of the liver reveals leukocytic infiltration, accompanied by degeneration and necrosis of hepatocytes. The damaged liver cells often include eosinophilic perinuclear material referred to as Mallory bodies or alcoholic hyaline.

The clinical management of patients with alcoholic hepatitis involves initial supportive therapy. The recommended regimen typically includes abstinence from further alcohol consumption, rest, and nutritional therapy. In addition, patients who present with severe complications, such as bleeding, ascites, or central nervous systems dysfunction, may require specific therapy directed at these disorders. Other therapeutic approaches have an uncertain benefit, including the use of corticosteroids, propylthiouracil, or colchicine.

CLINICAL DECISION-MAKING

The practicing physician is a problem solver whose clinical task is to maximize benefit to the patient by correctly diagnosing illness and instituting appropriate treatment. The problem-solving process in medicine involves:

(1) Collection and evaluation of diagnostic information.
(2) Formulation of diagnostic hypotheses.
(3) Consideration of alternative hypotheses.
(4) Appropriate use of an efficacious therapy or procedure.

This process is made difficult, in part, because of inherent uncertainty in the information both for diagnosis and for treatment. For example, information elicited from patients may be false, inconclusive, and of uncertain validity; signs often are not perfect indicators of the presence of specific diseases; and even laboratory and other diagnostic tests can yield misleading information—either false negative or false positive results. In addition, treatment modalities are far from perfect, and there always is uncertainty about how efficacious a therapy may be in an individual patient. This sea of uncertainty that bedevils the practice of medicine may be ameliorated, in part, by effective use and measurement of probabilities to assess the validity of diagnostic data and the efficacy of therapies, thus demonstrating that the practice of medicine is probabilistic—not deterministic—in nature.

An understanding of the derivation, calculation, and use of probabilities is important in making clinical decisions and, thus, is an important topic in clinical education. The subjects presented in this book have direct applicability to clinical decision-making. Although developed in populations, the concepts and measurements of disease frequency (incidence, prevalence, risk, and probability) have direct applicability to probability of disease in single patients. The sensitivity and specificity of information collected from the patient's history, the physical examination, and laboratory tests are probability measures that play a significant role in determining the diagnostic utility of the workup. In addition, the clinical trial assesses the efficacy of a therapy in terms of proportions of patients who benefit, so this probability of benefit derived from a population of patients can be used to predict the outcome of treatment in a single patient.

Formal decision analysis is an explicit process that utilizes information from epidemiologic and clinical studies to determine the preferred course of action when there are two or more alternative courses that could be followed—a frequent occurrence in medical practice. The process of formal decision analysis is, therefore, a powerful tool to assist in the process of making clinical decisions.

FORMAL DECISION ANALYSIS

Decision analysis is an explicit process that considers medical choices, medical outcomes, and the uncertainty in the clinical and test data used to make decisions. The process is explicit in that the medical alternatives present and the choices available in the management of a patient's care may be clearly specified and demonstrated to others: physicians, students and, with care, the patient. The elements in a formal decision analysis include:

(1) An underlying structure termed the decision tree (or decision diagram).
(2) The probabilities for uncertain events.
(3) The incorporation of test results.
(4) The medical outcomes of the alternative choices to be made.

Table 12–1 summarizes the considerations: the decision problem must be explicitly stated; the problem must be structured over time; the information about uncertainties and the value of outcomes must be characterized; and a preferred course of action must be demonstrated.

The important underlying structure of the process is the decision diagram or decision "tree" (Table 12–2). The diagram flows from left to right with choices being noted by boxes and probabilities by circles; out-

Table 12–1. Considerations for the analytic approach to decision-making.

I. Identify and set bounds for the decision problem:
  a. Identify alternative actions.
  b. Identify clinical information needed.
  c. Determine clinical states of the patient including possible outcomes of morbidity and mortality.
II. Structure the problem over time:
  a. Identify choices to be made.
  b. Identify uncertainties to be encountered.
  c. Identify possible outcomes.
  d. Draw a decision tree.
III. Characterize the information needed for the decision tree:
  a. Indicate probabilities for uncertain outcomes including risks and test characteristics.
  b. Assign values to outcomes.
IV. Choose a preferred course of action:
  a. Quantify uncertainties and values to determine expected values.
  b. Perform sensitivity analysis.

Table 12–2. Characteristics of decision trees.

I. Decision trees are based upon models that incorporate the following features of clinical practice:
   a. One must choose between alternative management strategies.
   b. The natural history of disease and effects of intervention for individual patients are uncertain, and can be represented in terms of likelihoods of outcomes.
   c. Tradeoffs often must be considered, which involves weighing the relative desirability of the outcomes under consideration.
II. Decision trees allow the systematic evaluation of components of a complex situation. On the other hand, all relevant features of a clinical situation may not always be adequately represented.
III. As a quantified display of clinical reasoning, decision trees allow consideration of both beliefs (about probabilities) and preferences (among the outcomes).
IV. Decision trees are tools to help in selecting a strategy for patient care that maximizes the expected value for the patient.

comes (often termed utilities) are inserted at the far right of the appropriate branches (Figure 12–1 and Figure 12–2). The tree, which should contain all appropriate outcomes and all uncertainties and choices, may be extensive in structure (available computer programs will allow several hundred branches). Appropriate numeric values for probabilities and values of outcomes are included in the diagram. Outcomes reflect (a) clinical events that may actually occur and may include complications, (b) probabilities of survival (or death), and (c) years of life expectancy and other measures of mortality and morbidity.

Alternative paths that may be chosen are termed clinical scenarios. For each path, an "Expected Utility" (expected outcome) is a numeric value that may be calculated as described below. The Expected Utility is interpreted as the average, or the expected result, if the decision maker follows a specific path (clinical scenario). The Expected Utilities for each clinical scenario can be compared, and the preferred medical choice can be selected. In this way, the uncertainty inherent in both medical information and in different outcomes of medical status can be considered when making the desired decision.

The numeric calculations used to derive the Expected Utility are simple in concept. At each chance node, the probabilities and numeric outcomes of each branch of the path are multiplied, and the results from separate branches are summed. This process is termed "averaging out." In this manner, calculations are performed from *right* to *left* to obtain the Expected Utility, which is always presented in the same numeric terms as the outcome. When certain pathways clearly will not, for medical reasons, be considered, the branch is "folded back" using double slash lines to indicate a path that is not considered appropriate. The calculations of Expected Utilities, which may become tedious to perform, are easily handled by available computer programs. The process of formal decision analysis is illustrated below for the situation described in the Patient Profile.

THE DECISION EXAMPLE

The patient had a history of heavy alcohol use and presented with fever, jaundice, and abdominal pain. The clinical presentation—along with laboratory findings of leukocytosis and elevated levels of bilirubin and liver enzymes—suggested a diagnosis of either cholangitis or alcoholic hepatitis. Beyond initial supportive care, surgical intervention would be warranted to relieve the biliary obstruction precipitating cholangitis, but surgery would be contraindicated for alcoholic hepatitis. This decision problem can be examined using the process of decision analysis. The various probabilities of uncertainty and outcome are presented in Table 12–3.

The structure of the tree (Figure 12–2) indicates the outcomes in terms of probabilities of survival for each

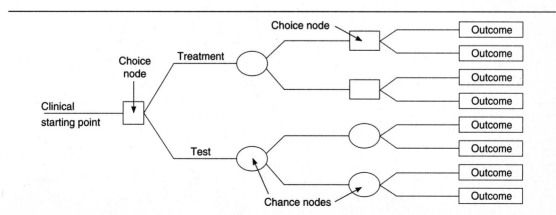

Figure 12–1. The decision diagram or decision "tree" flows from left to right, with choices being noted by boxes and probabilities by circles. Outcomes (often termed utilities) are inserted at the far right of the appropriate branches.

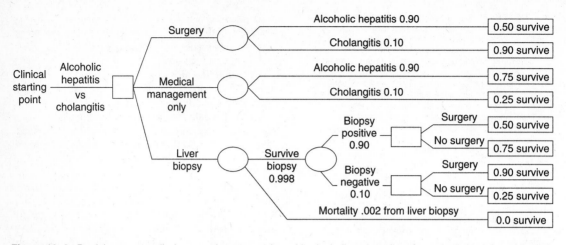

Figure 12–2. Decision tree applied to a patient presenting with alcoholism, jaundice, fever, leukocytosis, and an elevated alkaline phosphatase level. Initial options are to (1) go to surgery, (2) manage medically with supportive care, or (3) do a liver biopsy. For each of these potential decisions, probabilities are generated (arms of the respective chance nodes). The outcome of each probability is given in terms of probability of survival. Note that the value for the limb of a chance node is the probability that outcome or clinical state will occur, ie, there is a 0.9 (90%) chance of the patient's having alcoholic hepatitis and only a 0.1 (10%) chance of cholangitis. Note also that the sum of the probabilities about a chance node always equals 1.0 (100%).

alternative, as well as probabilities of each clinical state or test result (the branches of the chance nodes). Note that if a biopsy is done, the decision for surgery or no surgery awaits the biopsy result, exactly as it would in the clinical setting. Note also that the summation of all probabilities at any chance node *always* equals 1 (100%). Once constructed, the tree is "solved" by multiplying the outcome values (survivals in this case) by their respective probabilities. Around each chance node, the products of the branches are added to give the value at that chance node. After all the chance nodes from a single decision arm are summed, one has achieved the "Expected Value" of that decision (expected utility). This can be compared with the "values" of the other branches of the choice node; then the best numeric choice may be selected as the most favorable option. The other potential choices are excluded or "folded back" (by convention with double slash lines). Values of each chance node are shown in that node.

The calculations are straightforward. For example, the Expected Utility at the surgery node, expressed as the probability of survival, is calculated as:

Expected
Utility = **(likelihood of alcoholic hepatitis)**
× **(survival probability if alcoholic hepatitis)**
+ **(likelihood of cholangitis)**
× **(survival probability if cholangitis)**
= **(.9 × .5) + (.1 × .9) = .54**

In this model, although there is a small risk of mortality associated with performing a diagnostic liver biopsy, the information gained from the biopsy helps to optimize the subsequent treatment decision (see

Figure 12–3). On the basis of this probabilistic argument, the clinical preference would be to perform a diagnostic liver biopsy. Note, however, that using this approach does not *ensure* the best outcome for the patient, since there is a small (0.2%) but real risk of a fatal complication from the biopsy. Nevertheless, after weighing the relative risks and benefits of performing the diagnostic biopsy, the most favorable outcome is likely to be achieved if a liver biopsy is performed first. This is reflected in Figure 12–3 by the Expected Utility for liver biopsy (0.76), which exceeds that for either surgery (0.54) or medical management (0.70).

Table 12–3. The elements to be included in the clinical decision analysis problem.

I. A 50-year-old man with a history of heavy alcohol use, presenting with fever, jaundice, abdominal pain, leukocytosis, and abnormal liver functions.
II. Choices in initial clinical management:
  A. Surgery.
  B. Medical therapy.
  C. Further diagnostic testing with a liver biopsy.
III. Probabilistic events:
  A. 90% of patients who present with this clinical picture will have alcoholic hepatitis and 10% will have ascending cholangitis.
  B. 0.2% of patients undergoing diagnostic liver biopsy will have a fatal complication.
IV. Outcomes:
  A. 75% of alcoholic hepatitis patients without surgery survive.
  B. 50% of alcoholic hepatitis patients with surgery survive.
  C. 25% of cholangitis patients without surgery survive.
  D. 90% of cholangitis patients with surgery survive.

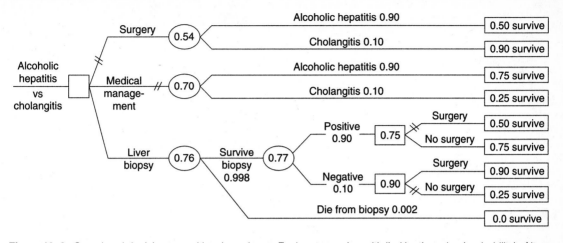

Figure 12–3. Completed decision tree with values shown. Each outcome is multiplied by the value (probability) of its respective chance node arm, and the sum of the two products about each chance node is obtained. For example, on the top or surgical decision limb, the value for the chance node is equal to (0.5 × 0.9) + (0.9 × 0.1) = 0.54. A value is likewise obtained for the other two decision limbs in similar fashion. Note that in doing the liver biopsy, one must take into account the possibility of a fatal complication of the biopsy itself (outcome value = 0.0). After biopsy is obtained, one must decide whether to do surgery. Note that at a choice node, only the highest-value limb is taken for the value of that choice node. The remainder of the "lower-value" limbs at that choice node are "folded back" (by convention with double slash lines) and discarded. A positive biopsy indicates the presence of alcoholic hepatitis, in which case surgery would not be indicated. A negative biopsy indicates cholangitis, and surgery is indicated.

This probabilistic approach contrasts with the traditional method of decision-making, in which the outcome is frequently the only criterion for assessing the method, so that good results may positively reinforce bad decision methods, and bad results may negatively reinforce good decision methods. It should also be noted that other outcomes could have been used, such as surgical morbidity, biopsy morbidity, and others. To the extent that morbidity parallels mortality, the optimal approach will remain the same. One can envision circumstances in which there may be discrepancies in Expected Utilities depending upon the choice of outcome, however. For this reason, it may be useful to consider different choices of outcome.

A criticism of formal decision analysis has been that the input data (probabilities) may not be verifiable, and the values may be subject to doubt. Data obtained through the conduct of large and well designed studies typically are the most reliable, and hence when available, are preferred for use in decision analysis. For many clinical scenarios, however, carefully designed studies have not been conducted, so one must rely upon data of less certain reliability and validity. The latter type of information can be collected by retrospective review of outcomes for a series of patients treated at a particular facility, and in the absence of any observational data, upon clinical impression based upon prior experience with treated patients.

The use of data that are little more than a "best guess" is subject to question. A method for handling this problem in decision analysis is called *sensitivity analysis*. The term sensitivity analysis should not be confused with the sensitivity of a diagnostic test. Sensitivity analysis involves substituting the reasonable maximum and minimum values of a particular probability in question into the decision tree. One then calculates an upper and lower bound on the outcome in question. If the preferred clinical scenario remains unchanged, then the analysis and results may be considered valid.

In applying sensitivity analysis to the problem illustrated above, eg, one may consider the impact of allowing the probabilities of death following surgery among patients with alcoholic hepatitis to range between 50% and 75%. When these values are inserted into the tree and the problem is solved, performing a diagnostic liver biopsy remains the preferred clinical scenario. One may conclude, therefore, that the inferences from the decision analysis are invariant to at least this range of post-surgical mortality probabilities for patients with alcoholic hepatitis.

Any of the variables (probabilities) may be subjected to sensitivity analysis, and if a reasonable maximum or minimum value changes the inference from the analysis, then this circumstance should be considered in choosing the preferred clinical scenario. Sensitivity analysis can be performed easily with a personal computer and appropriate software. The analysis may be done using either a spreadsheet program or a more specific program, of which there are several (see references). The computer allows rapid calculations over a wide range of probabilities, so that the answers are quickly available, often in easily understood graphs.

One must also consider that any test is less than 100% sensitive and specific in classifying disease. If the liver biopsy misses 5% of alcoholic hepatitis and incorrectly labels other diseases as alcoholic hepatitis 2% of the time, then these considerations must be included in the decision tree. The new tree will be slightly more complicated, but it can easily accommodate these differences. For this particular problem, sensitivity analysis of the possibility of alcoholic hepatitis using a wide range of values for sensitivity and specificity of the biopsy from 50–100% does not change the preference for performing the diagnostic test. The likelihood that the biopsy is positive has little influence on the decision to test over a wide range of probabilities.

In contrast, it can be shown that the preferred clinical scenario will vary somewhat with the probability of alcoholic hepatitis versus cholangitis. The results of a sensitivity analysis over a range of probabilities for alcoholic hepatitis from 0–100% is given in Table 12–4. Over most of the range of values (10–90%), there is clear benefit to obtaining the diagnostic liver biopsy. Only at the extremes of probability of alcoholic hepatitis is there any question about the value of the diagnostic biopsy. When it is virtually certain that the patient has cholangitis, proceeding directly to surgery offers an Expected Utility comparable with that of obtaining the diagnostic liver biopsy first. On the other extreme, when it is virtually certain that the patient has alcoholic hepatitis, proceeding directly to medical management offers an Expected Utility comparable with that of obtaining the diagnostic liver biopsy first.

As one might suspect, the estimated probability that the liver biopsy itself will produce a fatal complication also influences the decision of whether or not to test. The results of a sensitivity analysis using estimated probabilities of surviving a liver biopsy ranging from 90–94% are shown in Table 12–5. In this problem, the sensitivity analysis indicates that the preferred alternative is liver biopsy *unless* the risk of a fatal complication is greater than 8%.

SUMMARY

Reaching optimal decisions in clinical practice is complex, in part, because the decision may involve the use of information that is imperfect or of uncertain validity. The estimation of the degree of uncertainty in clinical information, based on the concept of probability estimates, and the use of these estimates in a logical structure are useful tools for making objective decisions in medicine. Formal decision analysis requires the specification of alternative management strategies and provides an explicit probabilistic method for choosing the most favorable anticipated course of action.

The elements of a formal decision analysis include the following: (a) identification of an underlying set of management options, (b) application of probabilities to uncertain events, (c) incorporation of test results, and (d) inclusion of anticipated clinical outcomes for alternative management options. Within the formal structure of the process, referred to as a decision diagram or tree, numerical values are inserted for the anticipated likelihoods of diagnoses, test results, and treatment outcomes. The clinical endpoints can be assessed in a variety of different ways, such as morbidity, mortality, or quality of life. The alternative management options within the decision diagram are referred to as clinical scenarios, each of which is associated with an Expected Utility (or outcome). The Expected Utilities of different scenarios are compared to arrive at the most favorable approach to management. In many circumstances, precise estimates of alternative diagnoses, test performance, or clinical outcomes are unavailable. In these situations, the impact of assuming different values for the unknown parameters can be be explored through sensitivity analysis.

Some clinicians may object to the use of probability estimates, arguing that their use may imply more precision than is warranted by the clinical information, that it dehumanizes the doctor-patient relationship, that it may somehow increase liability, and so on. While these concerns may limit the widespresd use of

Table 12–4. Sensitivity analysis varying the baseline probability of alcoholic hepatitis.

Probability (%) of Alcoholic Hepatitis	Expected Utilities			Preferred Decision
	Surgery	Medical	Biopsy	
0	.900	.250	.898	Surgery
10	.860	.300	.883	Biopsy
20	.820	.350	.868	Biopsy
30	.780	.400	.853	Biopsy
40	.740	.450	.838	Biopsy
50	.700	.500	.823	Biopsy
60	.660	.550	.808	Biopsy
70	.620	.600	.793	Biopsy
80	.580	.650	.778	Biopsy
90	.540	.700	.764	Biopsy
100	.500	.750	.749	Medical

Table 12–5. Sensitivity analysis varying the probability of surviving the liver biopsy.

Probability (%) of Surviving Biopsy	Expected Utilities			Preferred Decision
	Surgery	Medical	Biopsy	
94	.540	.700	.719	Biopsy
93	.540	.700	.712	Biopsy
92	.540	.700	.704	Biopsy
91	.540	.700	.696	Medical
90	.540	.700	.689	Medical

formal decision analysis, this technique can serve as a useful tool to aid in appropriate patient management. As the stethoscope aids an experienced clinician in making a diagnosis, decision analysis provides insight into alternative management strategies, taking advantage of clinical and epidemiologic methods; many of which are outlined in this book.

For the situation described in the Patient Profile, the clinical presentation suggested a diagnosis of either cholangitis or alcoholic hepatitis. Cholangitis requires surgery in order to relieve biliary obstruction, whereas surgery is contraindicated in alcoholic hepatitis. By framing this management problem in a formal decision analysis, performing a liver biopsy in order to reduce uncertainty about the diagnosis was shown to result in a more favorable outcome (in terms of mortality) than proceeding directly to either surgical or medical management.

Sensitivity analysis further demonstrated that the decision to perform an initial liver biopsy would be preferred under a fairly wide range of expected mortality probabilities for alcoholic hepatitis and test ac-curacy. There were only two circumstances in which an initial liver biopsy did not appear warranted: when there was minimal baseline uncertainty about the diagnosis and when the anticipated likelihood of a fatal complication of the biopsy reached an appreciable level. Using the available information, the physician in the Patient Profile would be justified in opting for a diagnostic liver biopsy before proceeding further in patient management.

STUDY QUESTIONS

Questions 1–4: For each numbered question below, select the most appropriate answer based on the decision diagram in Figure 12–4.

The diagram represents the decision to use medical therapy or bypass surgery in a 50-year-old patient with severe angina. The utilities are hypothetical outcomes scored from 0–100. Respective probabilities are also shown on the diagram. The preferred outcome is to survive as long as possible without angina.

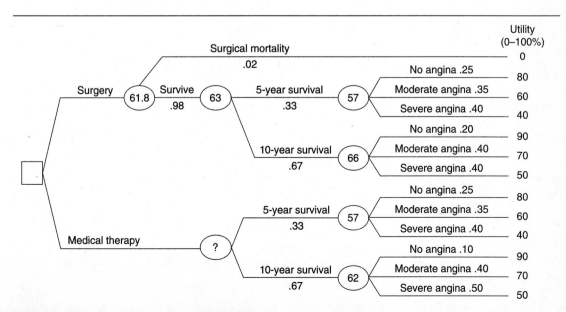

Figure 12–4. Decision tree for coronary bypass surgery.

1. In Figure 12–4, the expected utility for medical therapy is
   A. $57 + 62 = 119.0$
   B. $(57 + 62) \times (.67) = 79.73$
   C. $(57 \times .67) + (62 \times .33) = 58.65$
   D. $(57 \times .33) + (62 \times .67) = 60.35$
   E. $(57 \times .33) + (5\text{ yrs}) = (62 \times .67) + (10\text{ yrs})$
      $= 75.35$

2. If you were to base your decision on the Estimated Utility (EU) in Figure 12–4, what would be your preferred choice?
   A. Bypass surgery
   B. Medical therapy
   C. Observe the patient and consider bypass surgery in 6 months
   D. Observe the patient and consider bypass surgery in 9 months
   E. No rational therapeutic choice can be made based on the available data

3. Since the survival at 5 and 10 years is the same for surgery and medical therapy, what outcome event has led to the preferred choice in Question 2?
   A. A greater proportion of surgery patients have no angina at 10 years
   B. A greater proportion of surgery patients have no angina at 5 and 10 years
   C. A greater proportion of medical patients have no angina at 10 years
   D. A greater proportion of medical patients have no angina at 5 and 10 years
   E. An equal proportion of surgery and medical patients have no angina at 10 years

4. What is the mortality threshold ie, the probability of death associated with surgery that would necessitate a decision to change to medical therapy for the 50-year-old patient described above?
   A. .03
   B. .04
   C. .05
   D. .06
   E. .07

Questions 5–6: For each numbered question below, select the most appropriate answer based on the decision diagram in Figure 12–5, which represents the portion of a decision tree that depicts the use of a test to make a medical decision.

The probability that the test is positive is represented by p(POS), and the probability that the test is

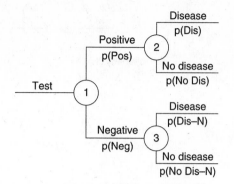

Figure 12–5. Portion of a decision tree that illustrates the use of test to formulate a medical decision.

negative is indicated by p(NEG). If the test is positive, the patient may have disease (ie, a true positive) or the patient may not have disease (ie, a false positive) with probabilities represented by p(DIS) and p(NO DIS), respectively.

The same disease outcomes are possible with a negative test. If the test is negative, the probability of disease is represented by p(DIS N) and the probability of no disease is represented by p(NO DIS N). N indicates that the test is scored as negative.

5. The probability that the test is positive can be easily determined based on the concept of predictive values discussed in Chapter 6. In Figure 12–5, consider TP, TN, FN, and FP as proportions, and Prev. as the pre-test prevalence, which is occasionally termed the pre-test probability. Which of the following calculations can be used to determine the probability p(POS) at the chance node 1?
   A. TP × Prev. + FN × Prev.
   B. TP × Prev. + TN × (1-Prev.)
   C. TP × Prev. + FP × (1-Prev.)
   D. TP × (1-Prev.) + FP × Prev.
   E. TP × (1-Prev.) + FN × (1-Prev.)

6. In Figure 12–5, consider PVP as the predictive value positive and PVN as the predictive value negative. At the chance node labelled 2, the probability of disease is given by which of the following?
   A. The PVP
   B. The 1 − PVP
   C. The PVN
   D. The 1 − PVN
   E. The TP × FP

FURTHER READING

Lipsett PA, Pitt HA: Acute cholangitis. Surg Clin North Am 1990;**70**:1297.

Weinstein MC, et al: *Clinical Decision Analysis*. W.B. Saunders Company, 1980.

REFERENCES

Boring JR, Francis JB, Simon DG: Analytic Medicine. In: *Medicine for the Practicing Physician.* 3rd ed, 1992. Hurst JW (editor-in-chief). Butterworth-Heinemann, 1992.

Sonnenberg FA, Parker SG: *Decision Maker,* Version 6.2. New England Medical Center, 1988.

Sox Jr. HC, et al: *Medical Decision Making.* Butterworths, 1988.

Interpretation of Epidemiologic Literature

PATIENT PROFILE

A 40-year-old accountant visited her family physician for a routine checkup. The patient's mother had been diagnosed with breast cancer in the past year, and the patient wanted advice about what she could do to reduce; her own risk of this disease. The patient had two children aged 6 and 8 years. She was in good health, with regular menstrual cycles, and she had a recent normal Papanicolaou smear and mammogram.

In responding to the patient's questions about breast cancer, the physician confirmed that a positive family history increases the risk of this disease. A number of other characteristics are associated with a reduced risk of breast cancer, such as early age at first full-term pregnancy and increasing number of pregnancies. Unfortunately, these factors are not easily susceptible to intervention, and the patient already had completed her childbearing. The physician was aware also of a controversy regarding the relationship between the intake of dietary fat and the occurrence of breast cancer. Before recommending that the patient reduce her fat intake, however, the physician wished to review the pertinent medical literature.

INTRODUCTION

The recommendations that physicians make to patients depend on the current state of knowledge available about diseases, the underlying pathophysiology, and the most effective treatment. The knowledge base of clinical medicine is continuously expanding, and physicians must therefore develop methods to seek out and apply new information. This process is complicated when inconclusive or conflicting results are found in the medical literature. The publication of articles, even in the most respected journals, does not guarantee that the investigators' conclusions are valid or, even if valid, relevant to the daily practice of a particular physician. The history of medicine includes countless examples of therapies that were once widely accepted but later were shown to be ineffective or even harmful to patients. Clinicians must develop skills that will allow them to update and reevaluate their knowledge to provide optimal patient care.

SEARCHING THE LITERATURE

The first step in acquiring new medical knowledge is to locate the appropriate literature. This is an increasingly difficult task as the number of medical journals increases each year. It is not possible for any physician to read everything relevant to his or her practice as it is published. Fortunately, help of various kinds is available to assist with literature searching when necessary. A search of the existing literature can be performed manually, by reviewing keyword listings in the annual published indexes of the medical literature, such as *Index Medicus*. Examples of keywords that might be searched in the present context include "breast neoplasms," "dietary fats," and "food habits." In reviewing listings in *Index Medicus,* one is limited to information about the authors' names, the titles of the articles, and the journal, volume number, and issue number, page numbers, and year of publication.

With the advent of computer technology, it has become possible to search the medical literature in an automated manner. For example, a search through a standard database, such as *Medline,* could be performed to assemble lists of articles that might be of interest. Again, the search process is based upon a few keywords chosen to recover articles on relevant subjects. Most computer databases include abstracts of articles from major journals, and some even include the entire text of articles from selected publications.

For example, a computer search for the title words "breast cancer and dietary fat" will retrieve a substantial number of journal articles over the previous 2-year period. These articles may include case series reports, ecologic studies, descriptive studies, case-control studies, cohort studies, randomized controlled clinical trials, and reviews, including meta-analyses.

CRITICAL REVIEW

Once the appropriate literature is identified, it is useful to apply a systematic approach to evaluate the articles. This process will encourage the reader to consider all aspects of a study before passing judgment on its validity and utility. The following sections provide one such approach to published studies. The steps in the review are presented in Figure 13–1 in the general sequence in which they should be considered. Each component of a review is dependent on the others to some extent, however, so that they are often considered collectively. The details of the review process are outlined in Table 13–1.

Research Hypothesis

It is important to consider the research hypothesis that is addressed by the study. In practice, this may be a difficult task. Authors often do not state the hypotheses they wish to test. Sometimes the goal of the study is stated as a research question, but occasionally a reader is left to infer the purpose of the study from a set of complicated analyses.

Once the purpose of the study is discerned, the reader should attempt to determine if the study addresses a question that has clinical importance. If the study does not, the results may have little relevance to clinical practice. For the physician who needs information in order to counsel a patient about the relationship of dietary fat and risk of breast cancer, it is necessary to identify articles that address that topic. A number of different kinds of hypotheses, however, may be relevant to the general topic. For example, a study of the effects of varying dietary fat composition

Table 13–1. Stepwise approach to critical appraisal of published medical research.

Step 1. Consider the research hypothesis.
Is there a clear statement of the research hypothesis?
Does the study address a question that has clinical relevance?
Step 2. Consider the study design.
Is the study design appropriate for the hypothesis?
Does the design represent an advance over prior approaches?
Does the study use an experimental or an observational design?
Step 3. Consider the outcome variable.
Is the outcome being studied relevant to clinical practice?
What criteria are used to define the presence of disease?
Is the determination of the presence or absence of disease accurate?
Step 4. Consider the predictor variable(s).
How many exposures or risk factors are being studied?
How is the presence or absence of exposure determined?
Is the assessment of exposure likely to be precise and accurate?
Is there an attempt to quantify the amount or duration of exposure?
Are biologic markers of exposure used in the study?
Step 5. Consider the methods of analysis.
Are the statistical methods employed suitable for the types of variables (nominal versus ordinal versus continuous) in the study?
Have the levels of type I and type II errors been discussed appropriately?
Is the sample size adequate to answer the research question?
Have the assumptions underlying the statistical tests been met?
Has chance been evaluated as a potential explanation of the results?
Step 6. Consider possible sources of bias (systematic errors).
Is the method of selection of subjects likely to have biased results?
Is the measurement of either the exposure or the disease likely to be biased?
Have the investigators considered whether confounders could account for the observed results?
In what direction would each potential bias influence the results?
Step 7. Consider the interpretation of results.
How large is the observed effect?
Is there evidence of a dose-response relationship?
Are the findings consistent with laboratory models?
Are the effects biologically plausible?
If the findings are negative, was there sufficient statistical power to detect an effect?
Step 8. Consider how the results of the study can be used in practice.
Are the findings consistent with other studies of the same questions?
Can the findings be generalized to other human populations?
Do the findings warrant a change in current clinical practice?

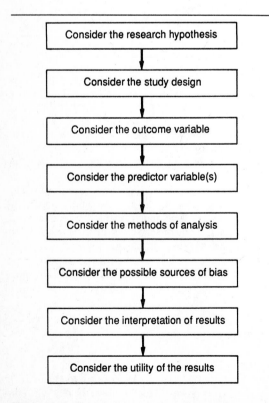

Figure 13–1. Steps in the evaluation of an epidemiologic study.

on the occurrence of mammary tumors in mice may be useful, because laboratory animal studies can be more tightly controlled than human studies. It may be useful to read a study on the effect of high-fat diet on circulating estrogen levels in women, since this may have relevance to the biologic plausibility of a potential relationship between dietary fat and breast cancer, and such research may yield information about the mechanism of disease development and prevention.

The various types of **significance** that may be ascribed to a research finding should be distinguished (Table 13–2). It is common practice to refer to results as significant if a statistical test indicates that the findings are unlikely to be attributable to chance alone. The evaluation of statistical significance—and therefore the likelihood of committing a type I (false-positive) error—is useful in the interpretation of results.

Even if a finding is statistically significant, however, one cannot infer that it is biologically or clinically important. For instance, a small difference in risk of breast cancer with increasing levels of dietary fat could be judged to be statistically significant if the finding were based upon a large number of observations. Nevertheless, this elevation in risk may be so small that an individual woman's risk of breast cancer would not be appreciably altered by changing her diet. As a result, a clinical recommendation to reduce dietary fat might not be supportable on the basis of the evidence. The biologic significance of a finding addresses yet another issue: Do the epidemiologic observations help to clarify the causal mechanism? This type of insight is most likely to be gained if the epidemiologic study involves biologic markers of exposure, susceptibility, and outcome.

Study Design

If the study question is of interest, the reader should then determine what type of study design was employed. As was noted in Chapters 7–9, certain designs may be more or less useful for answering specific kinds of questions. Another factor that may have determined the type of study design used by the investigator is the current state of knowledge. Early studies of a particular hypothesis may have a simple design, such as a descriptive study. As the hypothesis is refined, more definitive study designs can be utilized.

The appropriateness of the study design to the research question should be assessed. The incidence rate of the disease in question may be a determining factor. For example, although breast cancer is the most common form of cancer among women in the United States, this disease is diagnosed among only a small proportion of women during a short period of time. Accordingly, an appropriate choice of design for this disease would be a case-control study, since the sampling scheme for this type of study is efficient for including newly diagnosed women. In fact, studies of dietary fat intake and breast cancer have utilized several different designs, including descriptive, case-control, and cohort studies. The descriptive studies are most useful for hypothesis generation. The case-control and cohort designs provide more compelling evidence to test specific hypotheses. To date, all of the studies of dietary fat and risk of breast cancer have employed observational designs. An experimental study in which women are assigned randomly to groups receiving different levels of dietary fat and followed for the occurrence of breast cancer is underway, but results have not yet been published.

Outcome Variable

The outcome of interest in the Patient Profile is the development of breast cancer. In investigations of the relationship between dietary fat intake and risk of breast cancer, it is important to specify how the presence or absence of breast cancer was determined. There are several possibilities.

(1) Death certificates limit information to deceased subjects. In addition, a variety of studies have shown that information on death certificates may be incomplete or inaccurate, as discussed in Chapter 4.

(2) Self-reports require that subjects be alive or have relatives who can provide information on breast cancer. If the subjects are not medically sophisticated, they may mistake benign forms of breast disease for breast cancer.

(3) Medical records may provide more accurate information. However, it is possible that diagnostic criteria differ: (a) from physician to physician, (b) over time, or (c) across geographic regions or countries.

(4) Histopathologic diagnoses provide the most definitive information, but adequate tissue must be available for pathologic examination.

It is desirable to have the most definitive information possible on the presence of disease. This will tend to minimize the likelihood of misclassification of subjects. For breast cancer, it is possible that a small proportion of apparently healthy women may actually have occult (undiscovered) breast cancer. This could

Table 13–2. Types of significance in clinical research.

Type	Meaning	Assessment
Statistical	Exclusion of chance as an explanation for findings	Statistical test
Clinical	Importance of findings for changing current clinical practice	Magnitude of clinical response to an intervention
Biologic	Findings help to clarify mechanism of action	Compare findings to information from in vitro and in vivo laboratory experimentation

be evaluated by performing a screening test, such as mammography, on all apparently unaffected subjects. Since so few asymptomatic cancers are likely to be detected, however, study findings probably would not be affected greatly by limiting detection to routine histopathologic diagnosis.

It is also important to judge how precisely the investigator defines the outcome. In general, it is useful to specify a single disease entity when searching for causes. For example, a study of dietary fat and the risk of all cancers combined may produce misleading results, since different cancers have different causes, and only some causes may involve dietary fat. Restricting the study to breast cancer improves the likelihood of obtaining a definitive result for this disease of primary interest.

Predictor Variables

The predictor variable is the risk factor or exposure under investigation. Studies may involve a single risk factor of interest or several different predictor variables. If a number of exposure variables are included, they may or may not be closely linked.

In a study of the cause of breast cancer, an investigator might choose to examine a variety of exposure variables, including reproductive factors such as age at first full-term pregnancy, hormone levels, exposure to radiation, and dietary fat intake. While this sort of study may provide a more comprehensive picture of the causes of breast cancer, it may limit the ability to collect detailed information on each exposure of interest. Even if a study is focused on the question of dietary fat and the risk of breast cancer, it is necessary to collect some basic information on other possible determinants of breast cancer that could act as confounders.

The reader must determine whether the methods used to characterize the presence or absence of exposure are reliable and accurate. Possible ascertainment methods include subject or surrogate respondent reports, direct observation, or measurement of a biologic marker. Also, the reader should ask whether there are better ways to define the exposure levels of subjects.

The assessment of a dietary exposure can be especially difficult. One method is to ask subjects about their past dietary habits. This requires that the subjects remember the kinds and the amounts of foods that they ate. Various studies have indicated that such recall, while imperfect, may suffice to determine whether a subject consumed a relatively high, moderate, or low amount of dietary fat. Generally, it is desirable to have several levels of exposure defined, so that a dose-response relationship can be evaluated.

Another approach to determining dietary fat intake is to have subjects record what they currently eat. This can be done by keeping a diary or by checking off on a list of commonly eaten foods the meals and snacks the patient is ingesting. There are problems with this approach, however. Subjects may forget to record what they eat, or they may incorrectly estimate the size of portions. To help offset such problems, plastic models of different portion sizes are available to provide visual cues and reminders. It is important to remember that a subject's current diet may not accurately reflect past diet. In a case-control design based only upon current diet information, it is crucial to know if subjects with breast cancer changed their diets because of (a) the disease, (b) the side effects of treatment, or (c) the hope of influencing prognosis.

Another approach to collecting information on diet is to measure what subjects eat. This could be useful for a prospective cohort study in which subjects are followed to determine whether they develop breast cancer. This approach to measuring dietary intake would be extremely difficult in practice, however, as it would require a tightly controlled environment in which the investigator could observe the foods eaten by subjects.

Epidemiologists occasionally take advantage of a situation in which people maintain certain dietary habits for religious or other reasons. Thus, an epidemiologist may identify a group of people (eg, vegetarians) who consume very little fat in their diets. The frequency of occurrence of breast cancer in this group could be compared with the experience of another group whose members consume large amounts of fat. The problem of determining the precise intake of fat for subjects in both groups still remains, however. Furthermore, it is likely that the groups will differ in life-style factors other than intake of dietary fat.

The use of biologic markers of exposure has become more common in clinical research (see Chapter 10). Biologic markers are important because they can provide quantitative documentation of exposure in certain circumstances. No biologic markers of fat intake are currently available, but in order to assess long-term dietary fat intake, one might measure fatty acid content in biopsies of adipose tissue. Obviously, the utility of such a measure depends upon the extent to which it accurately reflects consumption patterns. The willingness of study participants to undergo a tissue biopsy must also be considered.

Methods of Analysis

The emphasis that is placed on a particular research finding often depends on the ability of the investigator to exclude chance as an explanation for the observed results. This is accomplished by the use of statistical tests. It is important for the reader to have a basic understanding of which statistical tests are appropriate for which types of analysis. The type of statistical test that should be used is determined by the goal of the analysis (eg, to compare groups, to explore an association, or to predict an outcome) and the types of variables used in the analysis (eg, categorical, ordinal, or continuous variables).

By convention, the 5% level of statistical significance is used as a standard in many biomedical studies. That is, the investigator is willing to accept a 1 in 20 risk that the observed effect is a result of chance variation alone. Care must be taken to avoid oversimplistic interpretations of *P*-values, however. One common mistake is to assume that a statistically significant result is biologically or clinically important. As discussed above, the clinical importance and biologic plausibility of results are not assessed by hypothesis tests.

A second common mistake is to dismiss a finding because it has not reached the predetermined level for statistical significance. A *P*-value of 0.08, eg, though not statistically significant in common practice, still represents a finding that is relatively unlikely to be attributable to chance. It would be unwise, therefore, to conclude on the basis of such a *P*-value that there is no relationship between dietary fat intake and breast cancer in a particular study. The heavy reliance upon *P*-values is particularly dangerous when the sample size of a study is small and the statistical power therefore is low as well. In such situations, even moderate differences between groups may fail to reach a conventional level of statistical significance, and the ability to reach a definitive conclusion is limited.

Possible Sources of Bias

A result must be examined also to determine whether it could be due to systematic errors related to the sampling strategy or to data collection procedures. A statistical test cannot address whether biases of one sort or another are responsible for the observed results. As discussed in Chapter 10, the consideration of potential bias often cannot be assessed in precise quantitative terms. Bias can occur in any study, although certain designs are more susceptible to specific types of bias. Regardless of the study design, the potential for three distinct types of bias should be considered (Table 13–3).

The first concern is whether the selection of subjects is likely to have distorted the results (**selection bias**). Few studies (if any) can examine an entire population. This means that the investigator must draw a sample in order to make inferences about the population. The reader must determine if the samples are likely to be representative of the population to which extrapolations are made.

The methods section of any published medical research paper should include details of how subjects were selected for the study. In a case-control study, selection bias could arise from the approach used to select cases, controls, or both. In the context of a case-control study of dietary fat and breast cancer, selection

bias might occur if prevalent (surviving) cases are used rather than newly diagnosed (incident) cases. This distortion would occur if prediagnostic nutritional status were related to disease prognosis. For example, if women who consumed high-fat diets before developing breast cancer survived longer than low-fat consumers, prevalent cases would overrepresent high-fat consumption, and the observed risk ratio may be biased toward larger values. The bias is presented schematically in Figure 13–2.

In a case-control study, the sampling of controls can be as great a source of selection bias as the sampling of cases. Consider a hospital-based sample of controls with diagnoses other than breast cancer. If the diseases of the controls are caused by dietary factors (eg, atherosclerotic heart disease) or, conversely, if the diseases influence dietary intake (eg, gastrointestinal disease) a biased case-control comparison may result. Sampling from the general population typically results in controls that better reflect the exposure patterns of persons without the disease of interest. Even general population sampling schemes can result in a distorted control group, however. For example, a telephone sampling technique might preferentially include higher-income women, because they are more likely

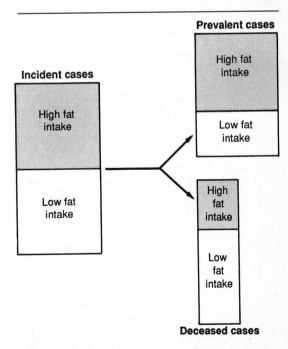

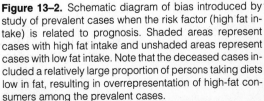

Figure 13–2. Schematic diagram of bias introduced by study of prevalent cases when the risk factor (high fat intake) is related to prognosis. Shaded areas represent cases with high fat intake and unshaded areas represent cases with low fat intake. Note that the deceased cases included a relatively large proportion of persons taking diets low in fat, resulting in overrepresentation of high-fat consumers among the prevalent cases.

Table 13–3. Types of bias in clinical research.

Bias	Source of Error
Selection bias	Sample distorted by selection process
Information bias	Misclassification of the variables
Confounding	An extraneous variable that accounts for the observed result rather than the risk factor of interest

than lower-income women to have telephones. Also, if higher-income women are less likely to work outside of the home, they would be more available when the sampling is performed. Since the diets of higher-income women may differ from those of other women, a biased case-control comparison may occur. In order to determine whether a telephone sampling scheme is likely to yield an unbiased sample of controls, one would want to know the completeness of telephone coverage of the target population. Also, multiple calls should be made to sampled residences, at varying times of the day and days of the week, to reach persons who work outside the home.

Cohort studies of the association between dietary factors and breast cancer also are subject to potential selection bias. The major source of selection bias in such studies is loss to follow-up during the study. If women who eat a high-fat diet and develop breast cancer tend to discontinue participation in the study for some reason prior to the diagnosis of cancer, the investigator will underestimate the risk for breast cancer associated with a high-fat intake. To date, cohort studies of this question have yielded conflicting results. An important consideration in such a situation is the extent to which bias due to loss to follow-up could explain the discrepancy.

Another source of bias can arise from systematic errors in measuring either the independent variable (exposure) or the dependent variable (disease). This type of bias is often referred to as **information bias** or **misclassification bias.** For example, in a case-control study, the validity of information on exposure may be questioned because the data are gathered retrospectively. Since the cases are aware of their disease and have undergone treatment for it, their reporting of past exposures may differ systematically from reporting of controls. This is referred to as **recall bias.** Studies of dietary risk factors may be susceptible to recall bias. For example, if breast cancer patients are wondering about the cause of their cancer, they may tend to overestimate past exposure to dietary fat, especially when the potential relationship has been widely publicized. Controls may be less concerned about past diet or may be worried about other problems such as obesity, which would tend to make them underreport exposure to dietary fat.

If recall bias occurred in a study, the investigator might overestimate the risk of dietary fat intake in relation to the occurrence of breast cancer. In fact, a number of studies have demonstrated problems of imperfect recall of dietary history. Only a few studies, however, have examined differential (biased) recall in cases vs controls by comparing prospectively collected dietary data with subsequent data collected retrospectively from the same subjects. In general, these investigations have not demonstrated differential recall of food intake in breast cancer cases compared with controls. This would suggest that recall bias is an unlikely explanation for inconsistent results reported

from case-control studies of the association of dietary fat intake and breast cancer.

It should be remembered, however, that even if cases and controls do not differ in the ability to recall dietary exposure, misclassification bias still could occur. Errors in reporting that are comparable between cases and controls give rise to nondifferential misclassification. If nondifferential misclassification occurs, it may reduce the estimated risk ratio. In other words, such misclassification tends to make it more difficult to detect any true differences between cases and controls.

The final consideration of bias is to determine whether **confounding** could account for the observed result. A confounder is an extraneous correlate of disease that, because of its association with the risk factor of interest, accounts for some or all of the observed association between the risk factor and the disease. In studies of dietary fat intake and breast cancer, it is important to determine if the investigator has accounted for the effects of known risk factors for breast cancer. These factors include age, race, reproductive characteristics (eg, age at first full-term pregnancy, number of pregnancies, duration of lactation), obesity among postmenopausal women, alcohol intake, and exposure to radiation. A schematic diagram for confounding of the relationship between dietary fat intake and breast cancer by number of pregnancies is presented in Figure 13–3. If women who eat a high-fat diet have fewer pregnancies than those who eat a low-fat diet, an apparent association between dietary fat and breast cancer could be attributable to the effects of reproductive history rather than to diet, per se.

In an observational study, confounding can be controlled in the following ways: (a) in the design of the study (by restricting subject inclusion to persons with a narrow range of the confounder values or by matching study groups on confounders) or (b) in the analysis of the results (through stratification by confounders or by regression techniques). All of these adjustment methods, however, are contingent upon knowing which variables are confounders. Since the known risk factors for breast cancer do not account for all occurrences of the disease, other unknown risk factors must

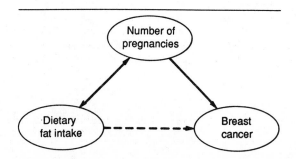

Figure 13–3. Schematic diagram of confounding of the dietary fat-breast cancer relationship by number of pregnancies.

exist. Any observed association between dietary fat and breast cancer could be explained, at least in part, in that way.

When the reader detects the potential for bias, it is important to try to estimate both the magnitude and the direction of the effect the bias could have on the results. In this way, the reader can determine if the bias is likely to have inflated the results or to have diminished the exposure's effect. In a case-control study, eg, if it is suspected that women with breast cancer are more likely than controls to remember and report fat intake, the risk ratio could be overestimated. In contrast, if it seems likely that breast cancer patients underreport their dietary fat intake in comparison with controls, the observed results may underestimate the true impact of dietary fat intake on the occurrence of breast cancer. In discussing the results, an investigator may attempt to convince the reader that the magnitude of bias would not be sufficient to skew the results, or that the true relationship is as strong as or stronger than that observed.

Interpretation of Results

If the investigator reports a statistically significant result that cannot be explained by bias, the reader must then decide whether the result is clinically important. Consider, eg, a study concluding that a 50% decrease in dietary fat intake is associated with a 5% decrease in risk of breast cancer. Even if this result is statistically significant, the magnitude of risk reduction is so slight in exchange for the major change required in diet that the finding is unlikely to lead to a useful clinical intervention—although it may still have biologic significance if it provides insight into the mechanism of carcinogenesis.

Conversely, when results are not statistically significant, one need not conclude that the findings are useless. Particularly when there is a small sample size or when the relationship between the exposure and the disease is weak, the possibility of a false-negative conclusion must be considered. The statistical power of the study to detect the observed effect may be too low to allow a definitive conclusion from the study.

Practical Utility of Results

When reviewing a published study, the reader must determine the practical utility of the results. The usefulness of a study finding depends on various factors, including the purpose of the study, limitations of the study population, the clinical and biologic importance of the results, and consistency with findings from other published studies. Clinical and epidemiologic research has various purposes. The clinical utility of a particular research finding must be viewed in the context of the type of question posed. As indicated in Table 13–4, a particular study may lead to findings relevant to disease causation, early detection of disease, the prediction of prognosis, or improved treatment. Studies of the relationship between dietary fat and breast cancer

Table 13–4. Clinical applications of various types of studies.

Type of Study	Application to Clinical Practice
Etiologic	Can risk be reduced among susceptible persons?
Diagnostic	Can accuracy and timeliness of diagnosis be improved?
Prognostic	Can prognosis be determined more definitively?
Therapeutic	Can treatment be improved?

relate to disease causation. Unfortunately, there is no standard by which to judge whether an association between a risk factor and a disease is clinically important. Clearly, the stronger the association (ie, the farther the risk ratio is from the null value), the greater the potential impact of eliminating the exposure. In assessing clinical utility, one must also consider how difficult it is to change the risk factor (in this case, to reduce dietary fat intake), and one must consider the amount of morbidity and mortality associated with the disease.

The ability to generalize the findings beyond the study population should be taken into account. For this purpose, the definition and limitations of the study sample must be understood. For example, some studies of risk factors for breast cancer have focused on postmenopausal women. This may limit the applicability of such studies to the premenopausal patient in the Patient Profile. Investigators are often forced to restrict the sample by age, race, or other factors. The reader must decide what effect these restrictions may have on the broader applicability of results.

In determining whether the findings of a particular study can be generalized to other populations, it is useful to assess whether similar results have been obtained in other studies. It often happens that the first evaluation of a risk factor, diagnostic test, or therapeutic regimen is favorable, whereas subsequent reports demonstrate more limited utility. One reason for this pattern is that initial assessments often involve selected populations that offer a best-case scenario. Subsequent attempts to broaden the applicability may prove less successful.

ESTABLISHING A CAUSAL RELATIONSHIP

Ultimately, the reader may question whether a causal relationship between a risk factor and a disease has been supported by the results of a study. Table 13–5 presents selected criteria that can be used to evaluate suspected causal relationships. The consideration of causality is based upon the findings of a particular study, within the context of what is already known about a disease process.

The **strength of the observed association** is a primary criterion to evaluate whether a risk factor causes

Table 13–5. Selected criteria for evaluating a suspected causal relationship.

Strength
Presence of a dose-response relationship
Correct temporal sequence
Consistency of results across studies
Biologic plausibility

a disease. The strength of the association is indicated by the distance of the risk ratio or odds ratio from the null value. When the association is very strong, it is less likely that the association can be explained by chance or bias. Weak associations also may be causal, indicating only a lower risk of disease development. With a weak association, however, it is more difficult to exclude other factors and biases that may account for the relationship.

It is useful to examine whether there is a **dose-response relationship** between the proposed risk factor and the disease. If there is, increased levels of the risk factor will be associated with a greater risk of disease development (or with protection in the case of a beneficial factor). For example, as the level of dietary fat intake increases, the risk of breast cancer would be expected to increase if a causal relationship exists (Figure 13–4). The absence of a progressive, graded dose-response relationship does not preclude a causal relationship, however. For example, there may be a threshold above which the level of the risk factor confers increased risk. In this case, risk of disease will not be affected by changes in exposure below a certain level, but risk does vary with exposure at higher levels.

With any association, it is helpful to compare the findings with the results of other studies. If other investigators studying different populations in differing

settings find similar results, a causal explanation is supported. However, the reader must be careful when judging consistency of results, because it is possible that the same flaw could lead to incorrect conclusions in several studies.

The proposed causal relationship should be consistent with what is currently known about biology and the disease process. This is often referred to as **biologic plausibility.** If the proposed cause-and-effect relationship is not in accordance with current knowledge, causality may be questioned. The assessment of biologic plausibility often requires a review of research on other human populations, as well as a review of research that involves laboratory animal models.

The temporal relationship between a suspected cause and an effect is important. That is, *a cause must always precede an effect in time.* This seems intuitive, but, in reality, factors that are suspected to be causes sometimes turn out to be effects of the disease. For example, a person with an early undiagnosed cancer may make a change in food choices because of unrecognized systemic effects of the cancer. Consequently, a dietary change may appear to be the cause of the later diagnosed cancer, rather than an effect of the cancer. Case-control studies of chronic diseases with long latent periods are especially susceptible to this problem. For a factor to be considered the cause of a disease, it is theoretically important that removal or modification of that factor will prevent the disease from occurring or will ameliorate the disease once it has occurred. This criterion may have been met for the example cited in Chapter 9, since the incidence of eosinophilia myalgia syndrome appears to have declined with the removal of L-tryptophan from the market. However, surveillance for eosinophilia myalgia syndrome is not as active, so unreported cases of eosinophilia myalgia syndrome may still be occurring. For example, cases of eosinophilia myalgia syndrome continue to occur in Canada where L-tryptophan is available only by prescription (Spitzer WO, 1995). This means that the true incidence of eosinophilia myalgia syndrome currently is not known; nor do epidemiologists know the extent to which the incidence may have changed.

In practice, the criterion of removal or modification of a suspected causal factor may not always be satisfied. There are some instances where a causal factor may set off a protracted chain of events. Once established, this sequence may no longer depend on the presence of the causal agent for progression. For example, many cancers are thought to develop in response to an initiating event, followed by promotional effects that occur for many years. If the risk factor of interest contributes to initiation only, removal of the exposure during the promotional phase will not affect the subsequent risk of cancer development. Thus, eliminating an initiating risk factor for cancer may not affect the incidence of this disease for many years into the future.

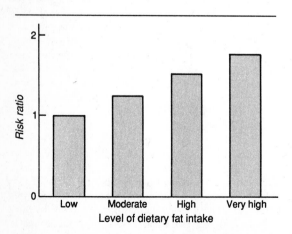

Figure 13–4. Hypothetical dose-response relationship between level of dietary fat intake and risk ratio of breast cancer. The reference category of exposure is low dietary fat intake.

DIETARY FAT
AND BREAST CANCER

As mentioned previously, the relationship between dietary fat intake and the risk of breast cancer was investigated in a variety of epidemiologic studies. These studies included case series reports, ecologic analyses, case-control studies, and cohort studies. To date, no randomized controlled clinical trial of a low-fat diet to prevent breast cancer has been published.

Ecologic or correlation studies have demonstrated a consistently strong relationship between dietary habits, as estimated by per-capita dietary fat, and breast cancer occurrence in different countries. Plots of these data have yielded a linear relationship, with increasing fat consumption associated with higher breast cancer occurrence. The problem with such studies is that they do not demonstrate that increased dietary fat in *individuals* is associated with breast cancer occurrence in the same individuals (ie, the **ecologic fallacy**) may be involved).

Case-control studies have yielded conflicting results on the question of diet and breast cancer. The reasons for these conflicting results are not clear. One criticism is that dietary data collected retrospectively are inaccurate (ie, dietary exposure is misclassified). General difficulties in recalling diet could contribute to nondifferential misclassification, and case-control differences in ability or motivation to recall dietary fat could result in differential misclassification. Another potential explanation is that the influence of dietary fat could have been exerted many years prior to breast cancer diagnosis. Most case-control studies have included diet information from the recent past but not from the remote past. Some reviewers have concluded that none of the studies, when viewed individually, had a large enough sample size to provide adequate statistical power. In other words, a true relationship between dietary fat intake and breast cancer risk might be missed because of inadequate discriminatory ability (ie, a type II error may be involved).

Some of these problems can be avoided with the cohort study design. Prospective cohort studies eliminate the potential for distortion of results from differential recall of dietary history. This type of study was used to investigate the question of fat in the diet and the risk of breast cancer. Again, the published results of cohort studies of this question have yielded conflicting results. Some studies have produced evidence of a relatively weak association, with risk ratios of approximately 1.4. Other cohort studies, however, actually have indicated that increased dietary fat intake may protect against the development of breast cancer.

In general, the dose-response relationship suggested by the ecologic studies has not been borne out in the case-control and cohort studies. Some reviewers have argued that the reason for this disagreement is that the range of dietary fat intake in the analytic studies is smaller than in the international ecologic studies and,

consequently, that there was too little variation in fat intake to demonstrate a dose-response relationship in the case-control and cohort studies. Others have argued that factors other than diet (ie, confounders) that could not be controlled easily in ecologic studies were the real explanation for the association between fat intake and breast cancer observed in correlation analyses.

In situations where the sample size is not adequate in individual studies to reach a firm conclusion, investigators sometimes combine the results of several studies. This pooling of data from several studies is referred to as a **meta-analysis**. Meta-analysis can be useful for achieving greater statistical power, but it cannot overcome the limitations and potential biases of individual studies. The investigator performing a meta-analysis must also be careful that selection of some studies and exclusion of others does not lead to a distorted conclusion. One meta-analysis of studies of diet and breast cancer combined the results from 12 case-control studies. No relationship between dietary fat intake and risk of breast cancer in premenopausal women was found, but an association between fat intake and breast cancer in postmenopausal women was detected, with a risk ratio of 1.5.

In the Patient Profile, the physician wanted to determine whether dietary fat intake is causally related to the development of breast cancer. The findings of studies were inconsistent, and the strength of association was modest at best, without clear evidence of a dose-response relationship. The temporal sequence of dietary fat intake and breast cancer appeared to be reasonable.

Was there biologic plausibility to the relationship? What pathophysiologic mechanism might be involved? Were there animal models that showed the relationship between fat in the diet and breast cancer? In fact, animal studies have found an association between fat intake and the development of mammary cancers in mice bearing the mammary tumor virus. Similar findings have been reported in other animal models. The pathophysiology involved in this process is less clear, but potential mechanisms have been discussed. It has been speculated that mammary neoplasms are controlled by endocrine balance, which in turn is affected by dietary factors, including fat intake. For example, women consuming high-fat diets have been shown to have more circulating estrogen than women on low-fat diets. In postmenopausal women, adipose tissue has been demonstrated to be a contributor to the production of estrogen. Dietary fat intake may also have modified DNA synthesis and cell duplication. If this were found to be true for breast tissue, this could be relevant to breast carcinogenesis. Therefore, there are some theoretical reasons to believe that a causal relationship exists between dietary fat intake and breast cancer.

The physician in the Patient Profile, however, is left without a firm answer to the question about the relationship between dietary fat and breast cancer. Even if research had demonstrated a small increase in risk with high-fat diets for postmenopausal women, the patient is premenopausal, so it is not clear that the results can be applied to this patient. On the other hand, it is only a matter of time before she undergoes menopause. Dietary habits presumably would be continued and could be protective in later life. The physician also may believe that a low-fat diet is justifiable for other reasons, including reduction of risk for cardiovascular disease. In addition, there are other cancers, such as colon cancer, for which the protective effect of a low-fat diet has been demonstrated more clearly.

This type of uncertainty is common in clinical medicine. Physicians often must weigh potential risks and benefits of an intervention and make decisions without complete information. The goal of medical research is to continue to provide better answers to important clinical questions. The best way to resolve the issue of the relationship of dietary fat and breast cancer is through large randomized controlled trials to compare breast cancer occurrence in women who are randomized to a low-fat diet vs those randomized to a high-fat diet. Clearly, this type of study would provide the most definitive evidence about a causal relationship between dietary fat and risk of breast cancer. Such a study would require a large number of subjects and a long follow-up period. It could be argued, therefore, that the resources required for this study would be better spent on studies of other questions where the evidence of a beneficial effect is stronger.

Much of the satisfaction derived from patient care relates to the ability to incorporate new knowledge into the practice of medicine. In order to update one's knowledge, it is imperative to develop the skills required for critical review of the medical literature. This is a difficult task, but the reward is enormous when it results in improved patient care.

SUMMARY

In this chapter, a structured approach to reviewing published epidemiologic studies was presented. The ultimate goal of this approach is to help integrate epidemiologic information into clinical practice. As a focus for discussion, the literature on dietary fat intake and risk of breast cancer is used to illustrate the evaluation process.

The initial step in reviewing the medical literature is to conduct a thorough search for relevant recent publications. Screening for appropriate articles can be accomplished through a manual or a computer-assisted approach. In either case, a correct choice of keywords calculated to retrieve pertinent articles is essential. Computer searches can save time and consequently are extremely popular.

The actual review of a publication begins with the stated purpose of the investigation. For the medical practitioner, a primary consideration is whether a particular study addresses a clinically important question. Are the results likely to influence the delivery of patient care? In the present context, clinical importance might be assessed in terms of whether the findings support a recommendation to lower dietary fat intake so as to reduce the risk of breast cancer.

The design of an investigation determines the types of inferences that can be drawn from it. The most compelling evidence for cause-and-effect relationships is derived from randomized controlled clinical trials. Among observational investigations, prospective cohort studies generally are least susceptible to bias, followed by retrospective cohort and case-control studies. Descriptive studies are useful for generating research questions but not for testing hypotheses.

The measurement of outcome (ie, development of disease) as well as the documentation of exposure to risk factors can be complicated in observational research. Emphasis must be placed on obtaining the most accurate information possible, recognizing that the ideal often cannot be achieved. Whenever possible, assessment should be performed in a blinded manner and should be based upon objective, standard criteria.

A distinction must be made between the concept of statistical significance, which can be evaluated by a hypothesis test, and clinical or biologic significance. P-values should not be used to indicate the importance of a finding but, rather, the likelihood that sampling variability can explain the results. Clinical importance relates to whether a difference in outcomes observed between study groups is large enough to warrant a change in clinical practice. Biologic significance refers to the extent to which findings help to elucidate the underlying biologic processes.

Systematic errors may arise in observational research from the approach to sample selection, information collection, or confounding. It is usually impossible to determine whether a particular bias actually has occurred. Attention, therefore, is focused on strategies to minimize the likelihood that systematic errors will affect the study conclusions. When bias is suspected in an investigation, the exact level of distortion generally is unknown. The direction of the systematic error (ie, a tendency to either overestimate or underestimate the strength of association) may be clear, however. The assessment of whether an observed association is likely to be one of cause-and-effect is based upon specific criteria, including strength of association, presence of a dose-response relationship, appropriateness of the temporal sequence of exposure and outcome, consistency of results across studies, and biologic plausibility.

When applied to the literature on dietary fat and breast cancer, this process of reasoning leads to an inconclusive assessment. The most consistent supporting evidence comes from the least compelling types of study. In situations where an association has been observed, the magnitude generally has been weak. Results have been inconsistent across studies, perhaps due in part to limitations of the study design and in part to the weakness of the relationship, even if it does exist.

The ultimate test of this hypothesis—a randomized controlled clinical trial—has not yet been published.

As with many issues in medicine, the dietary fat-breast cancer hypothesis remains unresolved. Since little harm probably results from restriction of dietary fat intake and because other benefits may accrue (ie, a reduction in risk of cardiovascular disease), it may be reasonable for the clinician in the Patient Profile to recommend this change in dietary habits to the patient. Until more definitive information is available, however, the patient should be counseled that the effect of restricting dietary fat intake on the risk of breast cancer is uncertain.

STUDY QUESTIONS

Questions 1–4: For each numbered situation below, select the most appropriate category of bias from the following lettered options. Each option can be used once, more than once, or not at all.

A. Selection bias
B. Random error
C. Information bias
D. Ecologic fallacy
E. Confounding
F. Birth cohort effect

1. Although national per-capita use of pesticides is associated with lymphoma mortality rates, patients with lymphoma do not have higher pesticide levels than persons without lymphoma.

2. In a cohort study of breast implants and the risk of connective tissue disease, 48% of the implanted patients are lost to follow-up.

3. In a case-control study of mouthwash use and risk of oral cancers, the cases tend to overreport the use of mouthwash.

4. In a cohort study of antioxidant intake and protection against atherosclerotic coronary artery disease (CAD), serum cholesterol is inversely correlated with antioxidant level and positively related to risk of CAD.

Questions 5–9: For each study, select the most appropriate study design from the following lettered options. Each option can be used once, more than once, or not at all.

A. Correlation study
B. Case-control study

C. Cohort study
D. Clinical trial
E. Descriptive study
F. Meta-analysis

5. A survey is conducted to determine the prevalence of mitral valve prolapse and correlates of occurrence within the general population.

6. The prior use of aspirin is compared among 500 patients with newly diagnosed colon cancer and 1000 healthy persons.

7. Prevention of lung cancer is studied within a population of 12,000 smokers who are assigned randomly to receive either vitamin E and beta carotene or an inert substance.

8. The reported national incidence rates of hepatitis B infection are associated with corresponding national mortality rates for liver cancer.

9. The results of several investigations of exposure to environmental tobacco smoke and risk of lung cancer are combined to reach a summary conclusion.

Questions 10–12: For each numbered situation below, choose the most appropriate criterion for establishing a causal relationship from the following lettered options. Each option can be used once, more than once, or not at all.

A. Strength of association
B. Presence of a dose-response relationship
C. Correct temporal sequence
D. Consistency of results
E. Biologic plausibility

10. In a case-control study of the association between occupational exposure to aluminum and risk of Alzheimer's disease, relative to no exposure, the odds ratios are: low exposure, 1.3 (95% confidence interval (CI): 0.9, 2.0); moderate exposure, 1.7 (95% CI: 1.4, 2.3); and high exposure, 2.3 (95% CI: 2.0, 2.9).

11. Five published case-control studies produce the following odds ratios: 1.4 (95% CI: 0.9, 2.4), 1.7 (95% CI: 1.3, 2.5), 2.4 (95% CI: 1.3, 4.6), 1.9 (95% CI: 1.5, 2.7), and 1.0 (95% CI: 0.8, 1.2).

12. At autopsy, the pathologic lesions within brains of Alzheimer's disease patients are shown to contain unusual levels of aluminum.

FURTHER READING

Hunter DJ, Willett W: Diet, body size, and breast cancer. Epidemiol Rev 1993;**15**:110.

REFERENCES

Dawson-Saunders B, Trapp RG: Reading the medical literature. In: *Basic and Clinical Biostatistics,* 2nd ed. Appleton & Lange, 1994.

Gehlbach SH: *Interpreting the Medical Literature,* 2nd ed. MacMillan, 1988.

Riegelman RK, Hirsch RP: Studying a study. In: *Studying a Study and Testing a Test,* 2nd ed. Little, Brown, 1989.

Sackett DL, Haynes RB, Tugwell P: How to read a clinical journal. In: *Clinical Epidemiology.* Little, Brown, 1985.

Spitzer WO et al: Continuing occurrence of eosinophilia-myalgia syndrome in Canada. Brit J Rheumatol 1995;**34**:246.

Glossary

Accuracy: the extent to which a measurement or study result correctly represents the characteristic or relationship that is being assessed.

Adjustment: a procedure for overall comparison of two or more populations in which background differences in the distribution of covariables are removed. (See also **Standardization.**)

Age adjustment: a procedure used to calculate summary rates for different populations in which underlying differences in the age distributions are removed. (See also **Age standardization.**)

Age-specific rate: a rate (usually incidence or mortality) for a particular age group.

Age standardization (direct): a procedure for obtaining a weighted average of age-specific rates in which the weights are selected on the basis of a standard age distribution (eg, the population of the United States in 1940).

Alpha error: see **Type I error.**

Analytic epidemiology: activities related to the identification of possible determinants of disease occurrence.

Analytic study: a research investigation designed to test a hypothesis that is often used in reference to a study of an exposure-disease association.

Antigenic drift: mutation of a pathogen (eg, Influenza A), such that the surface antigens differ from those of previously existing strains.

Association: the extent to which the occurrence of two or more characteristics are linked either through a causal or noncausal relationship.

Attack rate: the proportion of persons within a population who develop a particular outcome within a specified period of time.

Attributable risk percent: the percentage of the overall risk of a disease outcome within exposed persons that is related to the exposure of interest.

Beta error: see **Type II error.**

Bias: a nonrandom error in a study that leads to a distorted result.

Biologic marker: a measurable characteristic that either helps to classify level of exposure to a risk factor or susceptibility to (or presence of) a disease.

Birth cohort effect: an unusual age-specific rate (either incidence or mortality) within cross-sectional data that reflects the shared experience of persons born in specific years (birth cohort).

Blinding: assignment of treatment to individual subjects in such a way that subjects only **(single blinding)** or both subjects and treating physicians **(double blinding)** do not know the actual treatment allocation.

Case: a person who has a disease of interest (see also **Incident case** and **Prevalent case**).

Case-control study: an observational study in which subjects are sampled based on the presence (cases) or absence (controls) of the disease of interest. Information is collected about earlier exposure to risk factors of interest.

Case fatality: the proportion of persons with a particular disease who die from that disease within a specified period of time.

Causality: the extent to which the occurrence of a risk factor is responsible for the subsequent occurrence of a disease outcome.

Clinical scenario: one of two or more alternative paths of management available in a decision analysis.

Clinical trial: an experimental study that is designed to compare the therapeutic benefits of two or more treatments.

Cluster: a group of cases of a disease that are closely linked in time, place of occurrence, or both.

Cohort: a group of persons who share a common attribute, such as birth in a particular year or residence in a particular town, who are followed over time.

Cohort study: an observational study in which subjects are sampled based on the presence (exposed) or absence (unexposed) of a risk factor of interest. These subjects are followed over time for the development of a disease outcome of interest. (See also **Prospective cohort study** and **Retrospective cohort study**.)

Common-source exposure: contact with a risk factor that originates in the shared environment of multiple persons.

Concordant results: the same outcome status for two or more individuals, as in a pair-matched case-control study when both the case and the control are exposed (or unexposed).

Confidence interval: a range of values for a measure that is believed to contain the true value within a specified level (eg, 95%) of certainty.

Confounder: a variable that distorts the apparent relationship between an exposure and a disease of interest.

Confounding: a systematic error in a study that arises from mixing of the effect of the exposure of interest with other associated correlates of the disease outcome.

Control: in a case-control study, a subject without the disease of interest. See also **Adjustment.**

Control group: a population of comparison subjects in an analytic investigation.

Correlation study: a hypothesis-generating investigation in which the values of two or more summary characteristics are associated across different population groups.

Cosegregation: the tendency of alleles on the same chromosome to be inherited together.

Cross-sectional study: an analytic investigation in which subjects are sampled at a fixed point or period of time, and then the associations between the concurrent presence or absence of risk factors and diseases are investigated.

Cumulative incidence: the risk of developing a particular disease within a specified period of time.

Death rate: see **Mortality rate.**

Decision analysis: a formal probabilistic process for making clinical decisions which incorporates information on medical options, anticipated likelihoods of various outcomes and the uncertainty associated with clinical information.

Decision diagram: a flow chart used in decision analysis that identifies the clinical management choices, probabilities of events and likelihoods of outcomes.

Decision tree: see **Decision diagram.**

Dependent variable: see **Outcome variable.**

Descriptive epidemiology: activities related to characterizing patterns of disease occurrence.

Differential misclassification: incorrect categorization of the status of subjects with regard to one variable (eg, exposure) that is influenced by other characteristics of interest (eg, disease status).

Discordant results: different outcome status for two or more individuals, as in a pair-matched case-control study when one subject in a pair is exposed and the other individual is unexposed.

Disease outbreak: a sudden, unexpected increase in the occurrence of a disease within a relatively limited geographic area.

Dose-response relationship: an exposure-disease association in which the risk of disease varies with respect to the intensity or duration of exposure.

Ecologic fallacy: an association between summary characteristics across populations without actual linkage of the characteristics within individual persons.

Ecologic study: see **Correlation study.**

Emerging infectious disease: an infection that has newly appeared within a population or has existed but is rapidly increasing in incidence or geographical range.

Endemic rate: the usual rate of occurrence of particular events within a population.

Epidemic: a dramatic increase above the usual or expected rate of occurrence of particular events within a population.

Epidemiology: the study of the distribution and determinants of disease within human populations.

Excess risk: the extra risk of a particular disease occurring among persons exposed to a risk factor of interest. See also **Risk difference.**

Exclusions: persons who are eliminated from an analytic study because they do not satisfy the eligibility (inclusion) criteria.

Expected utility: a numerical value that represents the average result if the decision maker follows a particular path in a decision analysis.

Exposure: contact with or possession of a characteristic that is suspected to influence the risk of developing a particular disease.

External validity: the extent to which the conclusions of a study are correct for persons beyond those who were investigated. See also **Generalize.**

False-negative: a test result that is normal (negative) despite the true presence of a particular disease or a study result that incorrectly fails to identify a true effect (see also **Type II error**).

False-positive: a test result that is abnormal (positive) despite the true absence of the disease of interest or a study result that incorrectly suggests an effect, when in truth, the purported effect does not exist (see also **Type I error**).

Familial aggregation: the extent to which the occurrence of a particular disease tends to cluster within families.

Follow-up study: see **Cohort study.**

Generalize: the ability to extrapolate study results from the study subjects to other persons who were not investigated.

Genetic epidemiology: the use of epidemiologic techniques to study hereditary determinants of disease in human populations.

Historical cohort study: see **Retrospective cohort study.**

Historical controls: subjects in a clinical study who were previously treated with the standard therapy before the new experimental treatment was introduced.

Hypothesis-generating study: an exploratory investigation designed to formulate questions that are evaluated in subsequent analytic studies.

Hypothesis-testing study: an analytic investigation in which one or more specific refutable suppositions is (are) evaluated.

Inbreeding study: a study in which the degree of inbreeding is assessed with respect to risk of a particular disease.

Incidence density: see **Incidence rate.**

Incidence rate: the rapidity with which new cases of a particular disease arise within a given population.

Incident case: a person who is newly diagnosed with a disease of interest.

Incubation period: the time interval between contact with a risk factor (often an infectious agent) and the first clinical evidence of the resulting illness.

Independent variable: a factor that is suspected to influence the outcome of an analytic study.

Information (or observation) bias: a systematic error in a study that arises from the manner in which data are collected from participants.

Intention-to-treat: analysis of the results of a clinical trial based upon initial treatment assignment regardless of whether or not the subjects completed the full course of treatment.

Internal validity: the extent to which the conclusions of a study are correct for the subjects under investigation.

Latent period: time between exposure to a risk factor and subsequent development of clinical manifestations of a particular disease.

Lead-time bias: apparent increase in the length of survival with a disease as a result of earlier recognition of the disease through the use of a screening procedure.

Length-biased sampling: preferential detection of less aggressive forms of a disease through the use of a screening procedure.

Linkage analysis: a technique based upon use of marker alleles to assess the associations within pedigress of genetic factors with risk of a particular disease.

Linkage disequilibrium: an excess or deficiency of certain combinations of alleles at a gene pair.

Matching: a procedure for sampling comparison subjects based upon whether key attributes (ie, **matching factors**) are similar to those of subjects in the index group.

Median survival time: the duration from diagnosis to death that is exceeded by exactly 50% of subjects with a particular disease.

Medical outcome: See **Outcome.**

Misclassification bias: incorrect characterization of the status of subjects with regard to a study variable that leads to a distorted conclusion. See also **Information bias.**

Mortality rate: the rapidity with which persons within a given population die from a particular disease.

Natural history: the progression of a disease through successive stages that is often used to describe the course of an illness for which no effective treatment is available.

Negative predictive value: the probability that a person with a negative (normal) test result actually does not have the disease of interest.

Nondifferential misclassification: incorrect categorization of the status of subjects with regard to one variable (eg, exposure) that is unrelated to another characteristic of interest (eg, disease status).

Notifiable disease: a disease for which regular, frequent and timely information on individual cases is considered necessary for the prevention and control of the disease.

Null value: the point on the scale of a measure of association that corresponds to no association (eg, 1 for the risk ratio and the odds ratio, and 0 for the risk difference and the attributable risk percent).

Observation bias: see **Information bias.**

Observational study: a nonexperimental analytic study in which the investigator monitors, but does not influence, the exposure status of individual subjects and their subsequent disease status.

Odds: the probability that a particular event will occur divided by the probability that the event will not occur.

Odds ratio: the odds of a particular exposure among persons with a specific disease divided by the corresponding odds of exposure among persons without the disease of interest.

Outbreak: see **Disease outbreak.**

Outcome: clinical events that result from patient management decisions (eg, morbidity, complications, quality of life, or mortality).

Outcome variable: in an analytic study, the response of interest (eg, development of disease).

Pathogen: an agent responsible for the development of a particular disease.

Person-time: a unit of measurement used in the estimation of rates that reflects the amount of time observed for persons at risk of a particular event.

Person-to-person spread: propagation of a disease within a population by transfer from an affected person to susceptible persons.

Person-years of life lost: a measure of total life expectancy lost within a particular population because of premature death.

Placebo: an inert substance. The **placebo effect** occurs when persons affected with a specific illness demonstrate clinical improvement upon treatment with an inert substance.

Population at risk: persons who are susceptible to a particular disease but who are not yet affected.

Population-based study: an analytic study in which subjects are sampled from the general population.

Positive predictive value: the probability that a person with a positive (abnormal) test result actually has the disease of interest.

Power: see **Statistical power.**

Precision: the extent to which a measurement is narrowly characterized. **Statistical precision** is inversely related to the variance of the measurement.

Predictor variable: see **Independent variable.**

Premature death: a death that occurs earlier than would be expected in the absence of a particular disease.

Prevalence: the proportion of persons in a given population who have a particular disease at a point or interval of time.

Prevalent case: a person who has a disease of interest that was diagnosed in the past.

Prospective cohort study: a cohort study in which exposure status and subsequent occurrence of disease both occur after the onset of the investigation.

Randomization: procedure for assigning treatments to patients by chance.

Rate: the rapidity with which health events such as new diagnoses or deaths occur. See also **Incidence rate** and **Mortality rate.**

Rate ratio: the rate of occurrence of a specified health event among persons exposed to a particular risk factor divided by the corresponding rate among unexposed persons.

Recurrence risk: in genetic epidemiology, the risk of a particular disease experienced by relatives of a subject with that disease.

Relative risk: see **Risk ratio.**

Reliability: the extent to which multiple measurements of a characteristic are in agreement.

Response variable: see **Outcome variable.**

Retrospective cohort study: a cohort study in which exposure status and subsequent development of disease both occur prior to the onset of the investigation.

Risk: the probability that an event (eg, development of disease) will occur within a specific period of time.

Risk difference: the risk of a particular disease occurrence among persons exposed to a given risk factor minus the corresponding risk among unexposed persons.

Risk factor: an attribute or agent that is suspected to be related to the occurrence of a particular disease.

Risk ratio: the likelihood of a particular disease occurrence among persons exposed to a given risk factor divided by the corresponding likelihood among unexposed persons.

Sample: a subset of a target population that is chosen for investigation.

Screening: the use of tests to detect the presence of a particular disease among asymptomatic persons prior to the time that the disease would be recognized through routine clinical methods.

Segregation analysis: a complex statistical technique used to assess whether a particular disease has, at least in part, a genetic origin, and if so, the most likely mode of inheritance.

Selection bias: a systematic error in a study that arises from the manner in which subjects are sampled.

Sensitivity: the probability that a person who actually has the disease of interest will have a positive (abnormal) test result.

Sensitivity analysis: use of different values for an uncertain likelihood in a decision analysis in order to determine whether the preferred course of action remains unchanged.

Specificity: the probability that a person who actually does not have the disease of interest will have a negative (normal) test result.

Standardization: an analytic procedure for obtaining a summary measure for a population by applying standard weights to the measures within subgroups of the population.

Statistical power: the ability of a study to detect a true effect of a specified magnitude. The statistical power corresponds to 1 − Type II error.

Statistical significance: the likelihood that a difference as large or larger than that observed between study groups could have occurred by chance alone in a sample of the size investigated. Usually, the level of statistical significance is stated as a P-value (eg, $P < 0.05$.)

Surveillance: ongoing observation of a population for rapid and accurate detection of changes in the occurrence of particular diseases.

Survival: the likelihood of remaining alive for a specified period of time after the diagnosis of a particular disease.

Systematic error: see **Bias.**

True-negative: a test result that is normal (negative) when the disease of interest is actually absent.

True-positive: a test result that is abnormal (positive) when the disease of interest is actually present.

Twin study: a study of genetic susceptibility in which concordance for occurrence of a particular disease is compared between dizygotic (fraternal) twins and monozygotic (identical) twins, or between twins reared together versus apart.

Type I error: rejection of the null hypothesis when it is actually correct.

Type II error: failure to reject the null hypothesis when it is actually incorrect.

Underlying cause of death: (1) the disease or injury which initiated the train of morbid events leading directly to death, or (2) to the circumstances of the accident or violence that resulted in fatal injury.

Validity: the extent to which a measurement or a study result correctly represents the characteristics or relationship of interest.

Vital statistics: information concerning patterns of registered life events, such as births, marriages, divorces, and deaths.

Withdrawals: subjects who are initially included in a study but later voluntarily or involuntarily terminate participation.

Years of potential life lost (YPLL): a measure of total life lost to a particular age (eg, 65 years) within a population because of premature deaths.

Appendix A: Answers to Study Questions

CHAPTER 1

1. D
2. C
3. F
4. G
5. H
6. C
7. A
8. B
9. E
10. E
11. B
12. A

CHAPTER 2

1. G
2. C
3. E
4. K
5. D
6. B
7. E
8. A
9. B
10. A
11. A
12. B

CHAPTER 3

1. A
2. C
3. B
4. D
5. A
6. B
7. E
8. C
9. A
10. D

CHAPTER 4

1. C
2. D

3. C
4. E
5. B
6. C
7. D
8. A
9. B
10. A
11. B
12. A

CHAPTER 5

1. B
2. C
3. A
4. D
5. A
6. E
7. C
8. D
9. B
10. E

CHAPTER 6

1. F
2. G
3. D
4. H
5. F
6. C
7. B
8. F
9. D
10. C
11. A
12. E

CHAPTER 7

1. E
2. C
3. B
4. A
5. D

6. D
7. B
8. E
9. E
10. C

CHAPTER 8

1. A
2. B
3. D
4. A
5. C
6. D
7. A
8. C
9. B
10. E

CHAPTER 9

1. A
2. F
3. D
4. E
5. I
6. A
7. A
8. B
9. C
10. D
11. F
12. B

CHAPTER 10

1. D
2. C
3. A
4. B
5. A

6. B
7. C
8. D
9. C
10. D

CHAPTER 11

1. F
2. E
3. C
4. A
5. G
6. F
7. D
8. A
9. E
10. B

CHAPTER 12

1. D
2. A
3. A
4. C
5. C
6. A

CHAPTER 13

1. D
2. A
3. C
4. E
5. E
6. B
7. D
8. A
9. F
10. B
11. D
12. E

Appendix B: Estimation of Sample Size Requirements for Randomized Controlled Clinical Trials

The formulas used to estimate sample size requirements are provided in this appendix, along with illustrative calculations relative to the Diabetes Control and Complications Trial described in Chapter 7.

Prior to undertaking this study, the investigators specified an alpha level (0.05, or 5%), statistical power (90%, and thus a beta level of 10%), and the outcome difference that should be detected by the trial (a reduction in the proportion of patients diagnosed with diabetic retinopathy from 20% to 10%). The baseline proportion who would develop retinopathy is derived from previous literature. The amount of reduction in retinopathy is based on clinical judgment; the question was posed: "What would be a clinically important difference in the proportion of patients who would suffer this complication?"

The equation for sample size for a comparison of two proportions is as follows:

$$n = \left[\frac{z_\alpha\sqrt{2\pi_c(1 - \pi_c)} - z_\beta\sqrt{\pi_t(1 - \pi_t) + \pi_c(1 - \pi_c)}}{\pi_t - \pi_c} \right]^2 \quad (1)$$

where n is the number of subjects for each treatment group, π_c and π_t are the proportion of patients who develop retinopathy within 5 years in the control group (standard therapy) and treatment group (intensive therapy), respectively, and z_α and z_β are the values that include alpha in the two tails and beta in the lower tail of the standard normal distribution. These values can be determined from tables available in most statistical texts (see Dawson-Saunders and Trapp, 1994). The value for a type I error of 5% is 1.96, and the z_β value for a type II error of 10% is -1.28. As the acceptable level of error decreases, z_α and z_β increase.

Note that in equation (1), the larger the z_α and z_β—ie, the smaller the acceptable type I and type II errors—the larger the sample size required; also the smaller the difference in π_c and π_t, the larger the sample size required. What may not be so intuitively obvious is the relation of sample size to the distance of π_c from 0.5. The part of the equation $\pi_c(1 - \pi_c)$ is maximized, and therefore the numerator is greater

when $\pi_c = 0.5$. Movement of π_c away from 0.5 reduces the required sample size.

If one expected the proportion of patients on standard insulin therapy for diabetes to develop retinopathy by year 5 to be 0.20 and wanted this trial to be able to detect a reduction in retinopathy at 5 years from 0.20 to 0.10, then the sample size would be calculated as follows:

$$n = \left[\frac{1.96\sqrt{2 \times 0.2 \times 0.8} - (-1.28)\sqrt{(0.1 \times 0.9) + (0.2 \times 0.8)}}{0.1 - 0.2} \right]^2 \quad (2)$$

and $n = 305$. Therefore, a total of 610 subjects equally divided between groups would be required to answer the question: "Is there a reduction in the rate of retinopathy at 5 years from 20% to 10% using intensive rather than standard insulin therapy?" This can be restated as follows: If the true difference in rate of retinopathy at 5 years is 10% vs 20%, then the probability that the researchers will find no difference between the proportion of subjects developing retinopathy during the first 5 years of therapy with an equally divided sample size of 610 would be only 10%.

Since the diabetes trial had over 305 subjects in each group, the likelihood of not finding a true difference of this magnitude was actually less than 10%.

If average glucose levels 5 years after beginning therapy had been chosen to compare the two treatment groups, the required sample size could have been determined using the following equation:

$$n = 2 \left[\frac{(z_\alpha - z_\beta)\sigma}{\mu_1 - \mu_2} \right]^2 \quad (3)$$

where n is the number of subjects for each treatment group, $\mu_1 - \mu_2$ is the detectable difference between the means of the two groups, σ is the common standard deviation of each group, and z_α and z_β have the same meaning as in equation (1).

Again, without memorizing this formula, we can intuitively understand how its various components contribute to sample size. The greater the absolute values of z_α, z_β, and σ, and the smaller the difference in the means, $\mu_1 - \mu_2$, the larger the n, or sample size, required (Table 7–2). This makes sense, since smaller differences in means between groups would be harder to detect, and greater variability within the groups would tend to blur inter-group differences. As in all sample size calculations, the larger the values of z_α and z_β—ie, the smaller the acceptable type I and type II errors—the larger the sample size required.

Suppose the investigators estimated that the mean glucose levels at 5 years after the start of therapy would be 200 mg/dl for patients on standard insulin therapy and 175 mg/dl for those on intensive therapy, and the pooled standard deviation would be 45 mg/dl. The sample size for each group would be calculated using equation (3):

$$n = 2 \left[\frac{(1.96 + 1.28)45}{175 - 200} \right]^2 \tag{4}$$

and $n = 68$. This endpoint would have required far fewer patients to be enrolled in the trial. At the conclusion of the trial, however, treating physicians may not have considered a reduction in glucose a sufficiently important outcome to warrant a change to the more intensive therapy; whereas if the trial found that intensive therapy reduced the onset of retinopathy, intensive therapy would be judged to be a superior treatment regimen.

Appendix C: Method for Determining the Confidence Interval Around the Risk Ratio

An approximate 95% confidence interval (*CI*) around the point estimate of the risk ratio (*RR*) can be calculated using the following formula:

95% *CI*

$$= (RR) \exp [\pm 1.96 \sqrt{VAR(\ln RR)}]$$

where

$$\sqrt{VAR(\ln RR)}$$

$$= \sqrt{\frac{1 - A/(A+C)}{A} + \frac{1 - B/(B+D)}{B}}$$

where exp is the base of the natural logarithm raised to the quantity within the brackets and *A*, *B*, *C*, and *D* represent the numerical entries in the summary format in Table 8–6 and VAR(lnRR) is the estimated variance of the natural logarithm of the RR. This confidence interval is approximate because it is based on a computational short-cut for estimating the variance of the natural logarithm of the *RR*. For relatively large samples, this approximation yields confidence limits that are quite close to the exact values, which are much more difficult to calculate.

The 95% *CI* for the 10-minute Apgar score (0–3 versus 4–6) relationship to infant mortality desribed in Chapter 8 is:

95% *CI*

$$= (2.8) \exp \left[\pm 1.96 \sqrt{\frac{(1 - 0.344)}{42} + \frac{(1 - 0.125)}{43}} \right]$$

$$= (2.8) \exp \left[\pm 1.96 \sqrt{0.0156 + 0.0203} \right]$$

$$= (2.8) \exp (\pm 0.37)$$

Lower bound = (2.8) exp (−0.37) = 1.9

Upper bound = (2.8) exp (+0.37) = 4.1

Appendix D: The Odds Ratio as an Estimator of the Incidence Rate Ratio

To understand further the design of a case-control study, and why the odds ratio from a case-control study estimates the incidence rate ratio, consider first the occurrence of a particular disease within an underlying population that gives rise to the cases. This underlying cohort sometimes is called the source population. At the start of follow-up, all subjects are disease-free; P people are exposed, and Q are not. After following the cohort for t years, A of the P exposed and B of the Q unexposed subjects develop disease (Table D–1).

To calculate incidence rates for this cohort, as discussed in Chapter 2, one first calculates the person-years of observation (py) which is given by:

py = average size of source population × length of follow-up

This equation simplifies if few people develop disease during the follow-up period and the population undergoes no major demographic shifts, a situation termed the **"steady state."** If the steady state holds, the size of the source population is nearly constant and the equation above simplifies to:

py = size of source population × length of follow-up

Application of the latter equation to the hypothetical cohort yields $P \times t$ and $Q \times t$ person-years of observation, for the exposed and unexposed, respectively (Table D–1). Thus, the incidence rate in the exposed is $A/(P \times t)$, that in the unexposed is $B/(Q \times t)$, and the incidence rate ratio (IRR) is:

$$IRR = (A/P \times t)/(B/Q \times t) = (A \times Q)/(B \times P)$$

Now, turning to the case-control study design, cases arise from a clearly defined source population and the investigator then chooses controls from this same population. Thus, to conduct a case-control study using the source population described in Table D–1, one samples subjects with disease (cases) and subjects without disease (controls), then determines their respective exposure histories. Excluded from both the case and control groups are potential subjects known to have had disease when the study began—only newly diagnosed or **"incident"** cases are included. In practice, one may contact newly diagnosed cases and a sample from the general population, ask each subject about prior disease, and exclude those who were diagnosed prior to the study period. The data can be summarized as in Table D–2.

Cases and controls are selected without regard to exposure. For example, one might randomly sample cases from all those in the population who develop disease during the study period and randomly select controls from all those without disease. Sampling is "blind" to exposure, so that the proportion of cases in the study who were exposed should, on average, equal that of cases in the full cohort. Similarly, the proportion of controls in the study who were exposed should, on average, equal that of those without disease in the full cohort. Thus, the exposure odds among cases, a/b, is an estimate of A/B, the corresponding odds among new cases arising from the full cohort. In a parallel manner, the exposure odds among controls, c/d, is an estimate of P/Q, the corresponding odds among persons without disease in the full cohort. The cross-product or **odds ratio** (OR) is the odds that a case is exposed, a/b, divided by the odds that a control is exposed, c/d:

$$OR = (a \times d)/(b \times c)$$

Table D–1. Disease occurrence in a cohort by exposure status.

	Exposed	Unexposed
Number of new cases during follow-up	A	B
Person-Years of observation	$P \times t$	$Q \times t$
Incidence Rate	$A/(P \times t)$	$B/(Q \times t)$

Table D–2. Data from a hypothetical case-control study of a disease and a dichotomous exposure.

	Exposed	Unexposed	Total
Diseased	a	b	M_1
Not Diseased	c	d	M_2
Total	N_1	N_2	T

The odds ratio from the case-control study is, therefore, an estimate of the incidence rate ratio in the full cohort, which was shown above to equal: $(A \times Q)/(B \times P)$.

If exposure increases risk, more cases than controls will be exposed, so that $a/b > c/d$, or $OR > 1$. On the other hand, if exposure decreases risk, fewer cases than controls will be exposed, so that $a/b < c/d$, or $OR < 1$. Thus, an OR greater than one suggests that exposure is associated with higher incidence rates or risk, an OR less than one suggests that exposure is associated with lower incidence rates or risk and an OR near one suggests that exposure is not associated with higher or lower than average risk.

Appendix E: Method for Determining the Confidence Interval Around the Odds Ratio

An approximate 95% confidence interval (*CI*) around the point estimate of the *OR* for an unmatched case-control study can be calculated using the following formula:

$$95\% \; CI = (OR) \exp\left[\pm 1.96 \; \sqrt{\frac{1}{A} + \frac{1}{B} + \frac{1}{C} + \frac{1}{D}} \; \right]$$

where exp is the base of the natural logarithm raised to the quantity in the brackets, and *A, B, C,* and *D* represent the numerical entries into the summary format in Table 9–4. This confidence interval is approximate because it is based upon a computational short-cut to estimating the variance of the natural logarithm of the *OR*. For relatively large sample sizes, this approximation yields confidence bounds that are quite close to the exact values, which are much more difficult to calculate.

For the data in Table 9–5 relating L-tryptophan brand use to eosinophilia myalgia syndrome in an unmatched case-control study, the 95% *CI* was calculated as follows:

$$95\% \; CI = (7.5) \exp\left[\pm 1.96 \; \sqrt{\frac{1}{22} + \frac{1}{36} + \frac{1}{7} + \frac{1}{86}} \; \right]$$

$$= (7.5) \; \exp[\pm 0.94]$$

Lower bound = (7.5) exp[−0.94] = 2.9
Upper bound = (7.5) exp[+0.94] = 19.1

Similarly, an approximate 95% *CI* around the point estimate of an *OR* from a pair-matched case-control study can be calculated using the following formula:

$$95\% \; CI = (OR) \exp\left[\pm 1.96 \; \sqrt{\frac{1}{X} + \frac{1}{Y}} \; \right]$$

where exp is the base of the natural logarithm raised to the quantity in the brackets, and *X* and *Y* represent the numerical entries in the summary format in Table 9–6.

For the data in Table 9–7 relating L-tryptophan use to eosinophilia myalgia syndrome in a hypothetical pair-matched case-control study, the 95% *CI* was calculated as follows:

$$95\% \; CI = (11.4) \exp\left[\pm 1.96 \; \sqrt{\frac{1}{57} + \frac{1}{5}} \; \right]$$

$$= (11.4) \; \exp[\pm 0.91]$$

Lower bound = (11.4) exp[−0.91] = 4.6
Upper bound = (11.4) exp[+0.91] = 28.3

Index

Note: Page numbers followed by *t* or *f* indicate tables or figures, respectively.

L A N G E
medical books

Available at your local health science bookstore or by calling

Appleton & Lange toll free

1-800-423-1359

A smart investment
in your medical career

Basic Science Textbooks

Biochemistry
Examination & Board Review
Balcavage & King
1995, ISBN 0-8385-0661-5, A0661-7
Color Atlas of Basic Histology
Berman
1993, ISBN 0-8385-0445-0, A0445-5
1996 First Aid for the USMLE Step 1
Bhushan, et al.
1996, ISBN 0-8385-2597-0, A2597-1
Jawetz, Melnick, & Adelberg's
Medical Microbiology, 20/e
Brooks, Butel, & Ornston
1995, ISBN 0-8385-6243-4, A6243-8
Manual for Human Dissection
Photographs with Clinical
Applications
Callas
1994, ISBN 0-8385-6133-0, A6133-1
Concise Pathology, 2/e
Chandrasoma & Taylor
1995, ISBN 0-8385-1229-1, A1229-2
Introduction to Clinical Psychiatry
Elkin
1996, ISBN 0-8385-4333-2, A4333-9
Medical Biostatistics & Epidemiology
Examination & Board Review
Essex-Sorlie
1995, ISBN 0-8385-6219-1, A6219-8

Fundamentals of Medical Cell Biology
and Histology
Fuller
1996, ISBN 0-8385-1384-0, A1384-5
Review of Medical Physiology, 17/e
Ganong
1995, ISBN 0-8385-8431-4, A8431-7
First Aid for the USMLE Step 2
A Student-to-Student Guide
Go, Curet-Salim, & Fullerton
1996, ISBN 0-8385-2591-1, A2591-4
Medical Epidemiology, 2/e
Greenberg, Daniels, Flanders, Eley, &
Boring
1996, ISBN 0-8385-6206-X, A6206-5
Basic Histology, 8/e
Junqueira, Carneiro, & Kelley
1995, ISBN 0-8385-0567-8, A0567-6
Basic & Clinical Pharmacology, 6/e
Katzung
1995, ISBN 0-8385-0619-4, A0619-5
Pharmacology
Examination & Board Review, 4/e
Katzung & Trevor
1995, ISBN 0-8385-8067-X, A8067-9
First Aid for the Match
Le, Bhushan, & Amin
1996, ISBN 0-8385-2596-2, A2596-3
Medical Microbiology & Immunology
Examination & Board Review, 4/e
Levinson & Jawetz
1996, ISBN 0-8385-6225-6, A6225-5

Clinical Anatomy
Lindner
1989, ISBN 0-8385-1259-3, A1259-9
Pathophysiology of Disease
McPhee, Lingappa, Ganong, & Lange
1995, ISBN 0-8385-7815-2, A7815-2
Harper's Biochemistry, 23/e
Murray, Granner, Mayes, & Rodwell
1993, ISBN 0-8385-3562-3, A3562-4
Pathology
Examination & Board Review
Newland
1995, ISBN 0-8385-7719-9, A7719-6
Basic Histology
Examination & Board Review, 3/e
Paulsen
1996, ISBN 0-8385-2282-3, A2282-0
Basic & Clinical Immunology, 8/e
Stites, Terr, & Parslow
1994, ISBN 0-8385-0561-9, A0561-9
Correlative Neuroanatomy, 22/e
Waxman & deGroot
1995, ISBN 0-8385-1091-4, A1091-6

Clinical Science Textbooks

Clinical Neurology, 3/e
Aminoff, Greenberg, & Simon
1996, ISBN 0-8385-1383-2, A1383-7
Understanding Health Policy:
A Clinical Approach
Bodenheimer & Grumbach
1995, ISBN 0-8385-3678-6, A3678-8

(more on reverse)

Appleton & Lange • P.O. Box 120041 • Stamford, CT • 06912-0041 • 1-800-423-1359